Hospital for Special Surgery's Illustrated Tips and Tricks in Foot and Ankle Surgery

Hospital for Special Surgery's Illustrated Tips and Tricks in Foot and Ankle Surgery

EDITORS

Andrew J. Rosenbaum, MD
Assistant Professor
Director of Orthopaedic Research
Division of Orthopaedic Surgery
Albany Medical College
Albany, New York

David Levine, MD
Associate Professor
Division of Foot and Ankle Surgery
Department of Orthopaedic Surgery
Hospital for Special Surgery
New York, New York

Wolters Kluwer

Philadelphia • Baltimore • New York • London
Buenos Aires • Hong Kong • Sydney • Tokyo

Acquisitions Editor: Brian Brown
Development Editor: Sean McGuire
Editorial Coordinator: Ashley Pfeiffer
Editorial Assistant: Kate Sherryer
Marketing Manager: Julie Sikora
Production Project Manager: Sadie Buckallew
Design Coordinator: Joan Wendt
Manufacturing Coordinator: Beth Welsh
Prepress Vendor: S4Carlisle Publishing Services

9 8 7 6 5 4 3 2 1

Printed in China

Library of Congress Cataloging-in-Publication Data

Names: Levine, David (David S.), editor. | Rosenbaum, Andrew J., editor. | Hospital for Special Surgery, issuing body.
Title: Hospital for Special Surgery's illustrated tips and tricks in foot and ankle surgery / editors, David Levine, Andrew J. Rosenbaum.
Other titles: Illustrated tips and tricks in foot and ankle surgery
Description: Philadelphia: Wolters Kluwer Health, [2020] | Includes bibliographical references.
Identifiers: LCCN 2019008150 | ISBN 9781496365101
Subjects: | MESH: Foot—surgery | Ankle—surgery | Orthopedic Procedures | Atlas
Classification: LCC RD563 | NLM WE 17 | DDC 617.5/85059—dc23 LC record available at https://lccn.loc.gov/2019008150

shop.lww.com

RRS1903

Dedication

To my wife, Kristin, and my children, Charlotte and Madison. To my parents, Marc and Caren, and my sister, Caroline. You have all made sacrifices that have facilitated my maturation both personally and professionally. This book could not have been completed without your support. To David and Josh Dines, who have been committed to my growth for many years, and who are why I am an orthopedic surgeon. To my outstanding mentors from the HSS Foot and Ankle Service, Scott Ellis, Martin O'Malley, and John Kennedy, whose endless patience and devotion to my professional advancement have helped shape my practice, and, most importantly, to appreciate the importance of both clinical and academic orthopedic foot and ankle surgery. And lastly, to my residents, who regularly challenge me, humble me, and remind me of how special it is to teach and shape future generations of orthopedic surgeons.

Andrew J. Rosenbaum

Contributors

Mostofa Abousayed, MD
Chief Resident
Department of Orthopaedic Surgery
Albany Medical Center
Albany, New York

Curtis T. Adams, MD
Resident Physician
Division of Orthopaedic Surgery
Albany Medical College
Albany, New York

Maxwell C. Alley, Jr., MD
Resident
Department of Orthopaedic Surgery
Boston University
Boston, Massachusetts

Matthew Anderson, MD
Resident Physician
Department of Orthopaedic Surgery
Albany Medical College
Albany, New York

Kyle Angelicola-Richardson, MD
Orthopaedic Resident, Physician
Department of Orthopaedic Surgery
Albany Medical Center
Albany, New York

Afshin A. Anoushiravani, MD
Orthopaedic Resident, Physician
Department of Orthopaedic Surgery
Albany Medical Center
Albany, New York

Abdul Arain, MD
Physician, PGY3
Department of Orthopaedic Surgery
Albany Medical Center
Albany, New York

Samik Banerjee, MD
Chief Resident
Department of Orthopaedic Surgery
Albany Medical Center
Albany, New York

Keegan Cole, MD
Resident
Department of Orthopaedic Surgery
Albany Medical Center
Albany, New York

Jonathan T. Deland, MD
Associate Professor
Attending Surgeon
Department of Orthopaedic Surgery
Hospital for Special Surgery
New York, New York

Constantine A. Demetracopoulos, MD
Assistant Professor
Department of Orthopaedic Surgery
Hospital for Special Surgery
New York, New York

Khusboo Desai, MS, MD
Resident Physician
Department of Orthopaedic Surgery
Albany Medical Center
Albany, New York

Mark C. Drakos, MD
Assistant Professor
Division of Foot and Ankle Surgery
Department of Orthopaedic Surgery
Hospital for Special Surgery
New York, New York

Scott Ellis, MD
Associate Professor
Division of Foot and Ankle Surgery
Department of Orthopaedic Surgery
Hospital for Special Surgery
New York, New York

Akash Gupta, MD
Orthopaedic Surgeon
Eastside Orthopaedics and Sports Medicine
Portland, Oregon

Stefanos Haddad, MD
Resident Physician
Department of Orthopaedic Surgery
Albany Medical College
Albany, New York

MaCalus Hogan, MD
Associate Professor
Departments of Orthopaedic Surgery and Bioengineering
University of Pittsburgh
Pittsburgh, Pennsylvania

Christopher Johnson, MD
Resident Physician
Department of Orthopaedic Surgery
State University of New York—Upstate
Syracuse, New York

Mackenzie T. Jones, BA
Research Assistant
Division of Foot and Ankle Surgery
Department of Orthopaedic Surgery
Hospital for Special Surgery
New York, New York

Sydney C. Karnovsky, BA
Research Assistant
Division of Foot and Ankle Surgery
Department of Orthopaedic Surgery
Hospital for Special Surgery
New York, New York

Jillian Kazley, MD
Resident Physician
Department of Orthopaedic Surgery
Albany Medical Center
Albany, New York

John G. Kennedy, MD, MCh, MMSc, FFSEM, FRCS (Orth)
Attending Orthopaedic Surgeon
Department of Foot and Ankle Service
Hospital for Special Surgery
New York, New York

Hamza Murtaza, MD
PGY-1
Division of Orthopaedic Surgery
Albany Medical Center
Albany, New York

Casey M. O'Connor, MD
Resident Physician
Department of Orthopaedic Surgery
Albany Medical Center
Albany, New York

Martin O'Malley, MD
Associate Professor
Attending Surgeon
Department of Orthopaedic Surgery
Hospital for Special Surgery
New York, New York

Eric Perloff, MD
Resident Physician
Department of Orthopaedic Surgery
Albany Medical Center
Albany, New York

Andrew Posner, MD
Resident Physician
Department of Orthopaedic Surgery
Albany Medical Center
Albany, New York

Andrew J. Rosenbaum, MD
Assistant Professor
Director of Orthopaedic Research
Division of Orthopaedic Surgery
Albany Medical College
Albany, New York

Austin E. Sanders, BA
Research Assistant
Division of Foot and Ankle Surgery
Department of Orthopaedic Surgery
Hospital for Special Surgery
New York, New York

Rachel J. Shakked, MD
Assistant Professor
Rothman Institute
Bensalem, Pennsylvania

Yoshiharu Shimozono, MD
Orthopaedic Surgeon
Department of Foot and Ankle Service
Hospital for Special Surgery
New York, New York

Khusdeep S. Vig, MD
Resident Physician
Department of Orthopaedic Surgery
Albany Medical Center
Albany, New York

Joseph Young, MD
Resident Physician
Department of Orthopaedic Surgery
Albany Medical Center
Albany, New York

Preface

I am honored to serve as the editor of *Hospital for Special Surgery Tips and Tricks in Foot and Ankle Surgery*. This project would not have been possible without the daily experiences and interactions I had as a fellow at Hospital for Special Surgery. When I interviewed for the HSS foot and ankle fellowship, I immediately knew that I wanted to emulate the thought processes and technical skills of the faculty, many of whom are responsible for the treatment algorithms and surgical techniques used to treat the complex pathology we regularly see as orthopedic foot and ankle surgeons. My co-fellows, Stuart Saunders and Rachel Shakked, and I appreciated this unique opportunity and began taking notes immediately following cases, with technical pearls and diagrams recorded. We very quickly had an invaluable database of "tips and tricks" that have subsequently been passed on and used by each year of HSS fellows. I too have reviewed these notes countless times (and continue to do so as an attending surgeon). This experience brings back fond memories and reminds me of my roots and the invaluable experiences I had. I hope this text can similarly provide young foot and ankle surgeons with these useful techniques and the framework for a successful career.

Andrew J. Rosenbaum

Acknowledgments

This text would not have been possible without the dedicated faculty of the Hospital for Special Surgery foot and ankle fellowship. The "tips and tricks" shared in this book are a result of their tireless commitment to teaching and the advancement of foot and ankle surgery. I must also acknowledge the invaluable contributions from the many authors who have shared their expertise and passion in this work.

Andrew J. Rosenbaum

Contents

ANKLE ARTHRITIS

TENDON DISORDERS

STRESS FRACTURES OF THE FOOT AND ANKLE

ANKLE TRAUMA

FOOT TRAUMA

Section 1
Conditions of the Hallux

Chapter 1

Management of Hallux Rigidus

ABDUL ARAIN
KHUSBOO DESAI

Introduction

- Loss of motion of first metatarsophalangeal joint (MTPJ) in adults due to degenerative arthritis
- Associated with repetitive microtrauma and anatomic variations of the first metatarsal predisposing to arthritis
- Dorsal osteophyte formation leads to impingement, resulting in shoe irritation and limited dorsiflexion. Patients will also have increased pain and swelling with forced dorsiflexion of the great toe and decreased push-off strength.[1]

Chilectomy

- Sterile instruments/equipment
  - Tourniquet
  - Headlight
  - Dental picks and Freer elevators
  - Pointed reduction clamps
  - K-wires and wire driver/drill/saw
  - Skin hooks and Senn retractors
- Positioning
  - Regional ankle block consisting of a 1:1 mixture of 0.25% bupivacaine and 1% lidocaine without epinephrine
  - Intravenous (IV) antibiotics 30 to 45 minutes before the procedure
  - Supine with foot at distal edge of operating table
  - Prep and drape to lower calf.
  - Tourniquet around calf (optional)
- Approach
  - Dorsal approach to first MTPJ
  - Skin incision 3 cm proximal to MTPJ to middle of proximal phalanx (Figure 1-1)
  - Retract extensor hallucis longus (EHL) and dorsomedial sensory nerve laterally.
  - Carry incision down through dorsal capsule.
  - Reflect dorsal aspect of collateral ligaments to increase joint exposure.
  - Maximally dorsiflex hallux and resect osteophyte from base of proximal phalanx with flexible chisel (Figure 1-2).
  - Resect dorsal 25% to 30% of metatarsal head articular surface. Angle flexible chisel distal to proximally, exiting at the metaphyseal–diaphyseal junction.
  - Resect medial and lateral osteophytes as needed. Avoid destabilizing collateral ligaments.
  - Check metatarsophalangeal (MTPJ) range of motion after resection by maximally dorsiflexing (Figure 1-3). Resect additional bone as needed if residual impingement is encountered.

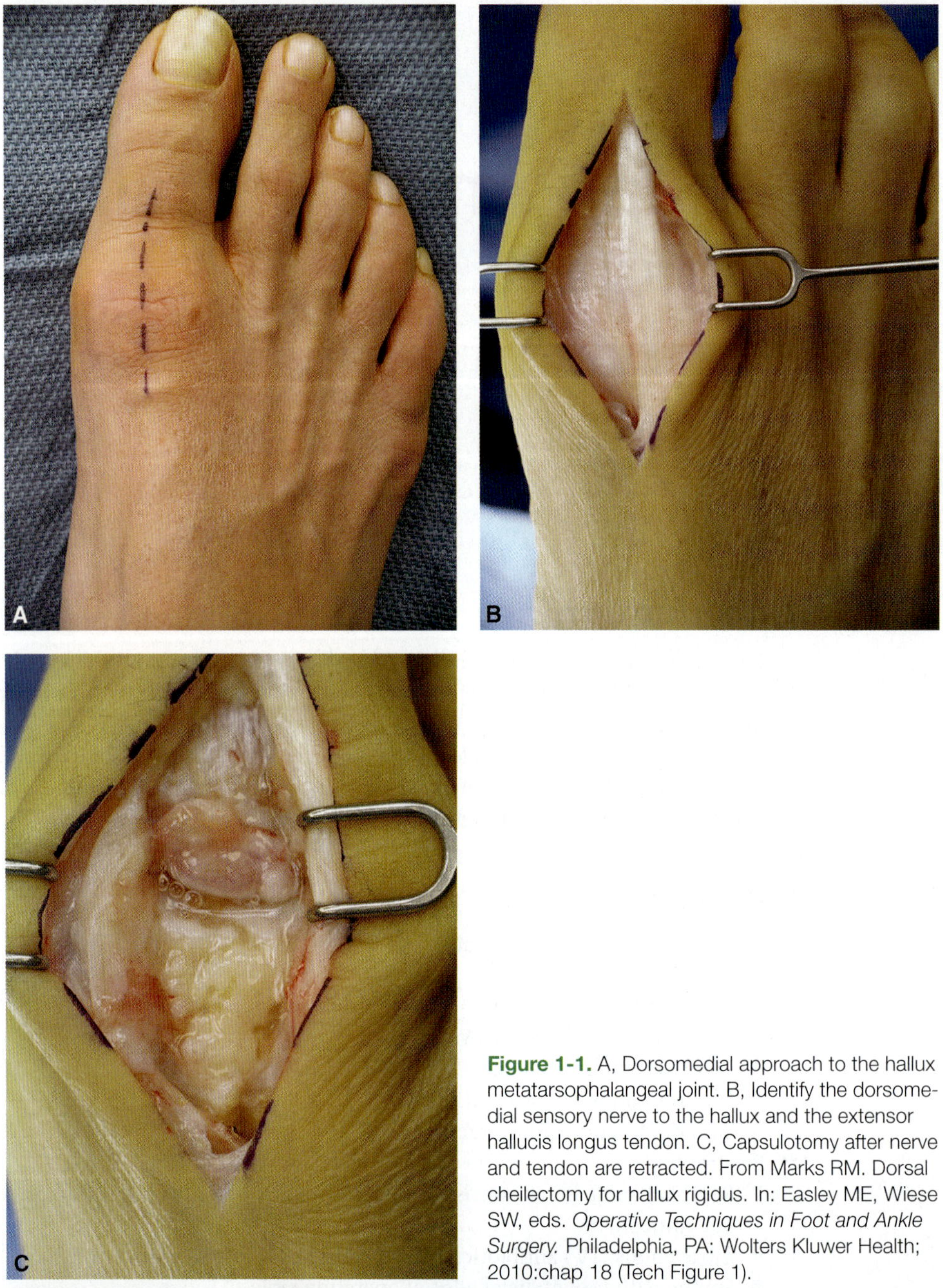

Figure 1-1. A, Dorsomedial approach to the hallux metatarsophalangeal joint. B, Identify the dorsomedial sensory nerve to the hallux and the extensor hallucis longus tendon. C, Capsulotomy after nerve and tendon are retracted. From Marks RM. Dorsal cheilectomy for hallux rigidus. In: Easley ME, Wiese SW, eds. *Operative Techniques in Foot and Ankle Surgery.* Philadelphia, PA: Wolters Kluwer Health; 2010:chap 18 (Tech Figure 1).

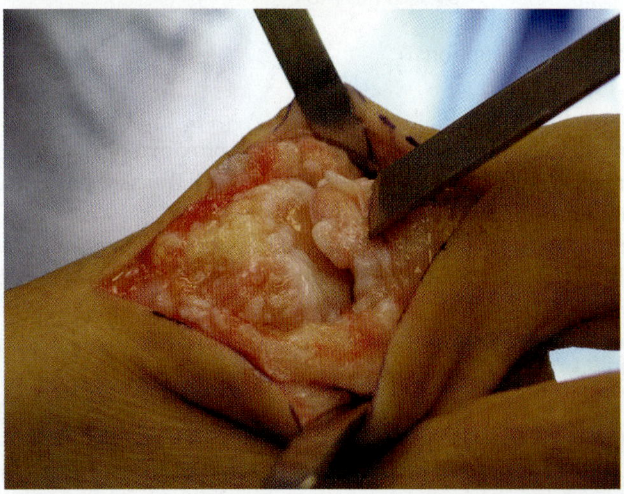

Figure 1-2. Resection of the dorsal osteophyte at the base of the proximal phalanx, performed with the hallux in maximal dorsiflexion, which will protect the remaining articular surface of the metatarsal head. From Marks RM. Dorsal cheilectomy for hallux rigidus. In: Easley ME, Wiese SW, eds. *Operative Techniques in Foot and Ankle Surgery.* Philadelphia, PA: Wolters Kluwer Health; 2010:chap 18 (Tech Figure 2A).

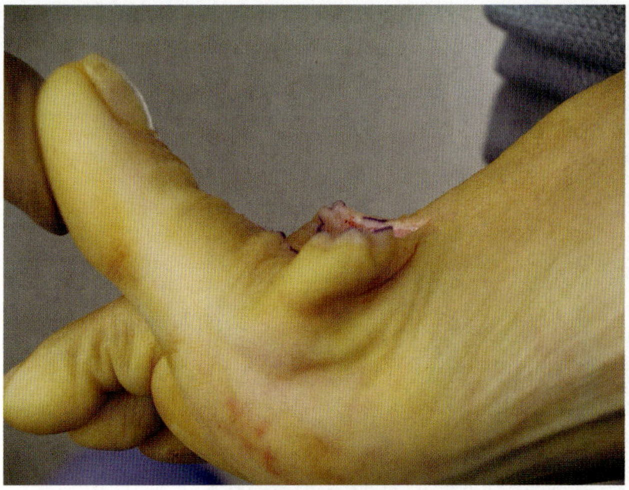

Figure 1-3. Assessment of hallux motion; should approach 90° of passive dorsiflexion. From Marks RM. Dorsal cheilectomy for hallux rigidus. In: Easley ME, Wiese SW, eds. *Operative Techniques in Foot and Ankle Surgery.* Philadelphia, PA: Wolters Kluwer Health; 2010:chap 18 (Tech Figure 2G).

- Completion
  - Irrigate wound.
  - Apply bone wax to cancellous bone of dorsal metatarsal.
  - Use a 2-0 absorbable suture to close capsule.
  - Use a 2-0 or 3-0 absorbable suture to close subcutaneous skin.
  - Close the skin with a 4-0 nylon.
  - Sterile compressive dressing
  - Heal weight-bearing in a postoperative shoe

Proximal Phalanx Osteotomy

- Sterile instruments/equipment
  - Tourniquet
  - Small Hohmann retractors
  - K-wires and wire driver/drill/saw
  - Skin hooks and Senn retractors
  - Small osteotomes
  - Rongeur
- Positioning
  - Tourniquet around thigh or calf (optional)
  - Regional ankle block consisting of a 1:1 mixture of 0.25% bupivacaine and 1% lidocaine without epinephrine along with IV sedation
  - IV antibiotics 30 to 45 minutes before the procedure
  - Position patient supine with a bump under the hip to bring foot to neutral.
  - Prep and drape to lower calf.
  - Have intraoperative fluoroscopy available.
- Approach
  - Mark a 5-cm dorsomedial incision, which is just medial to the EHL tendon.
  - Retract the EHL tendon laterally with a Hohmann retractor.
  - Protect and retract the dorsomedial nerve medially.
- Procedure
  - Complete cheilectomy.
  - Obtain exposure to the proximal phalanx (Figure 1-4).
  - Place a 0.062-in K-wire from medial to lateral and adjacent to joint surface. The wire should be placed approximately 3 mm distal to articular surface of the proximal phalanx.
  - Use a saw with small blade (0.5 cm) and start first cut. Avoid completing full osteotomy and keep plantar cortex intact.
  - Plan for second cut: 5 to 6 mm distal to the first.
  - Direct second cut proximally and plantarly such that it converges with the first cut (Figure 1-5).
  - Again, do not complete osteotomy and keep plantar cortex intact.
    - Allows for control of the osteotomy site and protects *flexor hallucis longus* (FHL) tendon.

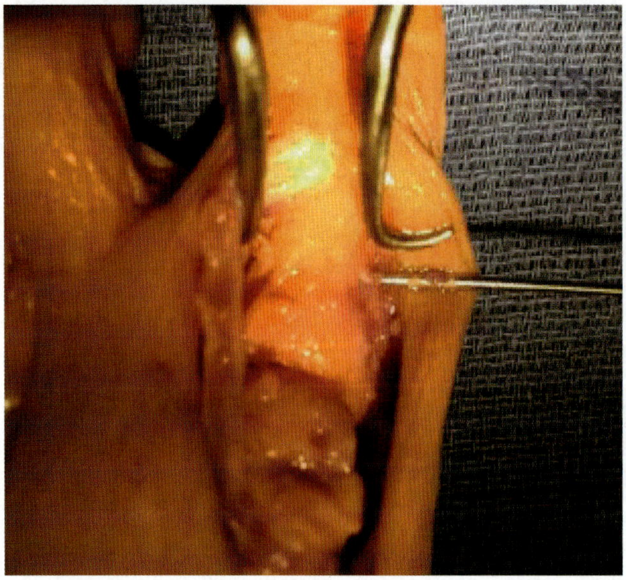

Figure 1-4. Exposure of the proximal phalanx.

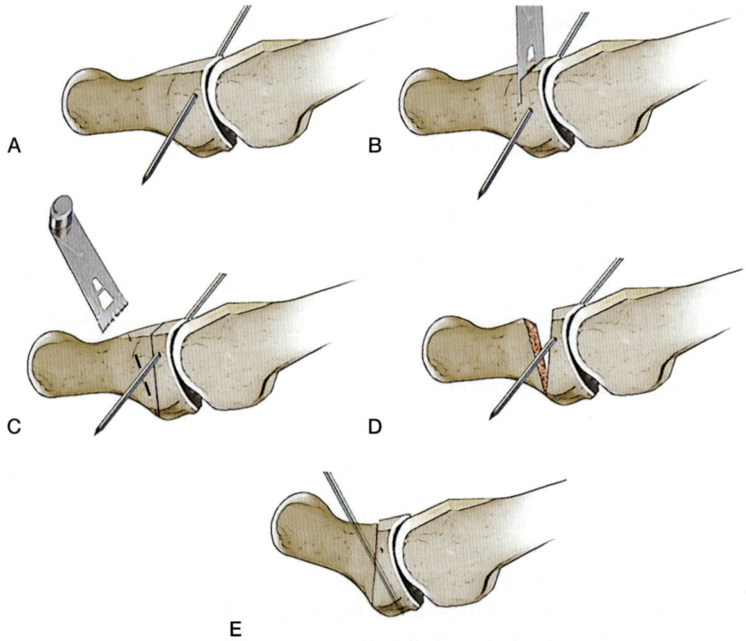

Figure 1-5. Diagram demonstrating saw trajectory for the Moberg osteotomy. A, A K-wire is placed approximately 3 mm distal to the MTP joint line. B, The first cut is made in a straight dorsal to plantar trajectory. C, The second saw cut is 5-6 mm distal to the first and is angled dorsal-distal to plantar-proximal. This ensures a dorsal wedge of bone is removed. D, The wedge is removed. The plantar cortex should ideally remain intact, allowing it to act as a periosteal hinge. E, Once manual pressure is used to close the osteotomy, provision stabilization is performed with a K-wire.

  - Complete wedge with small osteotome and use a rongeur or forceps to remove wedge.
  - Reduce the osteotomy site and fix with a wire suture, staple, or screw.
- Completion
  - Examine the MTPJ for stability.
  - Irrigate the wound.
  - Close the capsule with a 2-0 Vicryl.
  - Deflate tourniquet and obtain hemostasis.
  - Close the skin with a 4-0 nylon.
  - Apply a soft compressive dressing and place foot in hard-soled postoperative shoe.

MTPJ Arthrodesis

- Sterile instruments/equipment
  - Tourniquet
  - K-wires and wire driver/drill/saw
  - Small right-angle retractor or mini-Weitlaner

- Skin hooks and Senn retractors
- Fixation: interfragmentary cancellous screw, dorsal plate, or intramedullary Steinmann pins
- Rongeur
- Reamer

- Positioning
  - Tourniquet around thigh or calf (optional)
  - Regional ankle block consisting of a 1:1 mixture of 0.25% bupivacaine and 1% lidocaine without epinephrine along with IV sedation
  - IV antibiotics 30 to 45 minutes before the procedure
  - Position patient supine with a bump under the hip to bring foot to neutral.
  - Prep and drape to lower calf.
  - Have intraoperative fluoroscopy available.
- Approach
  - Mark a 5-cm dorsomedial incision, medial to the EHL tendon (Figure 1-1).
    - Start just proximal to interphalangeal joint and extend 5 to 6 cm proximally.
  - Sharply dissect and expose the first MTPJ.
  - Visualize both the medial and lateral aspects of the first MTPJ with small right-angle retractor or mini-Weitlaner.
  - Remove osteophytes over metatarsal joints with a rongeur.
- Procedure
  - With a small-blade saw, remove a 3-mm wafer off of the distal surface of metatarsal head. Cut should be perpendicular to the shaft (Figure 1-6).

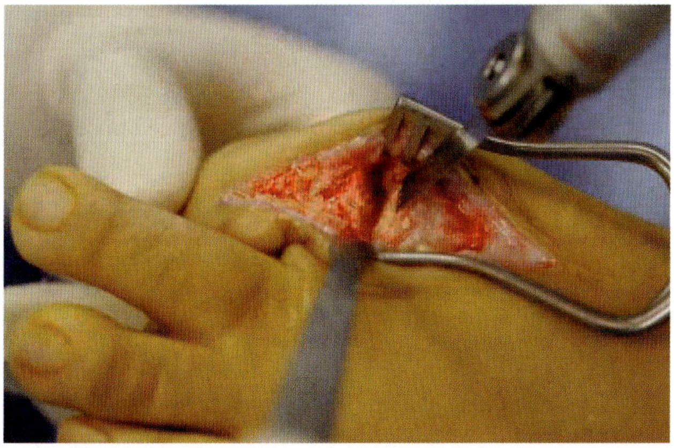

Figure 1-6. Trajectory of saw to prepare metatarsal head for arthrodesis.

  - Align hallux with first metatarsal.
    - Position: 15° of dorsiflexion to plantar surface of foot
    - 15° of valgus
    - Neutral rotation
  - With a small-blade saw, remove base of proximal phalanx parallel to the cut made on first metatarsal.
  - Prepare fusion site as follows:
    - With a K-wire, make multiple small drill holes at base of proximal phalanx and metatarsal head.
    - Place K-wire at center and ream surface or metatarsal head and base of proximal phalanx (Figure 1-7).
  - Excise extraneous soft tissue and protect FHL tendon.
  - Once proper alignment is achieved, temporarily hold with two 0.045 K-wires.
  - Place a 4-mm interfragmentary cancellous screw, dorsal plate, or intramedullary Steinmann pins for fixation (Figure 1-8).
  - Remove K-wires.
  - Inspect for areas of unopposed bone and place cancellous bone graft as needed.

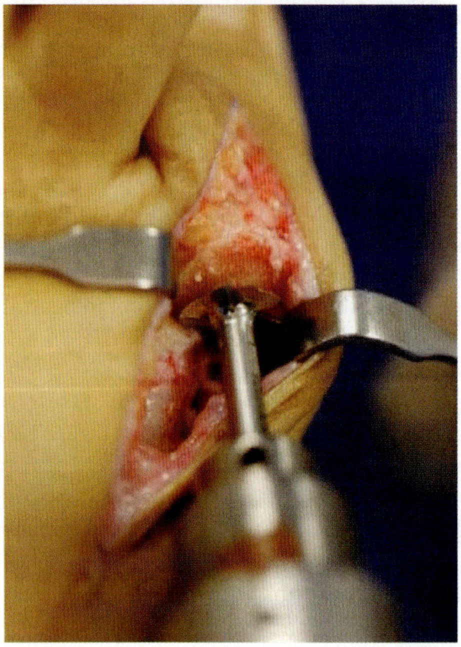

Figure 1-7. Joint preparation for hallux metatarsophalangeal arthrodesis with cone and cup reamer system.

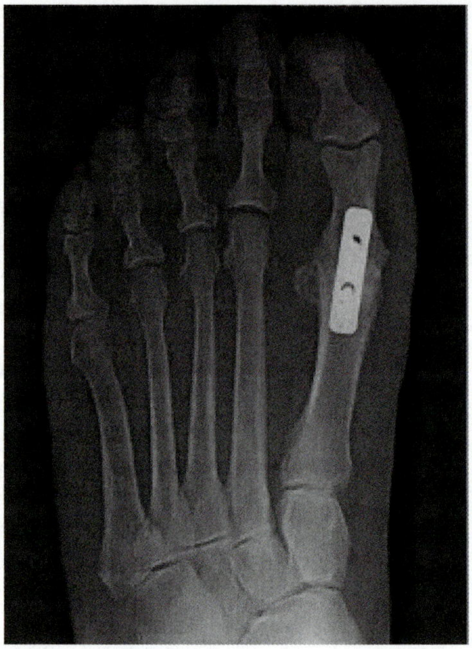

Figure 1-8. Plate fixation for hallux metatarsophalangeal fusion.

- Completion
  - Irrigate wound.
  - Close the capsule with a 2-0 Vicryl.
  - Close the skin with a 4-0 nylon.
  - Apply a soft compressive dressing and place foot in hard-soled postoperative shoe.

References

1. Shereff MJ, Baumhauer JF. Current concepts review-hallux rigidus and osteoarthrosis of the first metatarsophalangeal joint. *J Bone Joint Surg Am.* 1998;80(6):898-908.

Chapter 2

First Tarsometatarsal Joint Arthrodesis—Modified Lapidus Procedure and Akin Osteotomy

SAMIK BANERJEE
MOSTOFA ABOUSAYED
ANDREW J. ROSENBAUM

Modified Lapidus Procedure

Sterile Instruments/Equipment

- Pin distractor (Hintermann or Weinraub)
- Mini-Hohmann retractors
- 2-mm K-wires
- 2-mm drill bit
- 2.5-mm drill bit
- 3.5-mm drill bit
- Wire driver and drill
- Angled and straight curettes
- Small rongeur
- Flat lamina spreader
- Teethed lamina spreader
- Pointed reduction (Weber) clamps
- 2-mm ball-spiked or olive K-wires
- Allogeneic bone graft
- Implants
  - Plantar, medial, and dorsal locking and nonlocking plates (2.0/2.4/2.7)
  - 3.5-/4.0-mm cortical screws

Positioning

- The patient is positioned supine on a radiolucent cantilever-operating table (Figure 2-1).
- The patient is brought to the foot end of the bed for unrestricted access to medial and lateral sides and sole of the foot.
- Opposite leg bony prominences are padded, including greater trochanter, fibular head (common peroneal nerve), and elbow (ulnar nerve).
- A small bolster is placed under ipsilateral hip to position the ipsilateral patella neutral and pointing directly up.
- Anteroposterior, lateral, and oblique fluoroscopic views are obtained throughout the procedure.

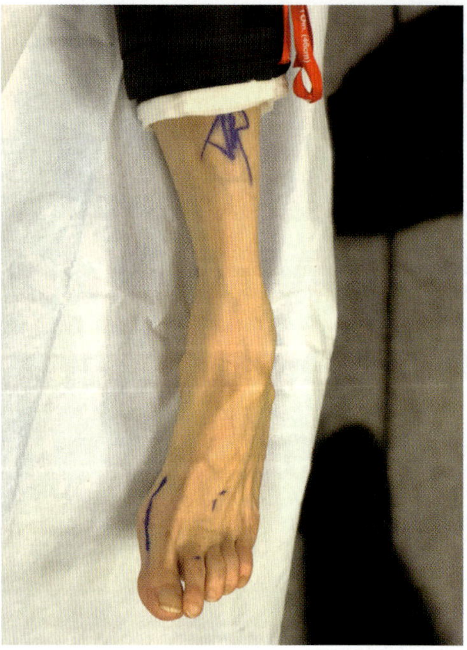

Figure 2-1. Patient positioned supine on a standard operating table with the foot placed to the edge of the table.

- Thigh or calf tourniquet (when applied low, particularly Esmarch-type, constricts the extensor tendons and may exaggerate correction)
- Regional block with sedation or general anesthesia is used for the procedure.

Surgical Approach

- The affected extremity is prepped and draped from mid-calf (if calf tourniquet is used; Figure 2-2) or mid-thigh downward (with thigh tourniquet).

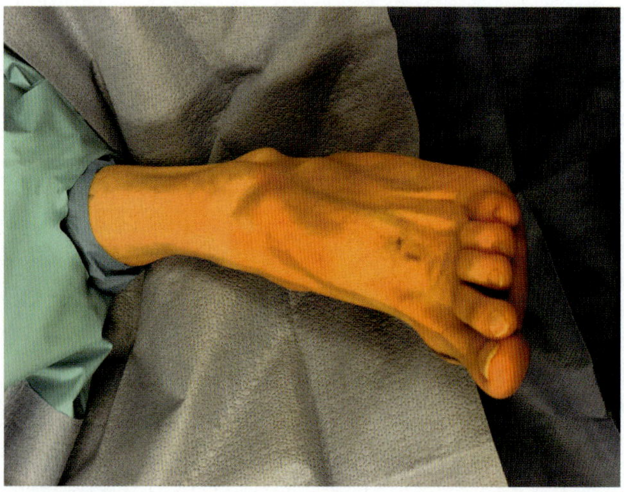

Figure 2-2. After prepping and draping.

- Three- to 6-cm dorsal longitudinal incision is made centering over the first tarsometatarsal joint (TMTJ) to approach the joint through the sheath of the extensor hallucis longus (EHL) tendon.
- The EHL tendon is retracted laterally, protecting the dorsalis pedis artery and the deep peroneal nerve.
- Longitudinal dorsal capsulotomy of the first TMTJ is made initially.
- The capsule of the first TMTJ is incised and elevated along the articular borders of the metatarsocuneiform articulation to visualize the articular surfaces medially, dorsally, and plantarly.
- A pin distractor (Hintermann or Weinraub) may then be used to pry open the metatarsocuneiform articulation after inserting 2.0-mm K-wires in the cuneiform and first metatarsal (MT) base.

Fusion Techniques

- Osteophytes, if present, are removed with rongeurs and the articular cartilage is removed with a combination of small straight and angled curettes. Utmost care is taken to avoid removing subchondral bone and unnecessarily cause first ray shortening.
- The first TMTJ may extend up to 3 cm plantarly, and thorough inspection and cartilage removal is essential for optimal preparation of the articulating surfaces for fusion. Adjusting the pin distractor and using an additional lamina spreader for adequate visualization are critical in this step of the procedure. Caution should be exercised when using a teethed lamina spreader to avoid crushing the bone surfaces.

Pearl

- Modified Lapidus procedure can potentially provide three-dimensional correction of adduction, plantarflexion, and rotational components of hallux valgus deformity.
- Dorsal malunion may result if the plantar cartilage is not completely removed.
- No wedges of bone are removed, because this shortens the MT.
- Plantarflexion of the MT may accommodate for the shortening from inadvertent bone removal.
- Caution is advocated, because as little as 3 mm of plantar bone removal may lead to 1 cm of plantarflexion of the MT.
- Denuding the cartilage is adequate for obtaining correction of the intermetatarsal angle (IMA).

- Once the MT base and the cuneiform are denuded of articular cartilage, the subchondral bone is fenestrated with a 2-mm K-wire or 2-mm drill bit. A 4-mm curved osteotome is then used to connect the perforations to allow bleeding from the cancellous bone.
- The frontal plane deformity is addressed next and the hallux is derotated out of valgus into a varus direction to get the nail plate parallel to the ground while stabilizing the hindfoot. Once this is achieved, the hallux metatarsophalangeal joint (MTPJ) is dorsiflexed, initiating the windlass mechanism, to compress the first TMTJ while simultaneously plantarflexing the first MT. All this is done while maintaining correction in the transverse plane.
- Additionally, the surgeon can use thumb pressure to manually reduce and maintain the first IMA in the transverse plane.

Surgical Tip

- The ledge of the MT and the medial cuneiform may need to be removed in order to achieve optimal compression across the arthrodesis site.
- Weber pointed reduction clamp or pin distractor may also be used at this stage to hold, reduce, and maintain correction of the IMA (Figures 2-3 and 2-4).
- Ensure that the sagittal relationship of the first and lesser MTs is maintained when using the pointed reduction clamps.

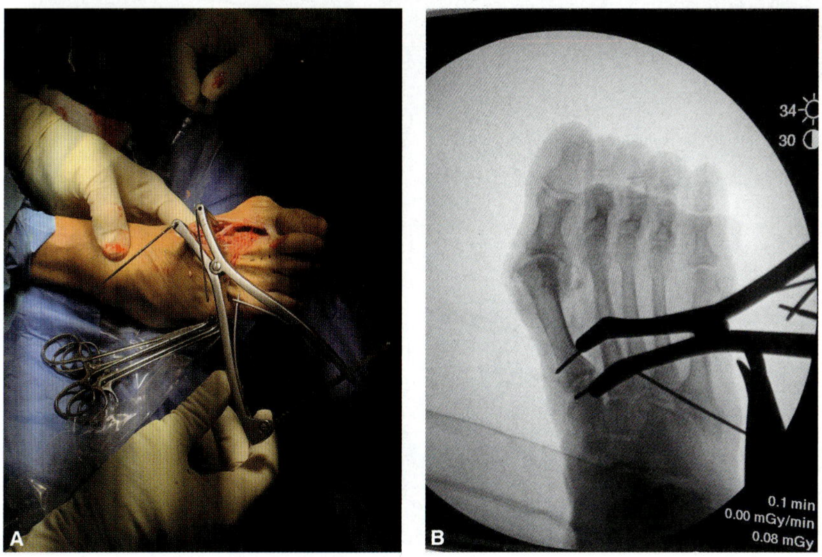

Figure 2-3. Clinical photograph (A) and radiograph (B) showing placement of the pin distractor for the Lapidus procedure.

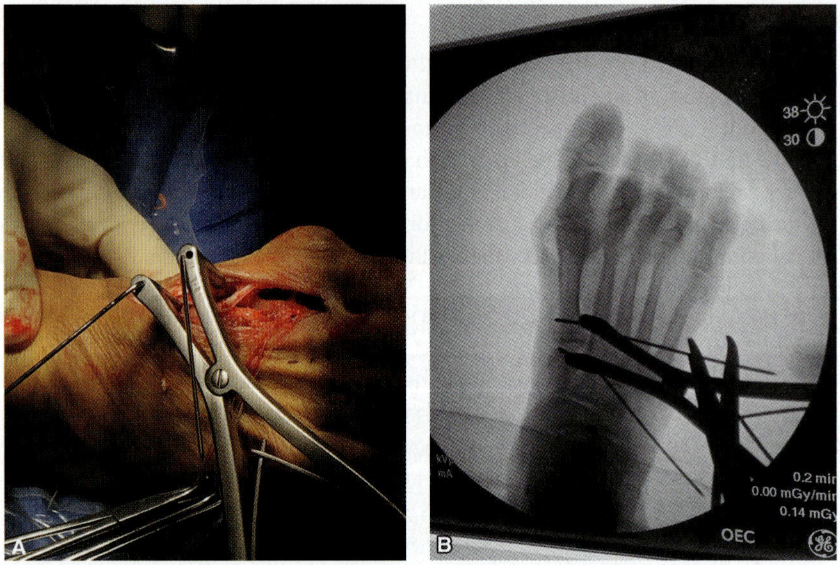

Figure 2-4. Clinical photograph (A) and radiograph (B) demonstrating correction of the intermetatarsal angle using the pin distractor as a corrective device.

- Temporary stabilization of the fusion is then performed with a K-wire or ball-spiked wire, and appropriate positioning of the arthrodesis is checked with gross inspection, fluoroscopy, and using a footplate to ensure plantigrade positioning of the hallux. It is ensured that the direction of the K-wire is away from intended path of the interfragmentary compression screws. A second K-wire may be introduced from the first MT head to the second while maintaining steady adductory pressure over the first MT. The sesamoid correction is particularly evaluated at this point.

Surgical Tip

- A graft may be used for filling bone voids and in the presence of a shortened first ray.
- An iliac crest autograft or a structural allograft may be used in revision cases for length restoration.

Fixation Techniques

- Plates, staples, or the screws-only technique may be used for stabilization of the arthrodesis site. A hybrid construct may also be used, if needed.
- When screws are used, a 3.5-/4.0-mm cortical screw is first inserted dorsolateral to plantar medial from a distal to proximal direction (Figure 2-5).

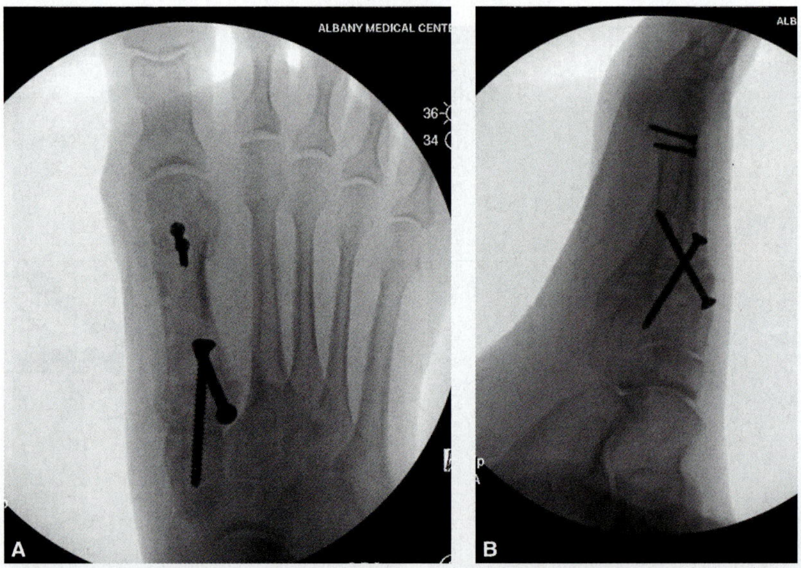

Figure 2-5. Home run screw distal to proximal screw (A) and additional proximal to distal perpendicular fixation (B) for first tarsometatarsal arthrodesis.

- Compression of the arthrodesis site is obtained by overdrilling the proximal cortex with a 3.5-mm drill bit for 3.5-mm screws and 4.0-mm drill bit for 4.0-mm screws. A 2.5-mm drill bit for 3.5-mm screws and 2.9-mm drill bit for 4.0-mm screws are then used for the distal cortices. The 4.0-mm cortical screws are generally used in larger individuals.

Surgical Tip

- The first screw is the most important screw and is termed the "home run screw"; it should have bicortical purchase.
- A trough or notch is created on the dorsal surface of the proximal one-third of MT base using a power burr. This notch is made deeper than one-half diameter of the screw head and is gradually tapered to the MT shaft in the same direction of screw insertion. This prevents splitting of the cortex during final tightening for maximal compression.
- The drill bit for the initial distal to proximal home run screw is directed toward the inferior medial aspect of the cuneiform, because the largest cross section of bone is in the medial cuneiform.
- A small dorsal gap at the TMTJ may appear after interfragmentary compression, and bone grafting may be necessary.

- Additional fixation with staples, screws, or plates may then be used without compromising the alignment of the first MT. If the screws-only technique is used, the second 3.5-mm cortical screw is inserted using an AO standard lag technique perpendicular to the home run screw. This is inserted proximal to distal from the medial cuneiform to the MT base in a dorsolateral to plantar medial direction for additional correction of the IMA.
- Plantar, medial, and dorsal plate fixation has also been described for stabilization of the arthrodesis.

Surgical Tip

- The first ray splay test may be used to determine whether transverse plane instability persists after first tarsometatarsal (TMT) arthrodesis. With the subtalar and the midtarsal joints placed in neutral alignment, transverse plane pressure is applied with the thumb and index finger to the first and second MT heads.
- IMA is persistently wide or the transverse plane instability exists after first TMT stabilization, a third 3.5-/4.0-mm screw may be inserted obliquely from the first MT to the base of the second MT. This provides additional rotational stabilization of the metatarsocuneiform fusion site as well as reduction of the IMA if inserted using a lag technique.
- Alignment relationships between the first and second MTs must be maintained during insertion of the intermetatarsal screw to avoid sesamoid pain or second MT transfer metatarsalgia.
- First to second MT fixation is used, and debridement of the first and second MT bases must be performed using a rongeur and small saw.

Additional Procedures

A medial eminence resection and medial capsulorrhaphy may be added to the modified Lapidus procedure for additional correction of hallux valgus deformity. The first TMTJ arthrodesis is a powerful procedure and overcorrection with a resultant hallux varus deformity may occur if combined with a distal lateral soft-tissue release. Akin medial closing-wedge osteotomy or a distal MT osteotomy may be combined with TMTJ fusion for increased hallux valgus interphalangeus or hallux valgus angle overall.

Pearl

- The overall length of the first must be assessed after completion of the procedure and compared with the second and third MTs. Typically, shortening varies between 2.7 and 2.9 mm after modified Lapidus procedures, with shortening up to 5 mm unlikely to lead to symptoms of transfer metatarsalgia and may not be clinically relevant.
- Weil shortening osteotomies of the second and third MT heads may be needed in the presence of substantial shortening of the first MT length or in the presence of preoperative pain and/or synovitis of these lesser MTs.

Akin Osteotomy

Equipment

- Tourniquet
- Microsagittal saw
- K-wires and wire driver
- Mini- and small-fragment screws (2.4/2.7/3.0 cannulated screws)

Positioning

- Supine position (all bony prominences should be well padded)
- A thigh or calf tourniquet can be used.
- A bump underneath the contralateral hip may aid exposure of the medial side of the foot by externally rotating the surgical extremity.

Surgical Approach

- An Akin osteotomy is typically performed in conjunction with other procedures for hallux valgus deformity.[1]
- The incision is usually an extension of the longitudinal medial incision performed for distal soft-tissue procedure (modified McBride) with or without distal bony realignment.
- The incision extends distally to the level of the interphalangeal joint to expose the proximal phalanx shaft (Figure 2-6).

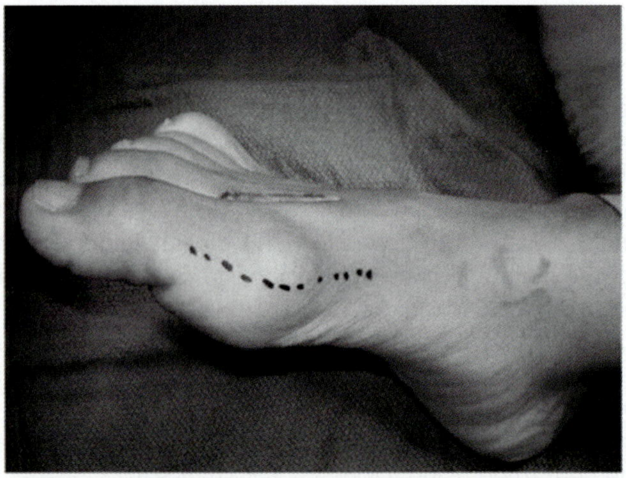

Figure 2-6. The medial incision for Akin phalangeal osteotomy.

- The medial dorsal cutaneous nerve and medial plantar sensory nerve should be identified and protected (Figure 2-7).
- The capsular incision done at the MTPJ for the modified McBride is carried distally along the shaft of the proximal phalanx.
- The first osteotomy is performed at the proximal phalanx base distal to the MTPJ angled from medial to lateral perpendicular to the long axis of the phalanx.
- The osteotomy can be done under fluoroscopic guidance to avoid penetration of the MTPJ and ensure adequate proximal bone for screw fixation.
- A K-wire could be placed under fluoroscopy just distal to the proposed osteotomy site to facilitate adequate osteotomy site.
- Care must be taken to avoid penetration of the lateral cortex (makes the osteotomy unstable). This can be aided by continuous fluoroscopic imaging.
- A second osteotomy about 2 to 3 mm distally is then performed at an angle to produce a closing wedge.
- Again, care must be taken to avoid penetration of the lateral cortex.

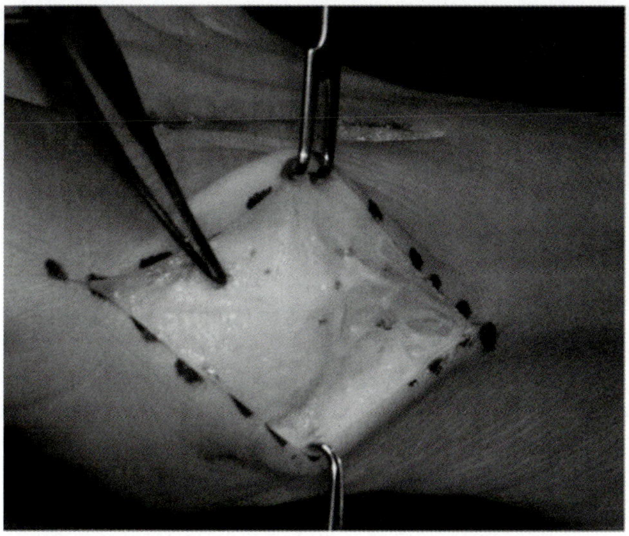

Figure 2-7. The medial dorsal cutaneous nerve identified and protected.

- Continuously irrigate with cool saline while performing the osteotomy.
- Alternatively, a biplane oblique osteotomy can be used.
- The first cut is started at the dorsomedial cortex at the mid-phalanx level. The osteotomy is then directed in a proximal, lateral, and plantar direction. Similarly, care must be taken to avoid penetration of the MTPJ or the lateral cortex (Figure 2-8A, B).
- A 2- to 4-mm wedge is then removed using the saw to create a closed wedge.
- The osteotomy is then hinged open and a temporary K-wire can be placed across the osteotomy for stabilization (Figure 2-9).

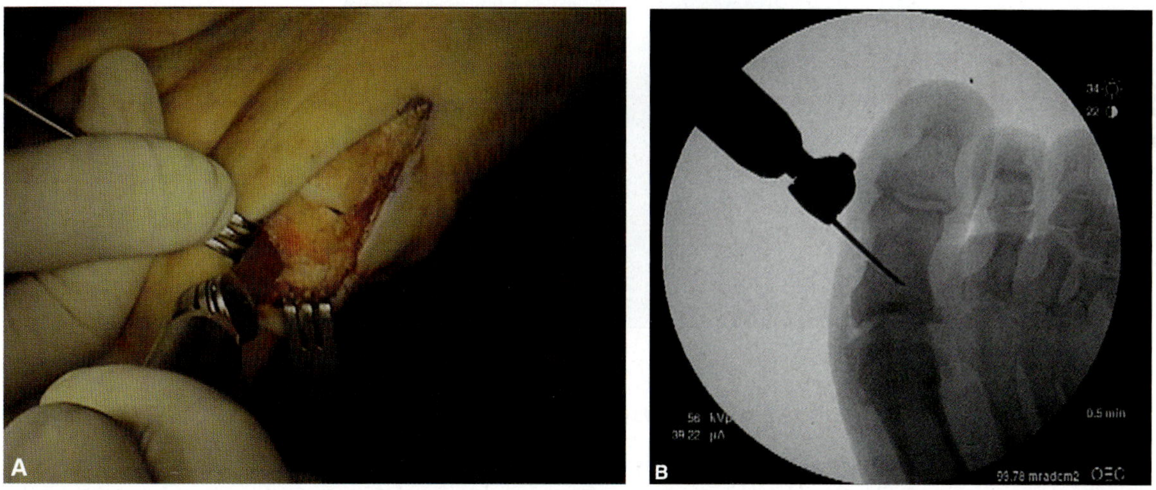

Figure 2-8. A, The first cut of the closing-wedge osteotomy is made starting at the dorsomedial surface of the proximal phalanx at the level of the mid-shaft. B, Under fluoroscopic guidance, the osteotomy is directed laterally exiting distal to the metatarsophalangeal joint.

- Before placement of the guidewire for screw fixation, ensure adequate visualization of the bone at the base of proximal phalanx by adequate dissection of the capsule to ensure proper seating of the screw.
- A guidewire for a small cannulated screw is placed across the osteotomy from plantar medial to dorsal lateral (this trajectory takes into account the normal inclination of the proximal phalanx).
- Guidewire placement should be checked under fluoroscopy before drilling.
- The drill should be advanced all the way to the lateral cortex.

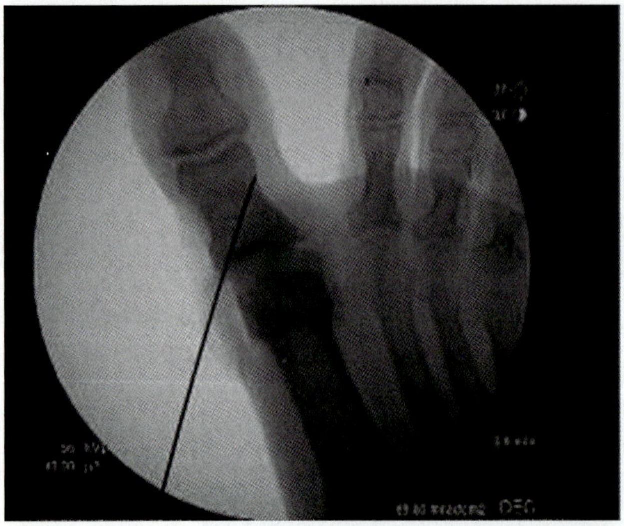

Figure 2-9. A guidewire is advanced across and perpendicular to the closed osteotomy.

- An adequate length screw is subsequently placed, which will close the osteotomy (Figure 2-10).
- The tourniquet is then released and adequate hemostasis is performed before closure.
- A 2-0 Vicryl suture is used to repair the capsulotomy.
- A 3-0 Vicryl can then be used for closure of subcutaneous tissue and 3-0 nylon for the skin.

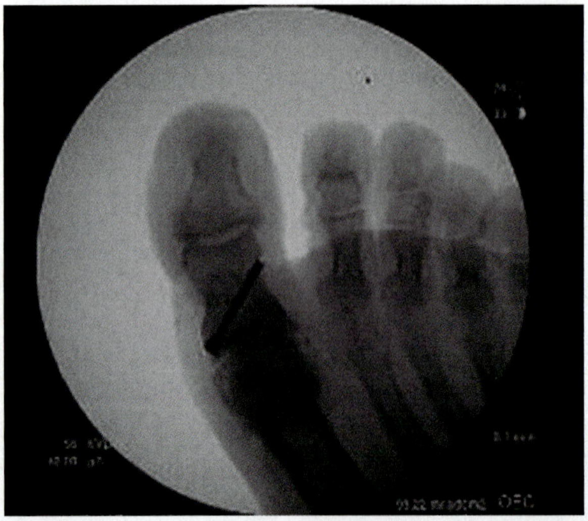

Figure 2-10. A screw is advanced across the osteotomy, resulting in stable compression of the osteotomy.

Postoperative Course

- The postoperative plan is typically dictated by other procedures done.
- For the Akin osteotomy, a soft bunion dressing is usually sufficient and patients can be weight-bearing as tolerated in a hard-soled shoe.
- At 10 to 14 days postoperatively, sutures are removed and patients are instructed to initiate range of motion exercises.
- Transition to regular wide-toe flexible shoe is usually permitted as swelling resolves and per patient comfort.
- At 6 weeks, if radiographs show adequate healing and alignment of the osteotomy, patients are encouraged to perform all activities as tolerated.

Reference

1. Frey C, Jahss M, Kummer F. The Akin procedure: an analysis of results. *Foot Ankle*. 1991;12:1-6.

Section 2
Metatarsalgia and Lesser Toe Deformity

Chapter 3

Management of Metatarsalgia and Equinus Contracture: Gastrocnemius Recession, Percutaneous Tendoachilles Lengthening, and Diaphyseal Metatarsal Shortening Osteotomy

RACHEL J. SHAKKED
MAXWELL C. ALLEY, JR.
CHRISTOPHER JOHNSON
ANDREW J. ROSENBAUM

Gastrocnemius Recession

- Instruments/equipment
  - Long-handled scalpel
  - Vaginal speculum
  - Right-angle retractors
- Positioning
  - The patient is positioned supine, with the leg in neutral or slightly externally rotated position.
- Surgical procedure
  - The author's preferred technique is a modified Strayer recession of the gastrocnemius (Figure 3-1).[1]
  - Identify the contour of the gastrocnemius muscle along the medial aspect of the lower leg (Figure 3-2).
  - A 3- to 4-cm longitudinal incision is made, medially centered over the musculotendinous junction as determined by visual inspection.
  - Identify the fascia and incise in line with the skin incision.
  - The musculotendinous junction should be visualized. Use blunt dissection to dissect the gastrocnemius fascia anterior and posterior to the gastrocnemius muscle just proximal to the musculotendinous junction.
  - Large right-angle retractors can be utilized for visualization.

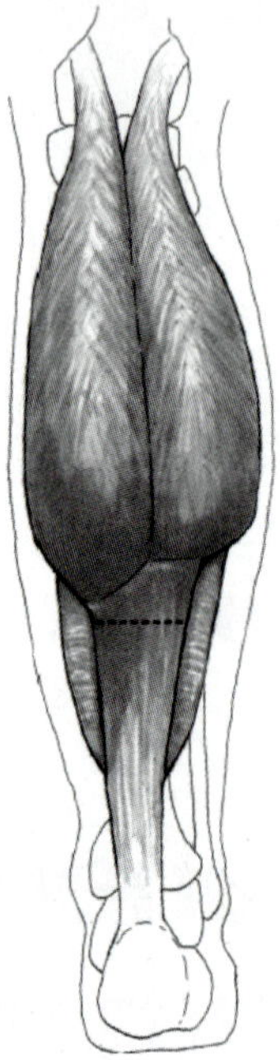

Figure 3-1. Cartoon depiction of the Strayer procedure demonstrating the location of the incision across the gastrocnemius fascia. Reprinted from Hsu RY, VanValkenburg S, Tanriover A, et al. Surgical techniques of gastrocnemius lengthening. *Foot Ankle Clin*. 2014;19(4):745-765. Copyright © 2014 Elsevier. With permission.

- Identify the sural nerve, which is typically midline and may be adherent to the posterior aspect of the gastrocnemius fascia. A small elevator can be used to gently sweep the nerve and its adventitial tissue away from the fascia.
- The plantaris tendon is tenotomized.
- A vaginal speculum can be used for optimal exposure (Figure 3-3). It is inserted to expose the gastrocnemius fascia and to protect the sural nerve.

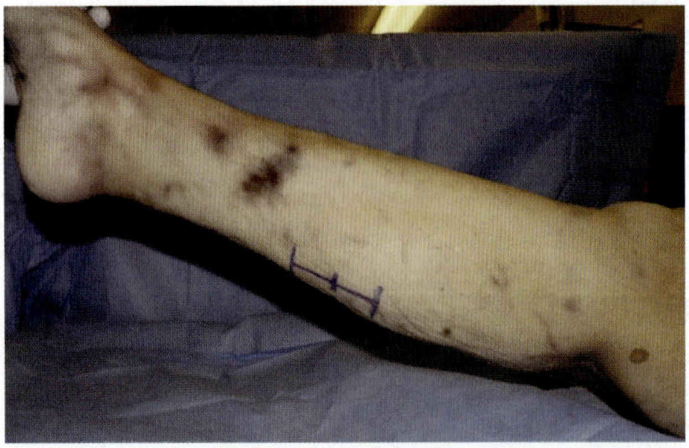

Figure 3-2. The incision is marked at the junction of the contoured gastrocnemius muscle and the most proximal portion of the Achilles tendon. Reprinted from Hsu RY, VanValkenburg S, Tanriover A, et al. Surgical techniques of gastrocnemius lengthening. *Foot Ankle Clin*. 2014;19(4):745-765. Copyright © 2014 Elsevier. With permission.

- Next, a long-handled scalpel or Mayo scissors can be used to incise the fascia from medial to lateral in line with the speculum (Figures 3-4 and 3-5). While performing this technique, an assistant holds the ankle in gentle dorsiflexion with the knee extended.
- Once the fascia is completely released, the speculum is removed and the sural nerve is visualized in the soft tissue posteriorly.
- After thorough irrigation, the superficial fascia is closed using a running, absorbable suture to prevent muscle herniation.
- Subcutaneous tissue is closed using interrupted 3-0 Vicryl sutures, and the skin is closed using 3-0 nylon sutures.

- Postoperative plan
    - When performed in isolation, the patient may weight-bear as tolerated in a fracture boot for 6 weeks. Stretching exercises may begin as soon as the incision is adequately healed, typically after the first postoperative visit at 2 weeks.

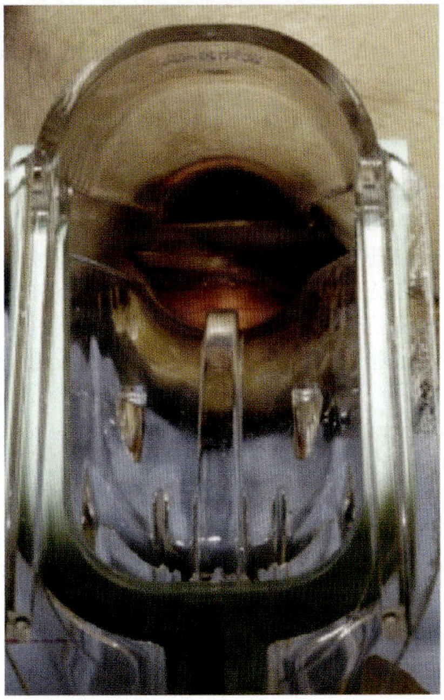

Figure 3-3. A vaginal speculum is used to isolate the gastrocnemius fascia from the muscle that lies anterior and the sural nerve that lies posterior. Reprinted from Hsu RY, VanValkenburg S, Tanriover A, et al. Surgical techniques of gastrocnemius lengthening. *Foot Ankle Clin*. 2014;19(4):745-765. Copyright © 2014 Elsevier. With permission.

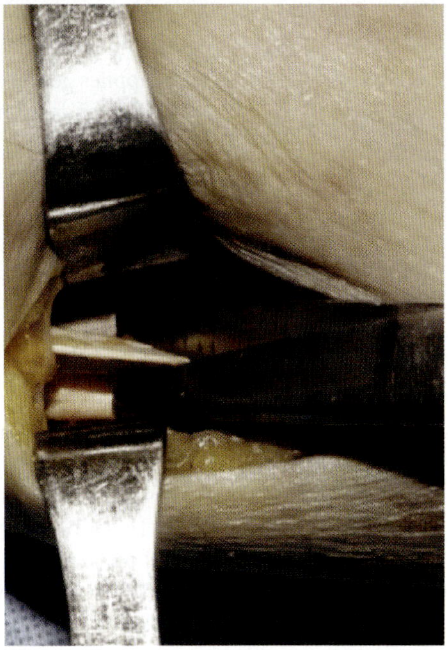

Figure 3-4. The fascia is incised using Mayo scissors. The gastrocnemius muscle and fatty adventitial layer containing the sural nerve are retracted out of the way. Reprinted from Hsu RY, VanValkenburg S, Tanriover A, et al. Surgical techniques of gastrocnemius lengthening. *Foot Ankle Clin*. 2014;19(4):745-765. Copyright © 2014 Elsevier. With permission.

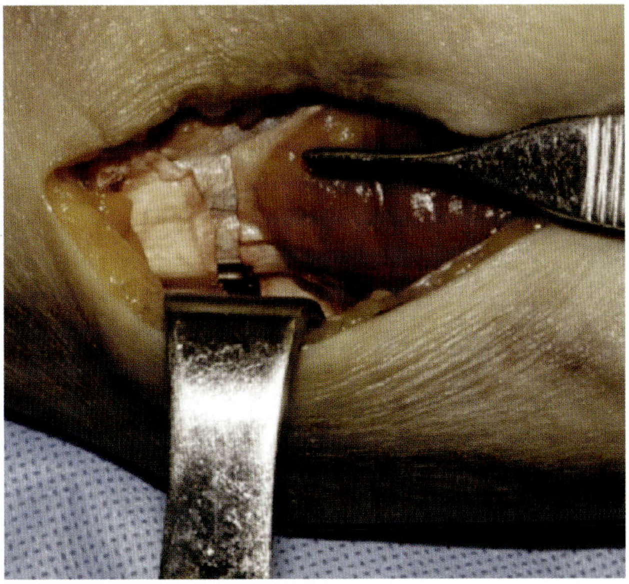

Figure 3-5. The gastrocnemius fascia is released and lengthened and the fascia of the soleus muscle is visualized in the surgical field. Reprinted from Hsu RY, VanValkenburg S, Tanriover A, et al. Surgical techniques of gastrocnemius lengthening. *Foot Ankle Clin*. 2014;19(4):745-765. Copyright © 2014 Elsevier. With permission.

Percutaneous Tendoachilles Lengthening

- Instruments/equipment
  - #11 scalpel blade
- Positioning
  - The patient is positioned supine because this procedure is typically performed in conjunction with other procedures that require the patient to be supine.
  - An assistant should be available to hold up the extremity.

- Surgical procedure
  - A tourniquet is not necessary. The assistant holds the lower extremity up for visualization and applies gentle dorsiflexion pressure to the foot while keeping the knee extended.
  - The tendon lengthening procedure, as popularized by Hoke, is the author's preferred technique (Figure 3-6).[2]
  - Three percutaneous incisions are made starting distally at about 2 cm proximal to the Achilles insertion and then spaced out by 2 cm each.
  - A #11 blade is used and inserted vertically through the skin and into the tendon in a midline position. The blade is then rotated to face medially and the tendon hemisection is completed percutaneously by applying digital pressure on the tendon through the skin.
  - The procedure is repeated 2 cm proximal in a lateral direction and then an additional 2 cm proximal in a medial direction.
  - The ankle is gently dorsiflexed to confirm adequate lengthening of the tendon.
  - The incisions are closed using 3-0 nylon sutures.
  - A sterile dressing is then applied.
- Postoperative plan
  - This procedure is typically performed in conjunction with other procedures that can affect the postoperative protocol.
  - When performed in isolation, the patient may be weight-bearing as tolerated in a tall fracture boot.

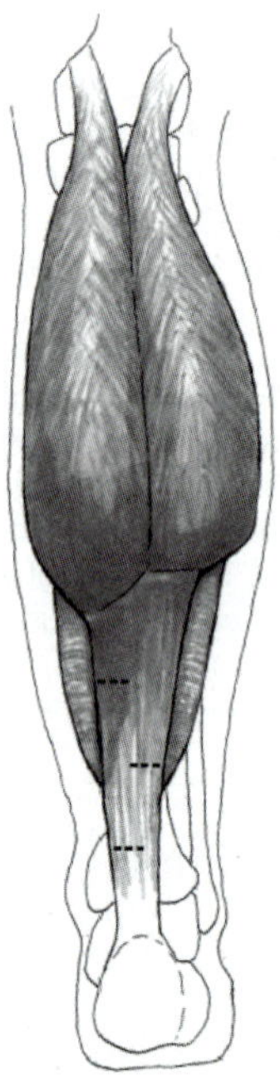

Figure 3-6. Cartoon depicting the percutaneous Z-lengthening procedure of the Achilles tendon as popularized by Hoke. Reprinted from Anderson JG, Bohay DR, Eller EB, et al. Gastrocnemius recession. *Foot Ankle Clin*. 2014;19(4):767-786. Copyright © 2014 Elsevier. With permission.

Diaphyseal Metatarsal Shortening Osteotomy

- Instruments/equipment
  - Microsagittal saw
  - A four-hole 2.4-mm locking compression plate (LCP)
- Positioning
  - The patient is positioned supine on the operating room table with a bump under the ipsilateral hip so that the toes are pointing toward the ceiling.
- Surgical procedure
  - The length differential between the operative metatarsal and its neighbors should be measured preoperatively to determine the degree of shortening to perform.
  - A dorsal longitudinal incision is made over the metatarsal shaft or in the interspace if more than one metatarsal is being addressed.
  - The extensor tendons are identified and retracted to expose the metatarsal shaft.

- Sharp dissection is used to incise the periosteum over the metatarsal shaft. Thick periosteal flaps are made medially and laterally and Hohmann retractors are used for exposure.
- A four-hole, 2.4-mm LCP is provisionally applied to the metatarsal and the position is checked on fluoroscopy. The osteotomy site should be diaphyseal and the plate should be extra-articular.
- Non-locking cortical screws are then placed bicortically in the distal two holes.
- A marking pen is used to delineate the osteotomy site, which should fall between the middle two holes of the plate.
- The more proximal of the screws is then removed and the distal screw is loosened to allow the plate to rotate out of the way of the osteotomy site.
- A microsagittal saw is then used to make a transverse osteotomy at the planned site. A second cut is made removing the planned length of bone, typically 2 to 4 mm.
- The plate is then repositioned and the distal screws are replaced and tightened.
- While holding the osteotomy site reduced, the proximal screws are drilled eccentrically, and non-locking, cortical screws are placed to achieve compression at the osteotomy site (Figure 3-7).

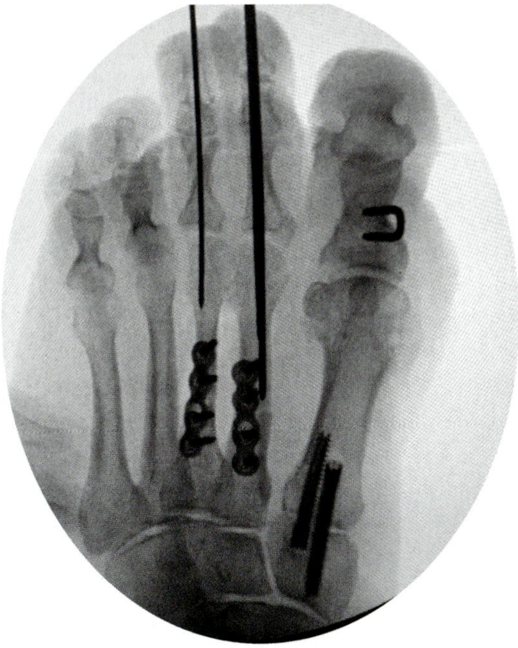

Figure 3-7. Postoperative radiograph demonstrating shortening osteotomies of the second and third metatarsals performed in conjunction with a forefoot reconstruction including Lapidus bunionectomy, modified McBride procedure, Akin osteotomy, and second and third hammertoe corrections.

- Manual palpation of the metatarsal heads is then performed to make sure the cascade has been reestablished.
- After thorough irrigation, the incision is then closed using a 3-0 Vicryl for the subcutaneous tissue and a 4-0 nylon for the skin. The patient is placed in a short leg plaster splint.

- Postoperative plan
  - Non-weight-bearing for 6 weeks. Ankle range of motion can be initiated upon transition to a tall fracture boot at the first postoperative visit. If radiographs demonstrate progression of healing at 6 weeks, the patient can initiate weight-bearing in the fracture boot.

References

1. Strayer LM Jr. Recession of the gastrocnemius; an operation to relieve spastic contracture of the calf muscles. *J Bone Joint Surg Am*. 1950;32A(3):671-676.
2. Hoke M. An operation for stabilizing paralytic feet. *J Orthop Surg*. 1921;3(10):494-507.

Chapter 4
Management of Lesser Toe Deformity: PIP Arthroplasty and Extensor Lengthening

RACHEL J. SHAKKED
MAXWELL C. ALLEY, JR.
CHRISTOPHER JOHNSON
ANDREW J. ROSENBAUM

Instruments/Equipment

- 1.6-mm and 1.25-mm Kirschner wires (K-wires) and wire driver
- Microsagittal saw
- Mini C-arm
- McGlamry Metatarsal Elevator
- Wire cutter

Positioning

- The patient is positioned supine, with a small bump under the ipsilateral hip to position the foot in neutral with toes pointing up to the ceiling.

Surgical Procedure

- A dorsal longitudinal incision is centered over the metatarsophalangeal (MTP) joint or in the webspace if more than one hammertoe is being addressed.
- First, identify the extensor digitorum longus (EDL) tendon and tenotomize as distal as possible. Next, identify the extensor digitorum brevis (EDB) and tenotomize as proximal as possible within the incision.
- Use a scalpel to make a transverse incision in the MTP joint capsule to release the dorsal capsule. Release the capsule medially and laterally along the metatarsal head, taking care to avoid the neurovascular bundles. Use a McGlamry Elevator to release the plantar capsule.
- Next, make a dorsal midline incision centered over the proximal interphalangeal (PIP) joint of the affected toe. Incise the extensor tendon in line with the incision and elevate subperiosteally medially and laterally to expose the joint. Release the collateral ligaments off the proximal phalanx.
- Excise the distal aspect of the proximal phalanx using a microsagittal saw oriented perpendicular to the shaft. Use the microsagittal saw to remove the cartilage from the middle phalanx.
- Use a small clamp to dissect plantarly and identify the three flexor tendons. Sequentially deliver each tendon, clamp, and then tenotomize on either side of the clamp to excise several millimeters of tendon.

- Pin toe in place using retrograde technique.
  - Drive a 1.6-mm K-wire through the middle phalanx out the tip of the toe leaving a small amount of wire exposed in the joint. Make sure to hold the distal interphalangeal joint extended to avoid plantarflexion deformity.
  - Reduce the PIP joint and insert the wire to the base of the proximal phalanx. Check the position of the wire under fluoroscopy.
  - Depending on the position of the existing K-wire under fluoroscopy, insert a 1.25 K-wire parallel and just medial or lateral for rotational stability (Figures 4-1 and 4-2).

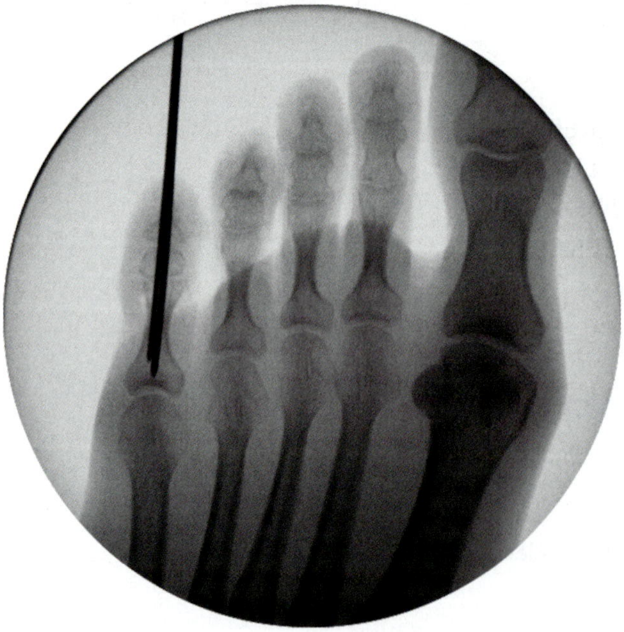

Figure 4-1. Intraoperative fluoroscopy demonstrating successful placement of a 1.6-mm K-wire and a 1.25-mm K-wire holding an acceptable reduction of the fifth proximal interphalangeal joint, as seen on the anteroposterior view.

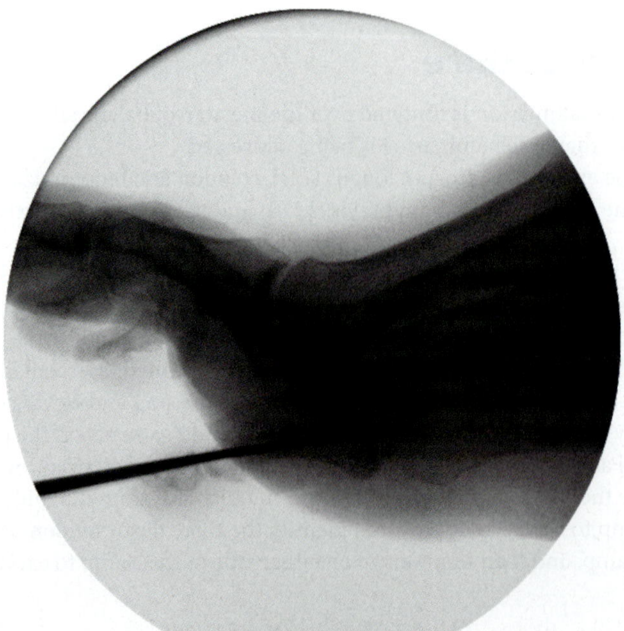

Figure 4-2. Intraoperative fluoroscopy demonstrating a lateral view of two K-wires within the fifth toe securing the proximal interphalangeal joint.

- If the MTP joint is still dorsally subluxated, the 1.6-mm K-wire can be passed across the MTP joint while holding it in a reduced position (Figure 4-3). If the joint is not easily reduced, or if there is more than subtle subluxation, then a metatarsal shortening osteotomy should be considered.

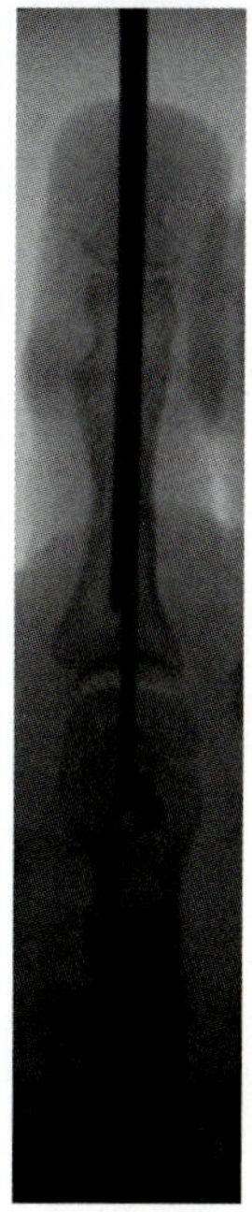

Figure 4-3. Anteroposterior view of a second toe that has undergone proximal interphalangeal resection arthroplasty for hammertoe. The patient also underwent a Weil shortening osteotomy with screw fixation. The 1.6-mm K-wire traverses the metatarsophalangeal joint to maintain a concentric reduction of the joint. The 1.25-mm K-wire placed for rotational stability is inserted only to the level of the proximal phalanx.

- The wires are then bent at the tip of the toe using a heavy needle driver and a metal suction tip. The wires are then cut short.
- After thorough irrigation, the EDL tendon is loosely reapproximated to the cut end of the EDB tendon using a 3-0 Vicryl suture.
- A layered closure is then performed using 3-0 Vicryl and 3-0 nylon sutures and a sterile dressing is applied.
- The tourniquet is let down while in the operating room to ensure adequate perfusion of the toe.
- If the toe is not perfused immediately, attempt the following:
  - Allow more time (up to 20 minutes) for reversal of vasospasm.
  - Apply warm saline to the toe.
  - Lower the foot relative to the rest of the body.
  - Remove skin sutures if tight and replace them more loosely.
  - Loosen the pin. If crossing the MTP joint, pull the pin back into the proximal phalanx and tape the toe in position.
  - Remove pin altogether.
  - Surgical exploration

Postoperative Plan

- If the wire traverses the MTP joint, then the patient must remain non–weight-bearing to avoid bending of the wire.
- If the wire does not traverse the MTP joint, then the patient may weight-bear as tolerated in a hard-soled shoe with crutches or a cane.
- Strict elevation is encouraged for the first 2 weeks postoperatively.
- Aspirin deep venous thrombosis (DVT) prophylaxis is typically provided if the patient is non–weight-bearing unless there are any additional risk factors for DVT.
- The wires are removed in the office at 6 weeks postoperatively.

Section 3

Adult Acquired Flatfoot Deformity

Chapter 5
Correction of the Flexible Flatfoot

JONATHAN T. DELAND
MACKENZIE T. JONES

Sterile Instruments/Equipment

- Tourniquet
- Cannulated drill 4.5, 5 mm
- Cannulated screws 4.5 mm
- Noncannulated screws 3.5, 4.0 cortical
- Pin distractor
- Blunt laminar spreader
- Two baby Bennett retractors
- Baby Wheatlander
- Tricortical allograft

Positioning

- The patient is placed in the supine position.
- Place a bump under the hip so that the toes point straight to the ceiling.

Surgical Approach

Medial Approach for Posterior Tibial Tendon and Flexor Digitorum Longus (FDL) Tendon

- Make an incision from the posterior tip of the medial malleolus to the inferior border of the navicular and first metatarsal tarsal joint distally (Figure 5-1).

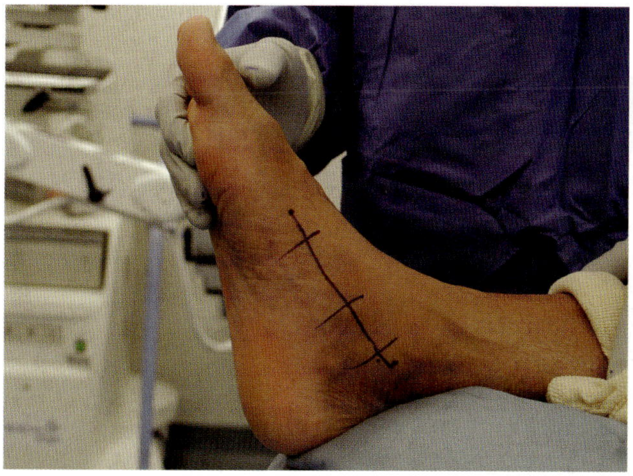

Figure 5-1. Incision for exposure of posterior tibial tendon and flexor digitorum longus tendon and possible spring ligament repair.

- This incision can be shorter if a Bio-Tenodesis screw is used for the FDL transfer. The screw allows for a shorter harvesting of the FDL tendon.

- Expose and examine the posterior tibial tendon (Figure 5-2).
  - If one-half of the diameter of the tendon is not severely degenerated, then retain the tendon and trim the most degenerated portion.
  - If the tendon is too degenerated, release it and leave a stump at the navicular. It can be useful to tie the transfer to at the end of the procedure.

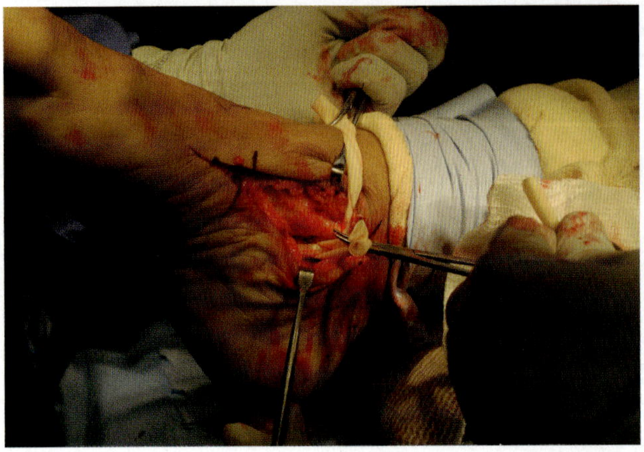

Figure 5-2. Exposure showing dorsal Penrose around posterior tibial tendon and inferior Penrose showing the flexor digitorum longus tendon.

- Incise the FDL sheath along a line that is parallel and just inferior to the posterior tibial tendon.
  - Moving lesser toes may allow palpation of the tendon through the sheath.
- Expose the FDL tendon down to a level distal to the navicular, staying on the inferior aspect of the navicular and medial cuneiform to avoid large veins.
- Release the FDL tendon at the level underneath the medial cuneiform.
  - The authors' preference is to expose the FDL underneath the metatarsal tarsal joint, which results in more dissection but allows for easier tensioning of the transfer at the end of the procedure (if the tendon is tied down at the dorsal exit of the navicular instead of using a Bio-Tenodesis screw).
- Underneath the metatarsal tarsal joint, expose the attachment of the flexor hallucis brevis, incise it longitudinally, and identify the flexor hallucis longus (FHL) tendon.
- Isolate the FDL tendon more laterally.
- Identify the interconnection from the FHL to the FDL and release the FDL tendon, but not the interconnection, and place a whipstitch in the proximal end of the tendon.
  - Do not release the interconnection of the FHL to the second and third toes.
- Expose the dorsal navicular and use an awl to mark the dorsal entry point for the guide pin in between the talonavicular and navicular cuneiform joints.
- Point the drill toward the medial inferior aspect of the plantar navicular and drill the guidewire through the awl hole from dorsal to plantar (Figure 5-3).
- Overdrill on the guidewire using a 4.5- or 5.0-mm hole according to the size of the tendon.

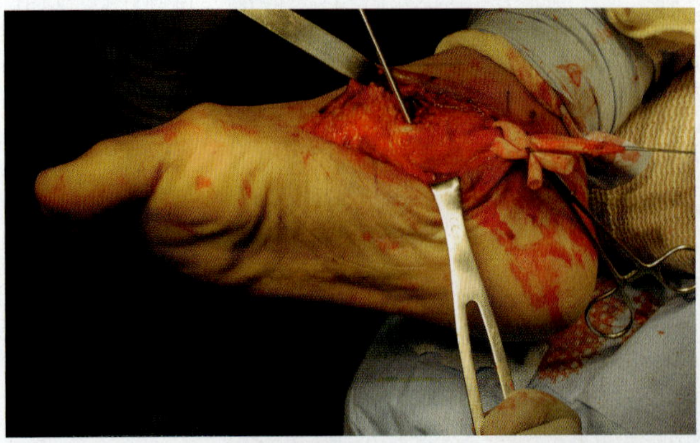

Figure 5-3. Guide pin for drill hole in navicular in place.

Dorsal Approach

If there is severe elevation of the first ray, a first metatarsal tarsal fusion is more effective than a Cotton osteotomy in bringing the first ray down and correcting metatarsus primus varus.

- Make an incision in between the first and the second metatarsals so that there is an adequate skin bridge if a long medial incision for the FDL transfer has been used (Figure 5-4).
- Expose the first metatarsal tarsal joint, being careful not to injure the superficial peroneal nerve proximally, place retractors, and open the joint dorsally.

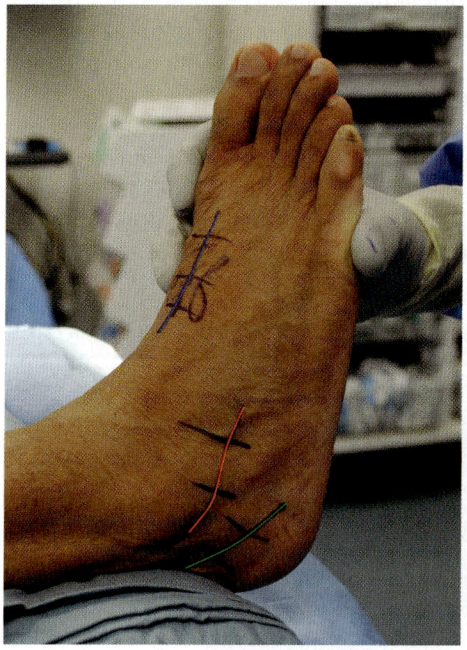

Figure 5-4. Incision for metatarsal tarsal fusion (blue). If Cotton osteotomy, just use the proximal one-third of this incision with a one sonometer proximal extension. The most posterior incision is for calcaneal osteotomy (green), with adequate skin bridge to the adjacent incision for lateral column lengthening (red).

- Remove the cartilage from the joint.
- Assess the amount of elevation of the first ray and metatarsus primus varus if present. Use saw cuts to take minimal bone (in the range of a millimeter) to correct the position of the metatarsal (Figure 5-5).
- After confirming that the joint is reduced in good position, perforate the fusion surfaces and oppose them, being careful to have excellent apposition along the fusion site, particularly plantarly.
- Using fluoroscopy, confirm good position of the first metatarsal and good apposition once the joint is pinned with K-wires.
- Confirm that the metatarsal head is slightly plantar or equal to the second metatarsal head.
- Do not place screws, because there is a small possibility that the position of the metatarsal may need to be adjusted after correction of the hindfoot. This is rare with experience.

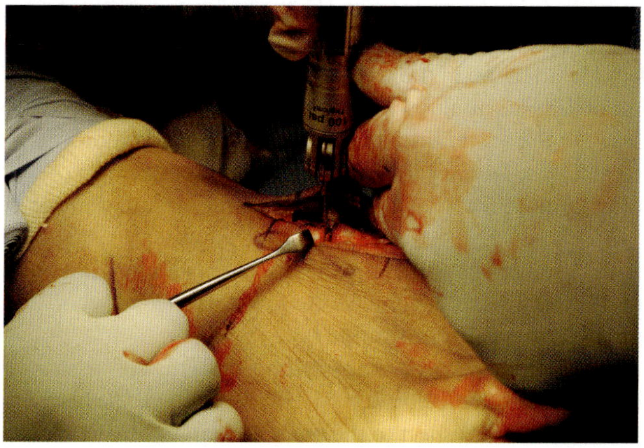

Figure 5-5. Saw cut for metatarsal tarsal fusion. Note minimal amount of bone being removed.

Cotton Osteotomy

If there is mild to moderate elevation of the first ray with minimal instability and no metatarsus primus varus, a Cotton osteotomy can be used, which is much simpler.

- Make an incision dorsally over the lateral border of the medial cuneiform (Figure 5-4).
- Blunt dissection is done while identifying and avoiding the dorsal branch of the superficial peroneal nerve.
- Expose the medial cuneiform dorsally.
- Place one 0.45 K-wire in the more distal aspect of the medial cuneiform and the other in the more proximal aspect, both perpendicular to the bone and allowing for the osteotomy in between.
- Check the lateral view of the medial cuneiform for good position.
- Once the position is confirmed, make a saw cut down to within 5 mm of the plantar cortex and hinge the osteotomy open with an osteotome dorsally.
- Using a pin distractor, adjust the amount of opening to correct the elevation of the first ray so that it is in good alignment with the second and fifth metatarsal head when the foot is plantigrade.
- Place a tricortical allograft according to the shape of the proper amount of the opening.
- A 2.4-mm screw is then used from the proximal dorsal cuneiform fragment to the plantar distal corner of the medial cuneiform (Figure 5-6).

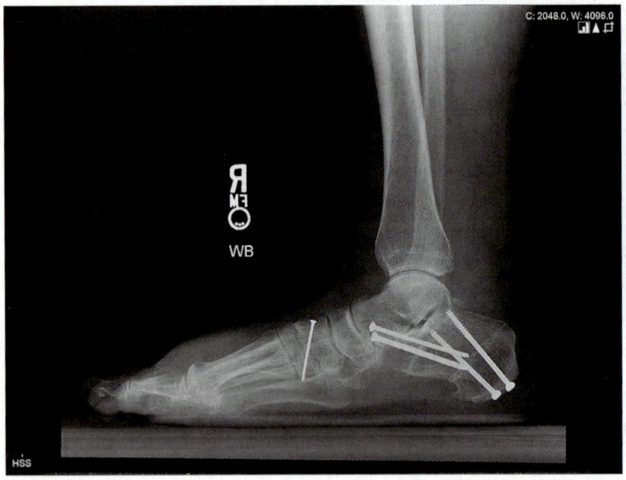

Figure 5-6. Post-op x-ray showing fixation with single screw of Cotton osteotomy. Plate fixation is too prominent.

Posterior Calcaneal Osteotomy

- Make a standard oblique incision from a soft spot that is just anterior to the Achilles tendon at the dorsal calcaneus to a soft spot that is just anterior to the plantar calcaneal tuberosity (Figure 5-4).
  - Keep the incision approximately 45° to the plantar aspect of the foot so that there is a good bridge between it and the sinus tarsi incision.
  - Make sure that the calcaneal incision is more vertical than the sinus tarsi incision, allowing for closure without excessive tension once the heel is slid.
- After blunt dissection down to bone, place a self-retaining retractor and two pins just in front of the posterior retracted skin flap.
  - Place the pins in the direction of the osteotomy, which is parallel to the skin incision.
- Check the position of the pins on fluoroscopy to confirm that the osteotomy site will be approximately midway between the posterior calcaneus and the subtalar joint.
- Use a saw blade to incise the lateral cortex, marking the osteotomy.
- Using a 12-mm osteotome, make a hatch mark in the midportion of the osteotomy line, perpendicular to it.
  - This mark will allow judgment of the proximal/distal position of the posterior fragment.
- Finish the osteotomy aiming slightly uphill as the saw goes medially, and incise the medial cortex by puncturing with two-handed control of the saw.
  - Control the saw with two hands so as not to plunge into the soft tissues.
- Slide the heel medially and hold the position of the heel, placing the foot in neutral and judging by an end-on view of the heel with respect to the posterior calf to obtain a "clinically straight heel."

- An equation using the hindfoot alignment x-ray, Saltzman view (Figure 5-7), can be used to predict the amount of heel slide.[1] Even if the equation is not used, having this x-ray is recommended so that the surgeon can visually estimate the amount of heel slide.
- Keeping the desired amount of heel slide, position the posterior fragment 2 mm distal to the hatch mark on the main body of the calcaneus and pin the heel.
- Confirm good position by end-on clinical heel view to posterior calf and lateral fluoroscopic view.

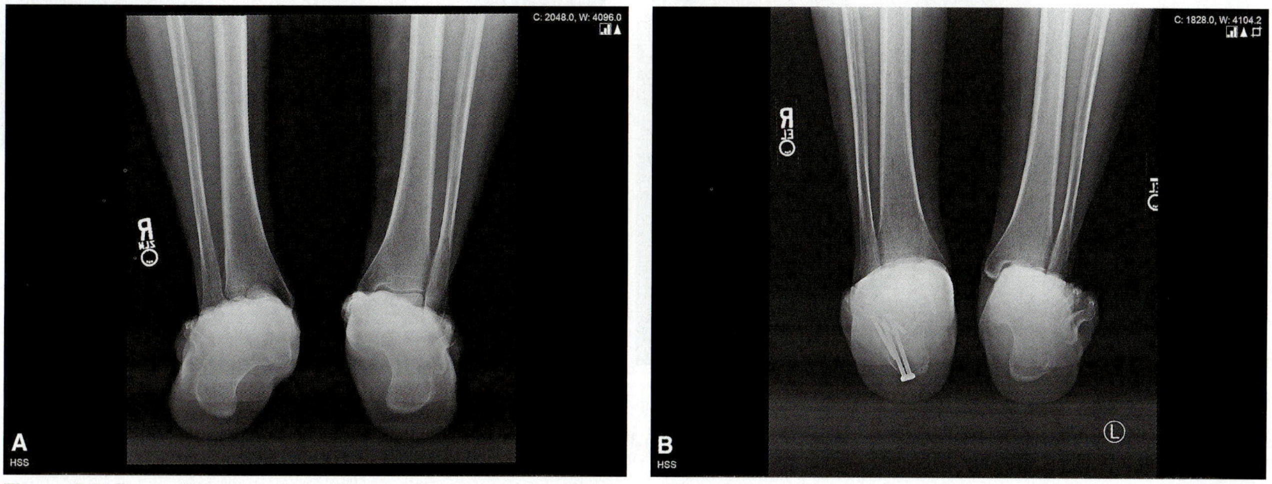

Figure 5-7. Pre-op (A) and post-op (B) heel alignment views showing correction of heel position in the right foot (on the left side of the image).

Sinus Tarsi Approach for Lateral Column Lengthening

- Make a longitudinal incision over the sinus tarsi from the tip of the fibula to the anterior process, staying just above the peroneal tendons and sural nerve (Figure 5-4).
- Expose the floor of the sinus tarsi and then laterally dissect along the surface of the anterior calcaneus, inferiorly exposing the whole lateral wall of the anterior calcaneus.

Technique No 1: Stepcut Osteotomy

A stepcut osteotomy has significant advantages in healing over an Evans osteotomy. Although presently unpublished data, I have found it to be quicker in healing and significantly less chance of nonunion than an Evans osteotomy. Clinical follow-up data of the stepcut osteotomy has been published.[2] It is more demanding for the surgeon, but not difficult with experience.

- If a stepcut osteotomy is used rather than a traditional Evans, it is necessary to expose more lateral wall, posterior and inferior to the peroneal tubercle.
- Also, it is recommended to dissect underneath the skin and to a level underneath the soft tissues surrounding the peroneal tendons and sural nerve so that a Penrose can be placed around them (Figure 5-8). In this manner, the tendons and the nerve can be retracted dorsally for the inferior vertical arm of the stepcut.
- At this point, retract the peroneal tendons and sural nerve inferiorly and posteriorly as much as possible and place a pin just anterior to them, holding them retracted (Figure 5-9).
- For a stepcut osteotomy, place a pin one-third of the way down the anterior calcaneus from the dorsal aspect approximately 11 mm from the calcaneocuboid joint (Figure 5-10).
  - Alternatively, a pin for the Evans osteotomy is made more proximally.
- Another pin is placed to mark the other end of the horizontal cut, 15 to 18 mm in a line going posterior and slightly plantar to the plantar aspect of the foot, ending at a point one-third the way up from the plantar cortex of the calcaneus.
- In this manner, the vertical saw cuts are made taking only a third of the distance from the horizontal cut to the dorsal or plantar cortex of the calcaneus, to avoid dangerous extensions of the vertical cuts.

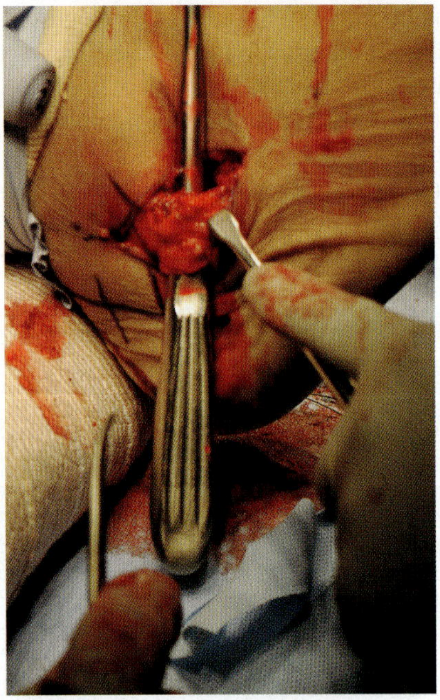

Figure 5-8. Subcutaneous dissection has been done to allow mobilization of both peroneal tendons and sural nerve as a unit for the inferior portion of the stepcut.

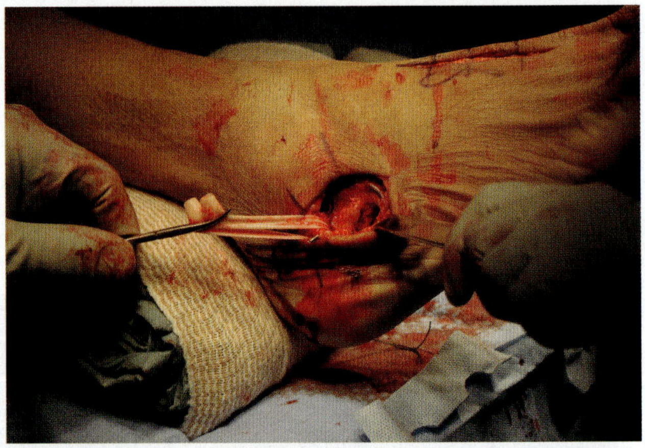

Figure 5-9. Exposure of lateral wall with pin, Penrose and baby Bennett retractors providing good exposure.

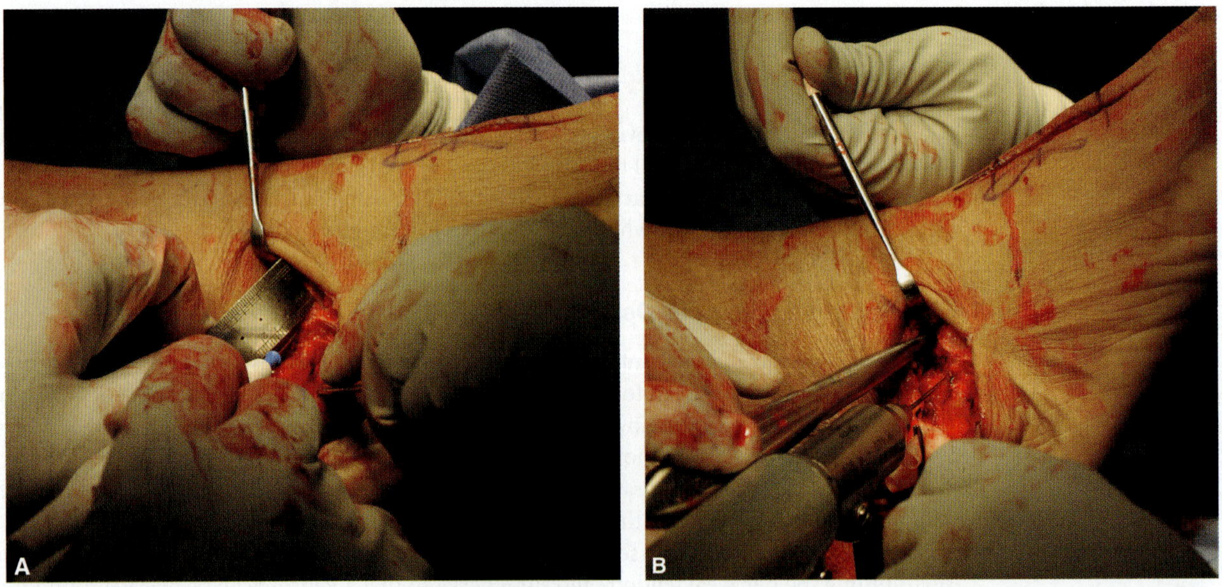

Figure 5-10. Marking 11 mm for location of anterior vertical limb of the stepcut (A) and placing a pin marking the corner of the cut (B).

- Using two-handed control and protecting the peroneal tendons with Bennett retractors, carefully make the horizontal cut. Use two-handed control to perforate rather than plunge through the medial cortex (Figure 5-11A).
- Make the anterior vertical cut, ensuring that the horizontal cut and the anterior cut are well connected and being careful not to plunge through the cortex medially or inferiorly. Make a complete cut through the medial cortex so the osteotomy will be mobile (Figure 5-11B).
  - Be careful that the saw does not whip down, from the hard sinus tarsi bone cutting the inferior two-thirds of the calcaneus.
- Similarly, make the posterior vertical cut being sure that the saw does not whip into the dorsal two-thirds of the calcaneus toward the subtalar joint (Figure 5-12).
  - The posterior cut can sometimes be made through this main exposure.

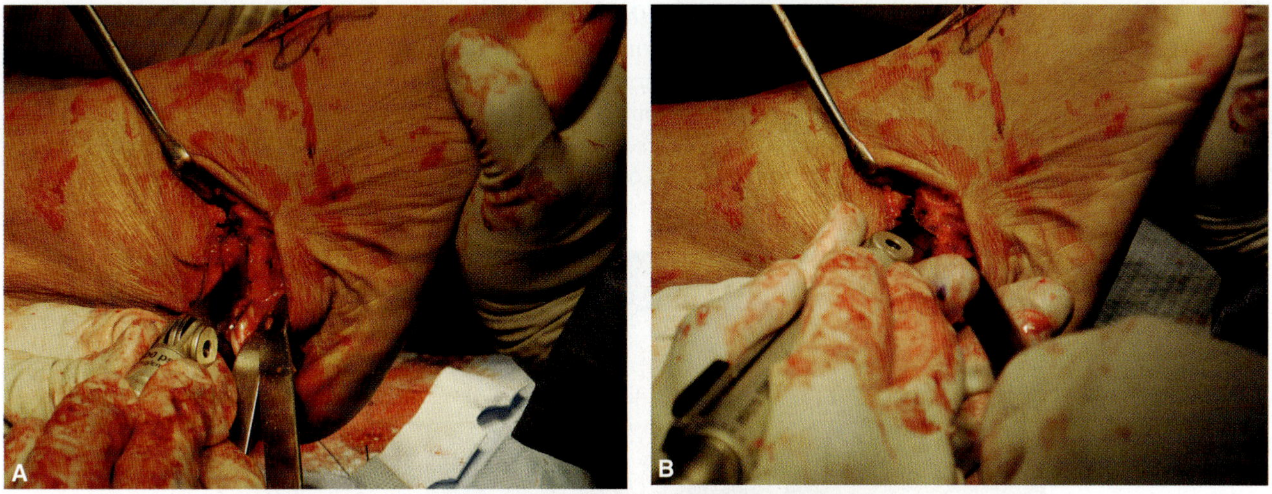

Figure 5-11. Saw with two-handed technique making the horizontal cut (A) and the vertical cut (B).

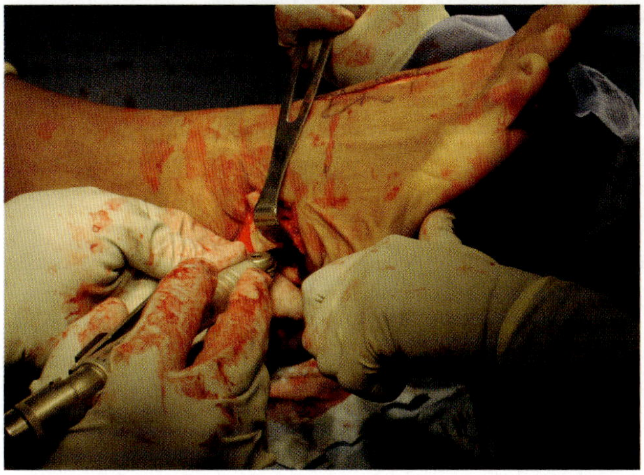

Figure 5-12. Retraction of peroneal tendons dorsally for the inferior vertical cut.

- Often, the pin retracting the peroneal tendons and sural nerve must be removed, and the tendons and nerve held retracted dorsally with an army–navy-type retractor and another right-angle retractor inferiorly. This creates a safe window for the posterior vertical cut.
- Make this cut, again being careful not to excessively plunge through the medial cortex and not to cut plantar soft tissues.

- If the osteotomy is not mobile, feel with the saw blade medially at the corners of the cut, because this is most often where the osteotomy is incompletely cut.
- Once good mobility of the osteotomy is obtained, place a pin distractor so that one pin is just inferior to the vertical cut and adjacent to the calcaneocuboid joint with the osteotomy reduced (Figure 5-13). Trying to use the pin distractor without having a mobile osteotomy can result in fracture.

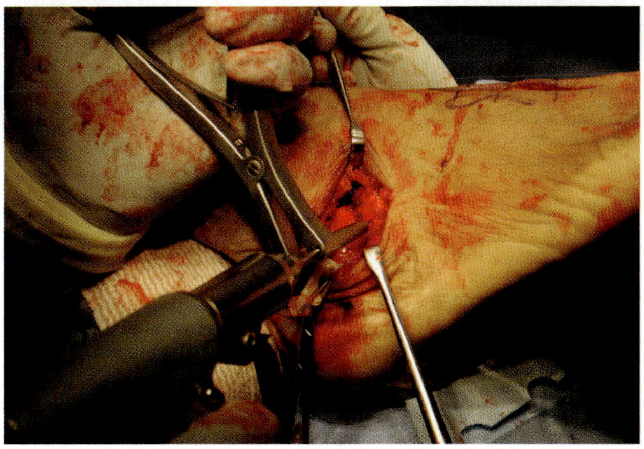

Figure 5-13. Placing pin adjacent to the calcaneocuboid joint for the pin distractor.

- Once the pins are in place, distract the osteotomy with the pin distractor (Figure 5-14).
  - This should be easy to do. If it is not, make sure the cuts of the osteotomy are complete.
- Spread the distractor to assess the amount of correction. Judge correction by obtaining an acceptable position of the talonavicular joint, as described later.
- The preference is to use trial wedges to assess the amount of correction in 1-mm increments because over- or undercorrection can occur from a 2-mm error in judgment.

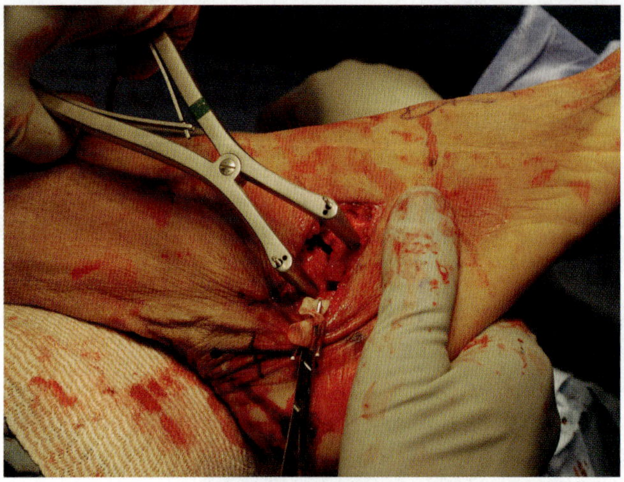

Figure 5-14. Distraction of the stepcut osteotomy, keeping the horizontal limb well reduced.

  - With a trial wedge in place, the position of the talonavicular joint is assessed and also that adequate near-normal position of the eversion of the hindfoot remains so as not to result in overcorrection and lateral overload. Also, if adduction is noted on a simulated weight-bearing anteroposterior (AP) fluroview in the operating room by everting the foot, then there is significant risk for lateral overload.[3]
- If bony impingement of the lateral talar process is noted after lengthening of the calcaneus has been done or is deemed likely, an ostectomy taking approximately 4 mm of the anterior lateral talar process at the anterior portion of the posterior facet makes impingement less likely (Figure 5-15).

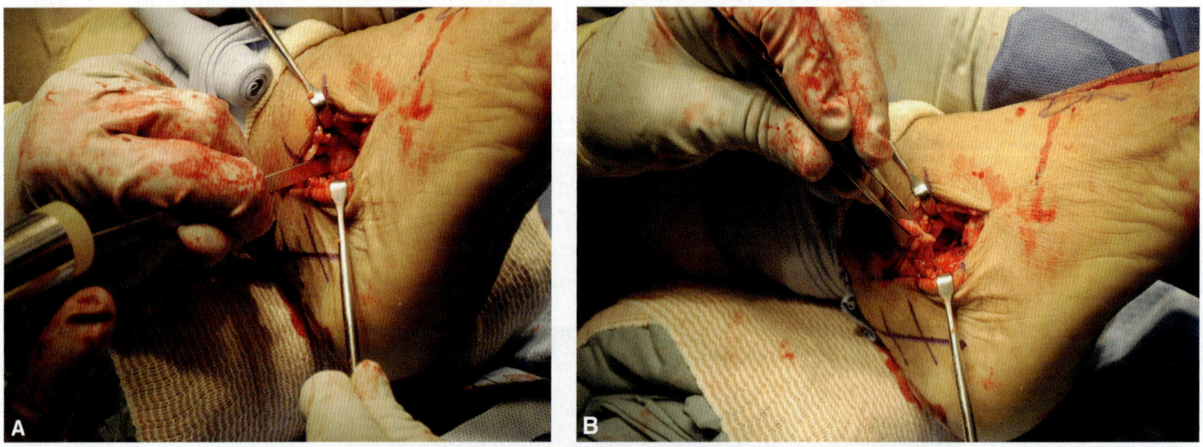

Figure 5-15. Ostectomy of talus with osteotome (A) to decrease chance of impingement if talar process comes close to the floor of the sinus tarsi after lateral column lengthening. Note the space created following the ostectomy (B).

Alternative Technique: Evans Osteotomy

An alternative is to do an opening wedge Evans osteotomy. This is a much simpler saw cut and easier. However, there is a small risk of loss of correction if nonunion occurs. The horizontal limb of the stepcut makes for non-bone graft–dependent healing, which can be faster and prevents loss of correction in the event of nonunion of the bone grafts. The bone graft using either allograft soaked in bone marrow concentrate or autograft from the iliac crest is shaped according to the opening of the osteotomy that has been determined to be the correct length. Trim the bone grafts accurately according to this space and trial them in the space with the osteotomy reduced. This step is done after the posterior calcaneal osteotomy and first metatarsal tarsal fusion is fixed in the next part of the procedure.

FINAL ASSESSMENT OF FOOT POSITION AND FIXATION OF OSTEOTOMIES/FUSION

- The alignment of the foot is judged with the lateral column lengthening temporarily held in position according to the lengthening desired, and the posterior calcaneus pinned with the desired amount of heel slide, and the first ray pinned in position with either the first metatarsal tarsal fusion or Cotton osteotomy.
- From an end-on view looking at the posterior calf, the heel should be clinically straight, neither in varus nor in valgus.
- The talonavicular joint position on AP view with eversion stress should show neither adduction at the joint nor noncoverage of the head. Assessment of the foot should also have equal plantar position of the first ray in comparison to the second and fifth metatarsals.
- Check again that there is near-normal eversion motion remaining in the hindfoot!
- Once good position has been confirmed clinically and radiographically, fix the osteotomies and fusion.

FIXATION OF OSTEOTOMIES/FUSIONS

- The posterior calcaneal osteotomy is fixed with two 4.5-mm screws first (Figure 5-16).
- Confirm good position of the guidewires for the cannulated screws on a lateral fluoroscopic view and an AP view of the foot in dorsiflexion showing that the guidewires are in proper position medially/laterally.

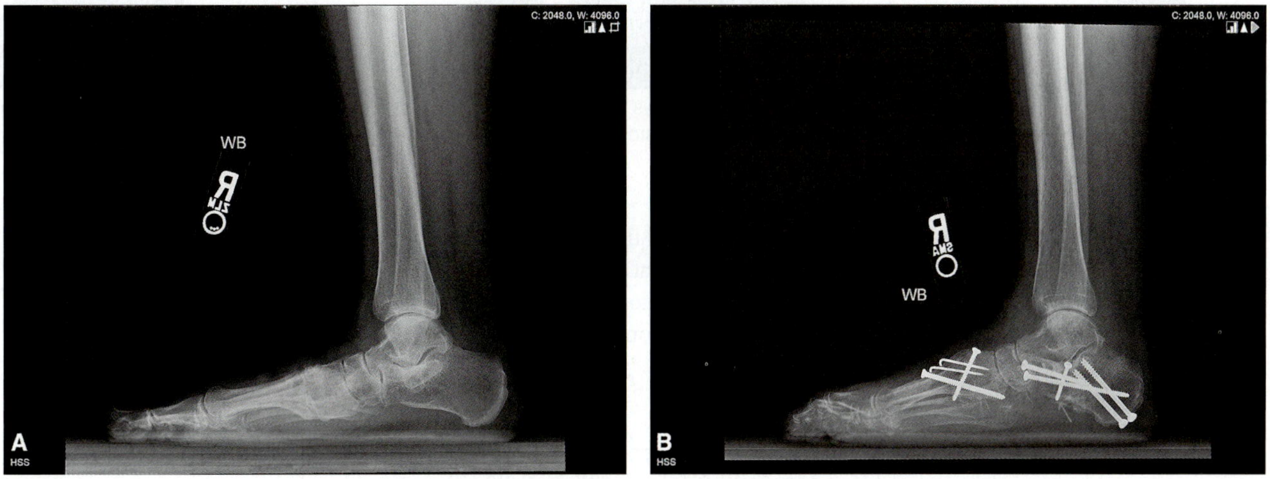

Figure 5-16. Pre-op (A) and post-op (B) lateral views showing correction and fixation of the hindfoot osteotomies. Note that there is a dorsal to plantar screw (see arrow) across the stepcut osteotomy, which is no longer used.

- Next, fix the first metatarsal tarsal fusion with two lag screws having cannulated drills over pins marking the position of the screws.
  - The proximal/dorsal to plantar/distal screw is placed first, with the distal exit in the first metatarsal plantarly close to the first metatarsal tarsal joint to allow for good plantar compression with the lag screw technique.
  - Then place the distal to proximal screw aiming for the plantar proximal corner of the medial cuneiform.
  - Confirm good position of the pins first with fluoroscopy before drilling.
- For the lateral column lengthening site, place the bone graft in this site, then compress and pin.
- Inspection should confirm excellent apposition both dorsally and along the lateral aspect.
  - There should be difficulty in placing a knife blade between the bone graft and the native bone in both the anterior and lateral sides.
- For the stepcut osteotomy, the anterior bone graft is placed first and the osteotomy compressed making sure there is good apposition along the horizontal limb as well.

- Temporary fixation with this osteotomy is with 2.06 K-wires placed in the anterior dorsal calcaneus to the posterior calcaneus.
  - Pins are placed so that they can be replaced by two 3.5-mm screws and the screwheads do not impinge on the cuboid with the motion of the calcaneocuboid joint. If there is not good apposition at the graft/natine bone interface, identify the prominent bone causing the distraction and trim it judiciously.
- Check a lateral and AP fluoroscopic view.
- With the osteotomy well reduced and well opposed, place a lag screw along the direction of one of the pins through the anterior calcaneus bone graft and into the posterior calcaneus, with the first screw being overdrilled in the proximal fragment to create compression (Figure 5-17A) .
- Then place the second screw just inferior to the first (Figure 5-17B) .

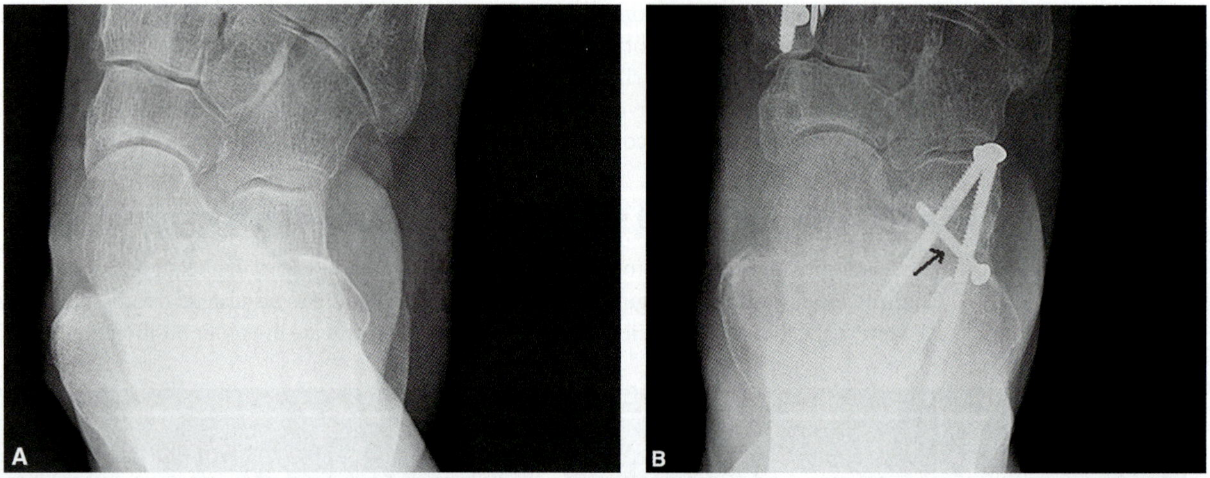

Figure 5-17. Pre-op (A) and post-op (B) anteroposterior views showing correction and fixation with stepcut osteotomy. Note that there is a dorsal to plantar screw (see arrow) across the stepcut osteotomy, which is no longer used.

- Finally, place the tricortical graft in the posterior vertical limb with good fit.
  - This graft should be cut after fixation of the anterior bone graft so the space can be accurately judged and the fit good. The fit does not need to be supertight. Placing a graft that distracts the ostectomy will disrupt the fixation.

References

1. Conti MS, Ellis SJ, Chan JY, Do HT, Deland JT. Optimal position of the heel following reconstruction of the stage II adult-acquired flatfoot deformity. *Foot Ankle Int.* 2015;36(8):919-927.
2. Demetracopoulos CA, Nair P, Malzberg A, Deland JT. Outcomes of a stepcut lengthening calcaneal osteotomy for adult-acquired flatfoot deformity. *Foot Ankle Int.* 2015;36:749-755.
3. Conti MS, Chan JY, Do HT, Ellis SJ, Deland JT. Correlation of postoperative midfoot position with outcome following reconstruction of the stage II adult acquired flatfoot deformity. *Foot Ankle Int.* 2015;36:239-247.

Chapter 6
Correction of the Rigid Flatfoot

JONATHAN T. DELAND
AUSTIN E. SANDERS

Sterile Instruments/Equipment

- Tourniquet
- Cannulated drills and guide wires
- Cannulated screws (6.5 and 4.5)
- Compression staples
- Straight and curved osteotomes
- Pin distractor
- 0.062 K-wires
- Bone graft (autograft or allograft)

Preoperative Planning

- Anteroposterior (AP), lateral, and oblique x-rays of the foot (Figure 6-1)
- Bilateral Saltzman views of the hindfoot (Figure 6-2)

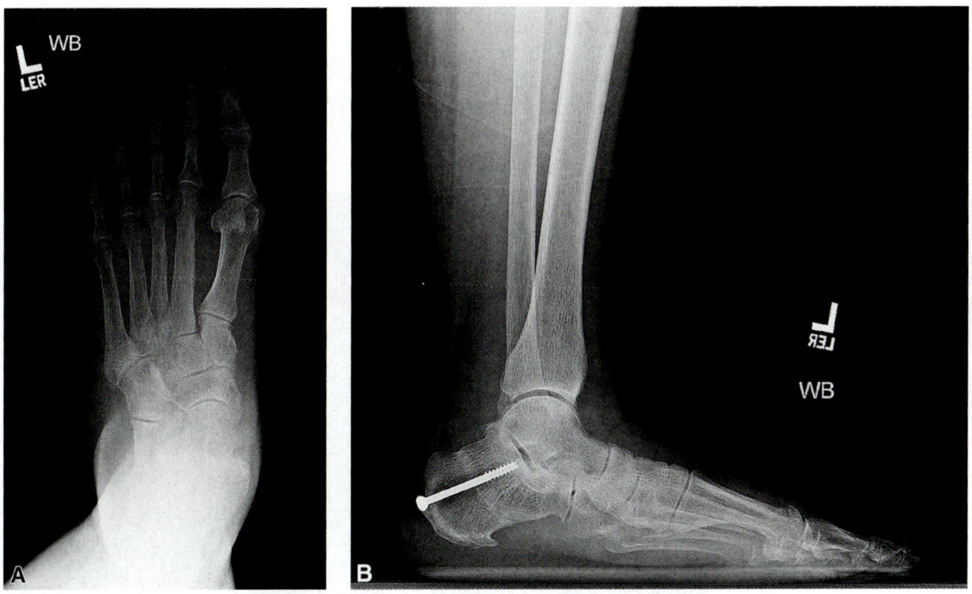

Figure 6-1. Standing anteroposterior view of the foot (A) and lateral view of the foot (B).

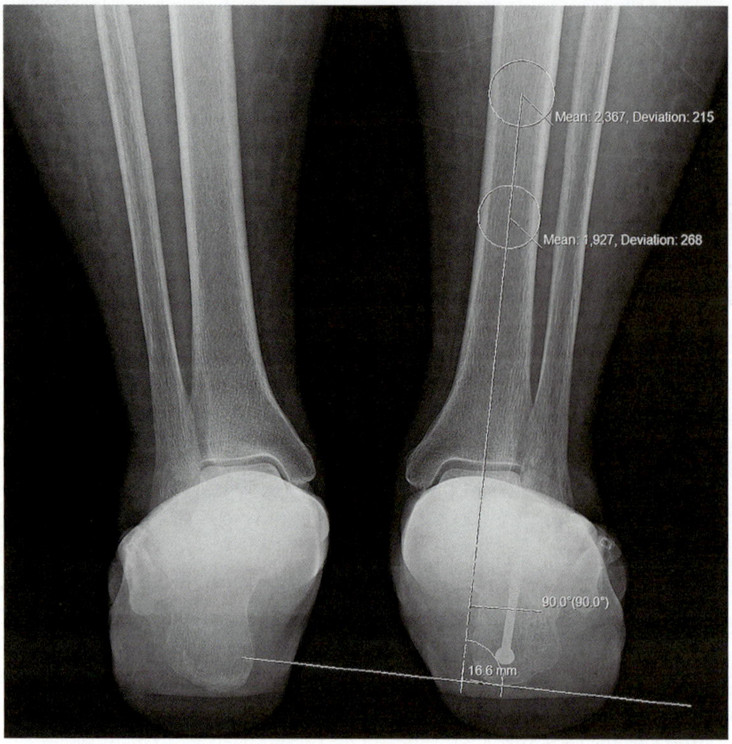

Figure 6-2. Hindfoot alignment view. Patient had previous surgery and the measurements are marked.

Positioning

- Supine, with a bump under the hip to make toes straight to the ceiling

Surgical Approaches

Medial Talonavicular Joint

- Incision and deep dissection is in between the posterior tibial tendon and anterior tibial tendon, retracting the saphenous vein and nerve dorsally.

This patient had previous surgery, with an incision that ended inferior and posterior to the medial malleolus. This old incision was resected. Otherwise, the incision would have been as marked in black in Figure 6-3.

Dorsal Talonavicular Joint

- The incision, as shown in green in Figure 6-4, and deep dissection is carried out just medial to the neurovascular bundle at the medial border of the extensor hallucis longus (EHL) tendon, directly over the talonavicular joint.

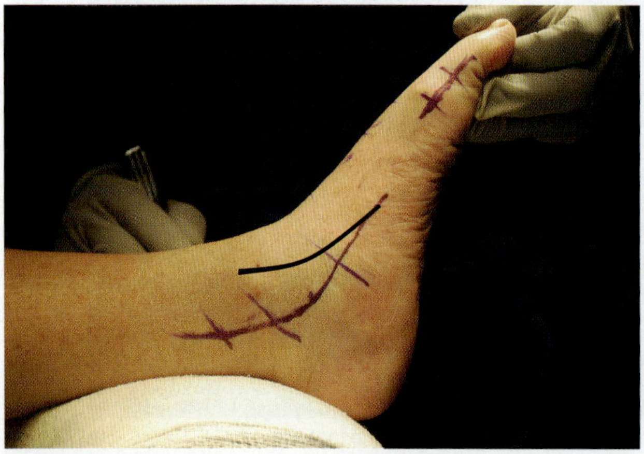

Figure 6-3. Medial approach to the talonavicular joint.

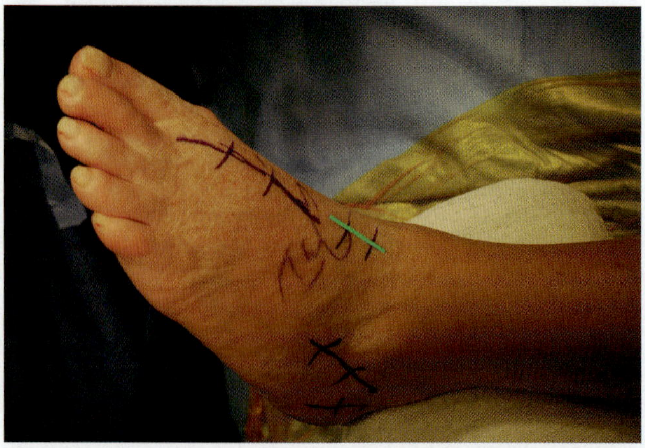

Figure 6-4. Dorsal approach to the talonavicular joint and the approach for the first metatarsal tarsal fusion.

- The neurovascular bundle is just lateral to the EHL tendon, so deep dissection laterally is carried out underneath the EHL tendon and neurovascular bundle.

Lateral Subtalar Joint

- Use the sinus tarsi approach just dorsal to the peroneal tendons and sural nerve from the distal tip of the fibula to the anterior process of the calcaneus. Incision is marked in blue (Figure 6-5).

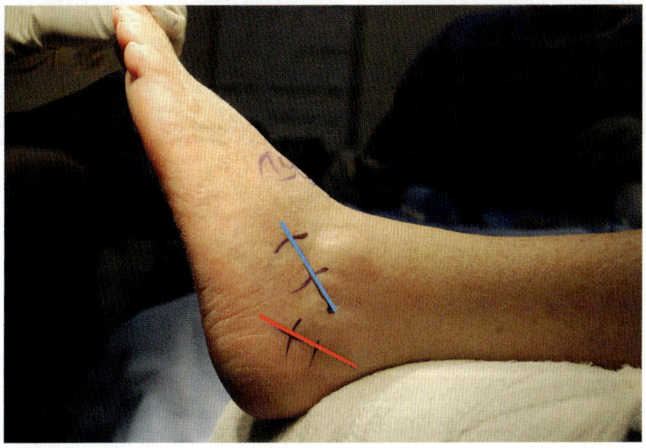

Figure 6-5. Sinus tarsi incision for subtalar fusion (blue) and posterior calcaneal osteotomy incision (red).

Combined Talonavicular and Subtalar Medial Approach

- In cases of severe valgus deformity, where correction of deformity can place excess tension on the lateral skin, the subtalar joint, as well as the talonavicular joint, can be approached medially.
- The incision is a long, oblique one from the tip of the navicular to the posterior aspect of the medial malleolus.[1]
- In addition, the dorsal talonavicular approach could also be used. The most commonly used approach is the lateral subtalar approach; if a posterior calcaneal osteotomy is needed, an additional oblique incision is made.

Posterior Calcaneal Osteotomy Approach

- If there is significant valgus deformity of the hindfoot and the surgeon believes that a posterior calcaneal osteotomy will be needed, a posterolateral approach for the osteotomy is made.
- The standard lateral oblique incision is made over the calcaneus at least two fingerbreadths posterior to the subtalar incision and somewhat more vertical than the subtalar incision (marked in red in Figure 6-5). Being more toward the vertical, there is less tension, and a somewhat larger skin bridge is achieved.

Preparation of Joints

Talonavicular

- Place pins for a medial pin distractor by holding the distractor over the joint, visualizing the proper placement of the pin paths.
- A pin is placed dorsomedially in the navicular and talus. The pins are bent over the shafts of the distractor and the joint is distracted (Figure 6-6).
- Standard preparation of joint surfaces is to remove any remaining cartilage in the joint with a curette.
- Lightly burr the bone, maintaining the shape and taking minimal bone (1 mm). Then make multiple perforations of each bony surface with a 0.062 K-wire (Figure 6-7).
- The lateral one-third of the joint is similarly prepared via the placement of a pin distractor dorsally.
- Pins are placed dorsally in the navicular and talus and the joint distracted.

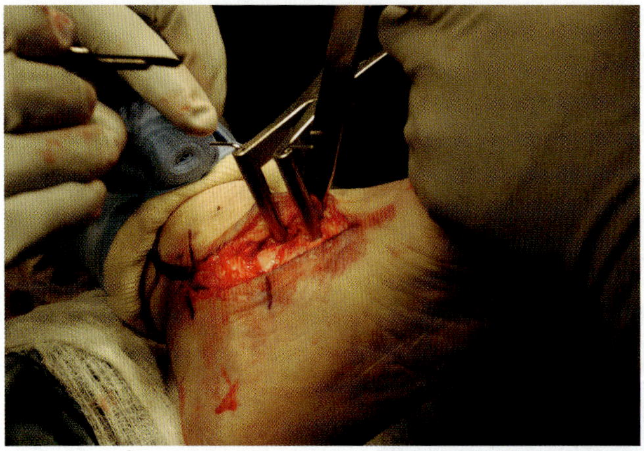

Figure 6-6. Placement of pin distractor for the talonavicular joint.

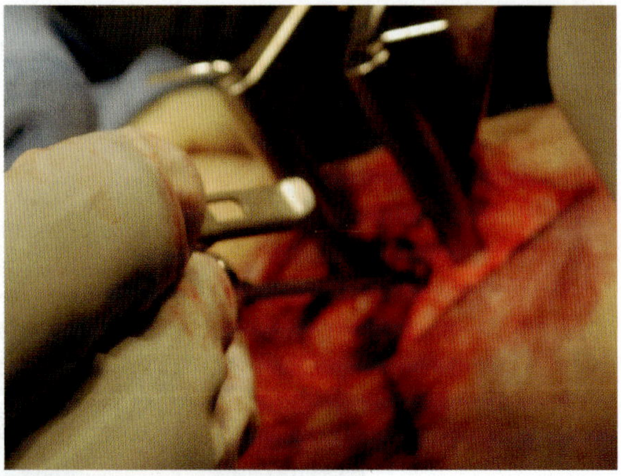

Figure 6-7. Burring of joint from the medial incision; same is done from the dorsal incision.

Lateral and Medial Subtalar Joint

- Via the sinus tarsi approach, place pins in the calcaneus and body of the talus through the distractor angled so that a nearly vertical distraction of the joint is achieved (Figure 6-8).
- An alternative is a tooth laminar spreader, which can work well in a joint that is not tight.
- For the medial subtalar approach, pins are also helpful to vertically distract the joint; distraction is not done too aggressively because of the nearby neurovascular structures (Figure 6-9).

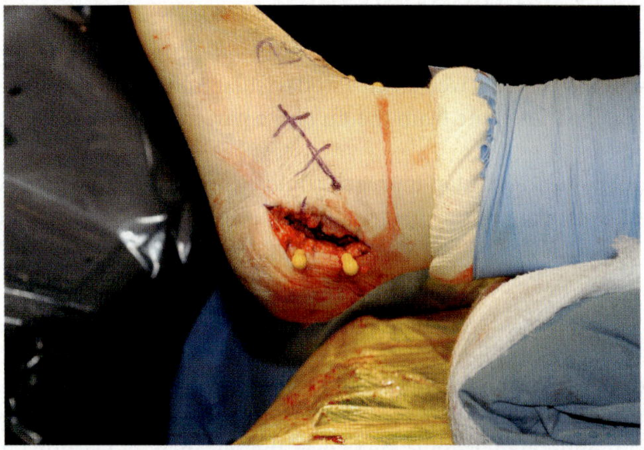

Figure 6-8. Approach for the posterior calcaneal osteotomy with pins defining a plane in front of which the osteotomy is made.

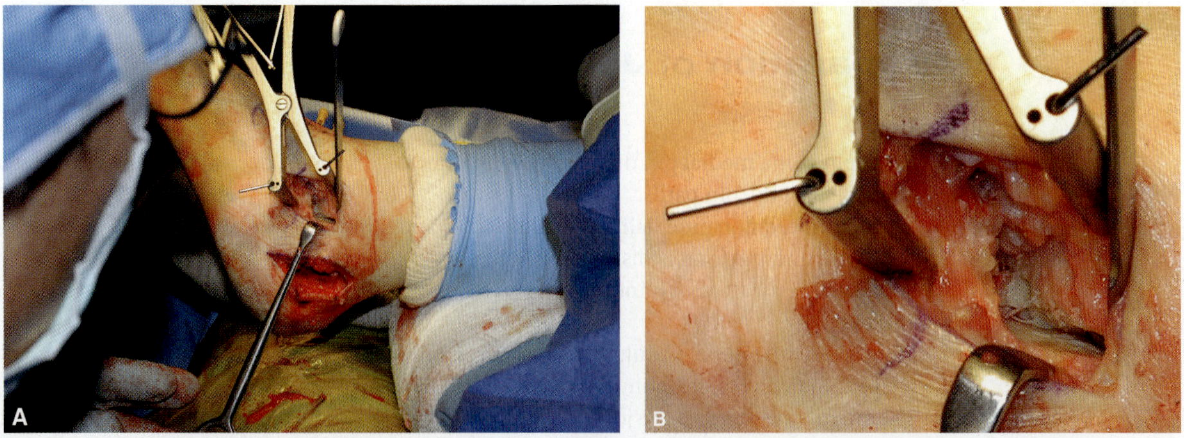

Figure 6-9. Approach to the subtalar joint with pin distractor in place (A) and close-up showing distraction of the joint (B).

- Be careful to avoid the medial tendons when placing the talar pin, and the flexor hallucis longus/ neurovascular bundle when placing the calcaneal pin.
- The posterior and medial facets of the subtalar joint are prepared in the standard manner, as described earlier.

Lateral Calcaneus for Posterior Calcaneal Osteotomy

- Just in front of the retracted posterior skin edge of the incision, place two pins from medial to lateral.
- The osteotomy is made just anterior to these pins. Under fluoroscopy check the position of the pins, which should be placed to allow an osteotomy midway between the subtalar joint and posterior border of calcaneus.
- Using the saw or osteotome, make a hatch mark perpendicular to the proposed osteotomy. This is so once the osteotomy is completed, the distal/proximal migration of the posterior fragment can be judged (Figure 6-10).
- Once the osteotomy is slid medially and temporarily fixed, the hatch marks and fluoroscopy should indicate that the posterior fragment has been moved distally a few millimeters to allow for any proximal migration during fixation (Figure 6-11).
- Check the placement of the pins under fluoroscopy before making the osteotomy.

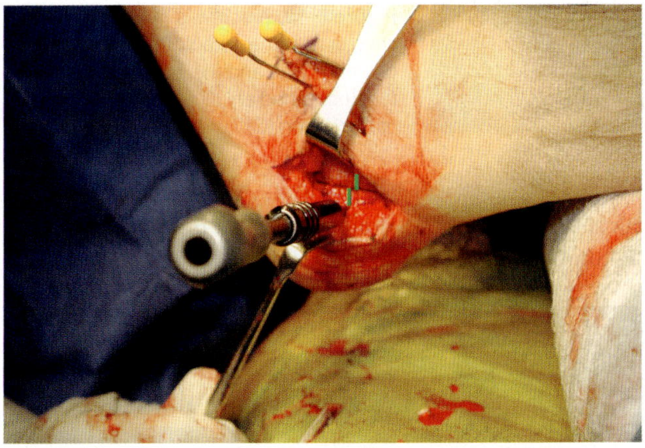

Figure 6-10. Posterior calcaneal osteotomy with hatch marks (green lines) to judge proximal or distal migration of the posterior calcaneal fragment.

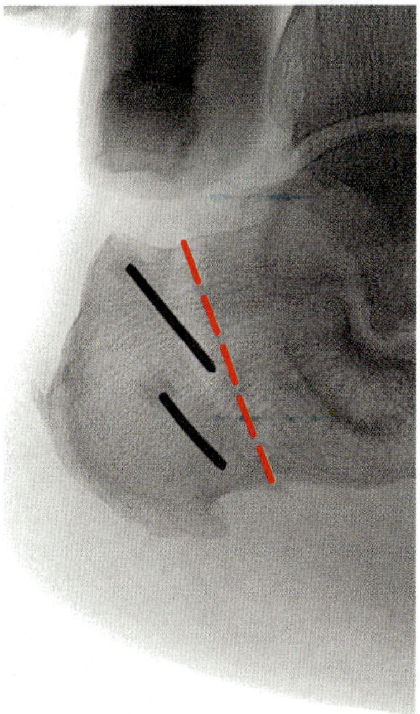

Figure 6-11. Fluoroscopy view with guide pins (black lines) in place before osteotomy cut. Patient had a previous posterior calcaneal osteotomy (dotted line) and needed further medial translation of the posterior calcaneus.

Calcaneocuboid Joint

- This joint is normally not included in the fusions because it is not necessary for correction or relief of symptoms.

Correction With Calcaneal Osteotomy

- A helpful technique, when a large amount of slide (11-15 mm) is needed, is to place a screw in the posterior fragment.
- This allows the surgeon to push the mobile fragment of the calcaneus as medial as possible (Figure 6-12).

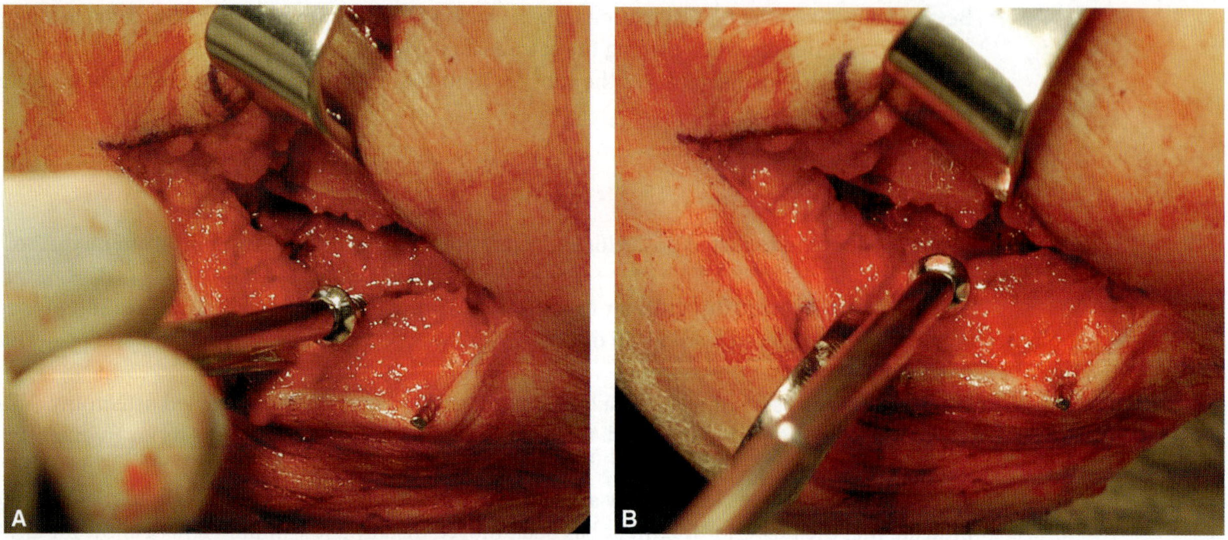

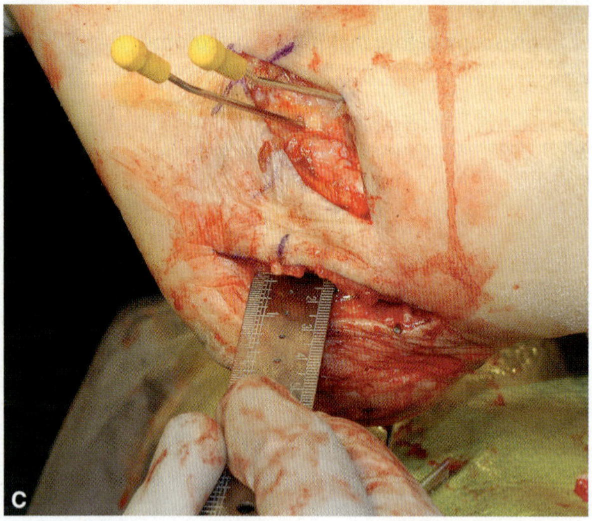

Figure 6-12. A screw is placed in the posterior tuberosity of the calcaneus after the osteotomy is performed (A). The screw is tightened down to bone and the screw driver is used to translate the calcaneal tuberosity medially (B). A ruler is then used to measure the amount of translation (C).

Bone Graft

- If performing a calcaneal posterior osteotomy, bone graft is harvested from the superior lateral edge once the osteotomy has been slid medially and fixed (Figure 6-13).

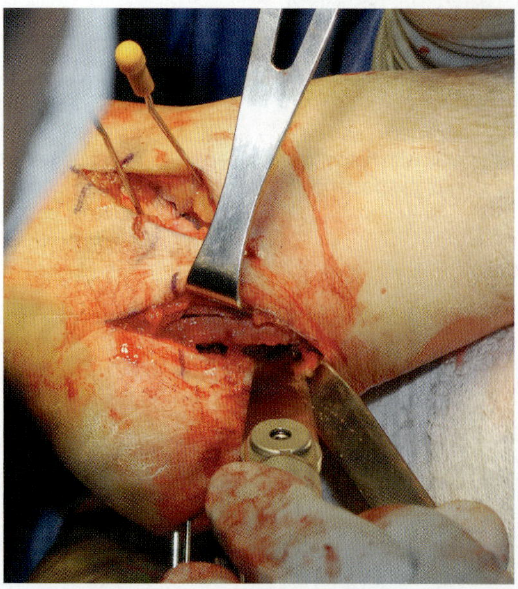

Figure 6-13. Bone graft harvest by trimming the prominent lateral ledge with a saw.

- Use a saw to cut a cortical cancellous block from the superior lateral rim.
- This is most commonly done after the heel is slid and provisionally fixed.
- After removing the block, more cancellous graft can be removed with a rongeur (Figure 6-14).
- Finally, the remaining prominent rim is smoothed down with a burr.
- An alternative to this bone graft is cancellous allograft chips mixed with bone marrow concentrate.

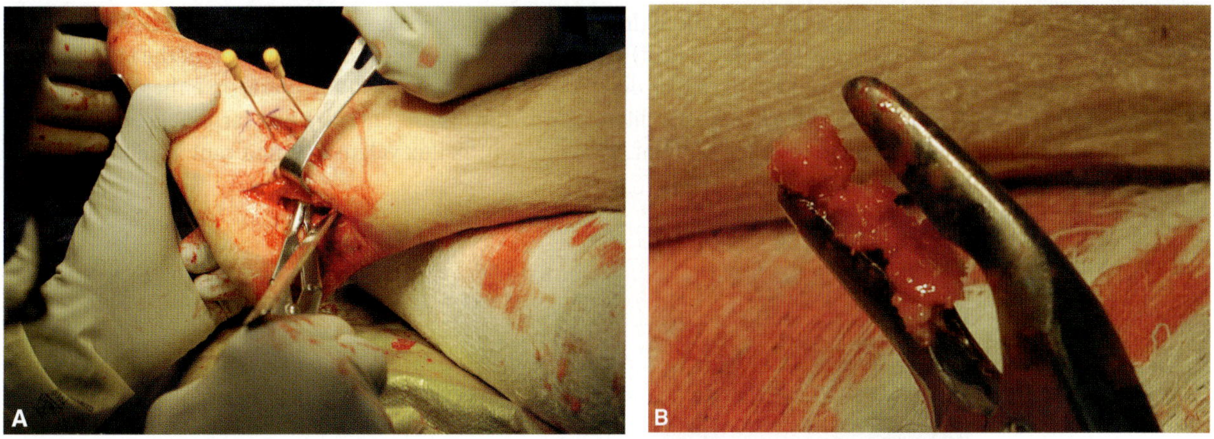

Figure 6-14. Rongeur harvest of cancellous graft (A). Note the large amount of autograft obtained (B).

Final Joint Preparation

- Fishscale the bony surfaces of the fusions so that the scales maintain their attachment to the bone but allow small bits of cancellous graft to be placed in the apex of the scales (Figure 6-15).
- These fishscales should be made so that they can mostly close when the fusion is reduced and not distract the joint.

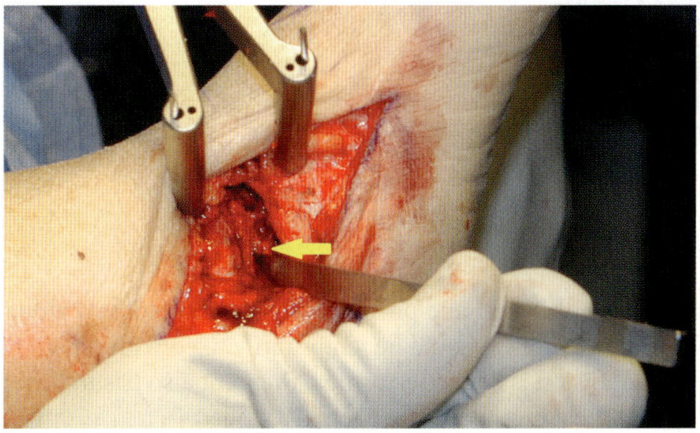

Figure 6-15. Fishscaling talar head, note the space for cancellous graft just to the cutting edge of the osteotome (arrow).

Reduce the Deformity

- Reduce the talonavicular joint into anatomic position first. Manually position and compress the talonavicular and subtalar joints.
- For reduction in the case of severe pronation deformity, bring the navicular medially and plantarly so that the medial border of the foot and first ray is in good position (navicular out of the abducted and medially elevated position).
- Check that the subtalar joint is well opposed at the posterior facet. Most often, it is helpful to hold and compress the subtalar joint and the talonavicular joint before pinning.
- While compressing the joints and holding them in good position, place the pins across the medial and dorsal talonavicular joints, respectively.

- By direct visualization and fluoroscopy, confirm good compression of both the medial and lateral talonavicular joint and subtalar joint.
- If good position is not confirmed, repeat the process after inspecting the joints for prominences that may be holding them distracted (Figure 6-16).
- Slide the medial calcaneal osteotomy so that the heel is directly underneath the calf and ankle when viewed from the end of the operating room table ("a clinically straight heel," not normal valgus or clinical varus).
- Within the osteotomy, check the lateral fluoroscopic view and clinical correction of the heel.
- If the first ray (first metatarsal) remains elevated despite good reduction of the talonavicular joint, having brought the navicular down out of its elevated position, perform either a Cotton osteotomy (if no hallux valgus or instability of the first ray is present) or a first tarsometatarsal fusion (if the first metatarsophalangeal joint is incongruent/hallux valgus or significant instability of the first ray is present).

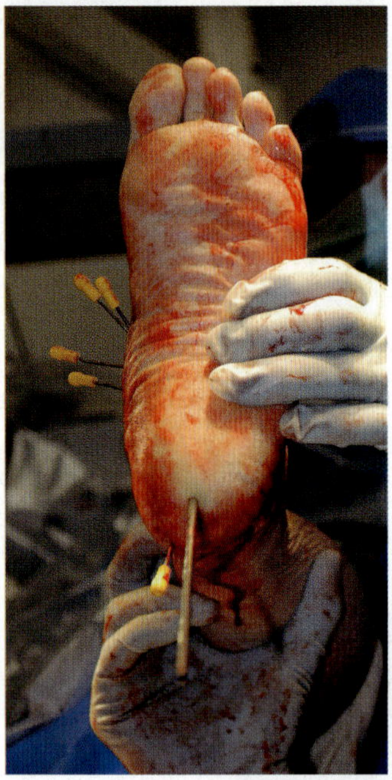

Figure 6-16. Heel in correct, straight position with guide pin in place for fixation of calcaneal osteotomy and subtalar joint.

Fixation

- At this point, the talonavicular joint and posterior calcaneal osteotomy along with a subtalar fusion and posterior calcaneal osteotomy should be temporarily fixed with pins.
- If a first tarsometatarsal fusion is being performed, the joint also has to be pinned in advance. This allows the alignment of the entire foot to be properly judged.
- Confirm the position of the first ray with respect to the rest of the foot that has been reduced.
- The plantar position of the first metatarsal head should be approximately equal to or slightly prominent in comparison to the second and fifth metatarsal heads.
- If the choice of a Cotton osteotomy has been made, the osteotomy has been done but with the bone wedge not yet placed.
- Determine the amount of distraction of the Cotton osteotomy with the use of the pin distractor, checking the position of the first metatarsal head plantarly.
- Place tricortical allograft bone of the proper wedge size in the osteotomy and fix the osteotomy with a 2.4-mm screw.

Subtalar and Posterior Calcaneal Osteotomy Fixation

- Place guidewires for two 6.5 cannulated compression screws across the calcaneal osteotomy and subtalar fusion, as shown in Figure 6-17.

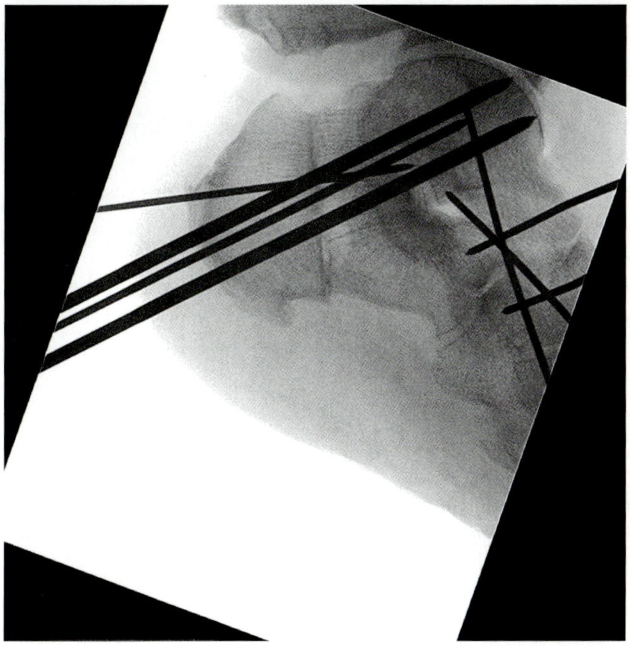

Figure 6-17. Fluoroscopic view showing placement of large guidewires for cannulated screws.

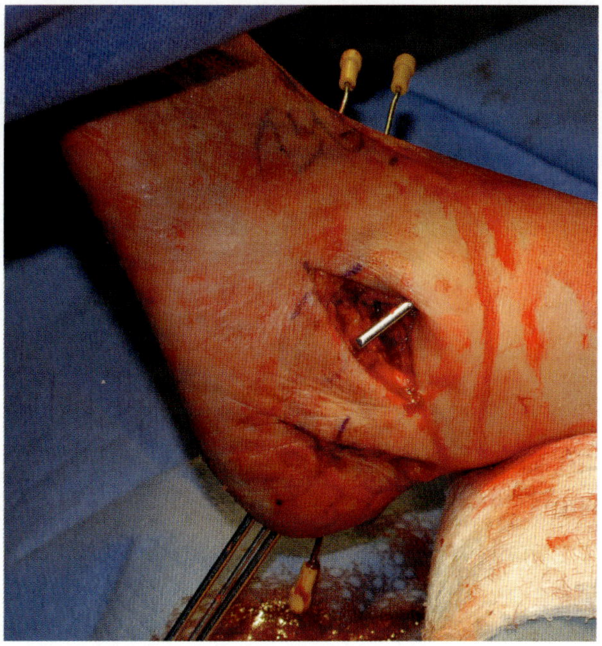

Figure 6-18. Initial placement of lateral compression staple across the posterior facet of the subtalar joint.

- Be sure that the pins are directed medial enough to end in the center of the body of the talus on the AP ankle fluoroscopy view. These pins can easily end up too laterally in the talus or in the distal talofibular joint.
  - Do not start too medially in the plantar calcaneus.
  - If the pins end up too medially, the medial tendons and neurovascular bundle are at risk.
- Additional compression of the subtalar joint can be gained by a lateral compression staple placed via the sinus tarsi (Figure 6-18).
- It must be placed at the very anterior aspect of the posterior facet into the talus and calcaneus. Although the staple is good for compression directly at the joint, it can be too prominent or hit the fibular with dorsiflexion of the ankle. The position of the staple should be so as not to hit the fibula or peroneal tendons.
- Compress the screws most of the way, then place and compress the staple and finally finish tightening the screws (Figure 6-19).

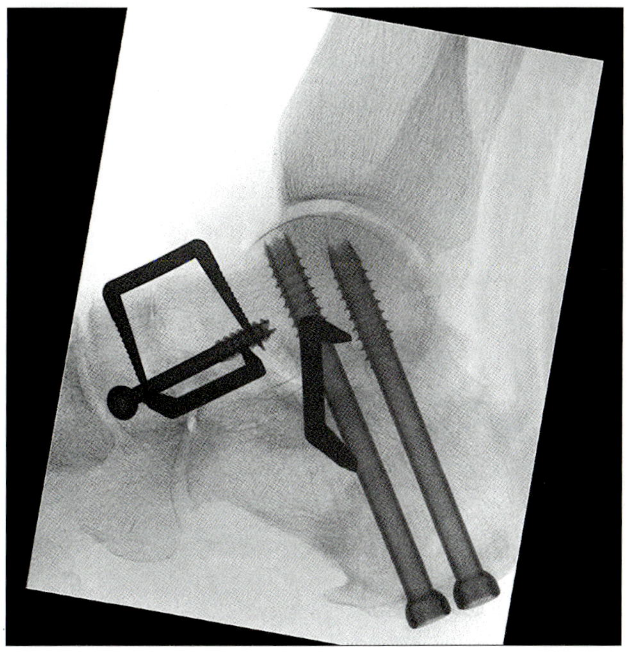

Figure 6-19. Final fixation of posterior calcaneal osteotomy, subtalar joint, and talar navicular joint.

Talonavicular Fixation

- Confirm plantar, medial, and lateral compression.
- Both visual inspection and AP and lateral fluoroscopic views should be checked.
- Start with a compression staple or 4.5-mm compression screw medially, but only lightly compress the joint. Then start a dorsal compression staple or screw compressing the joint laterally.
- Once good compression of both the medial and lateral joints is confirmed, finish compressing medially and laterally with the fixation.
- A third point of fixation, a medial screw started more dorsally, can be added.
- Check the direction of the prongs of the staples or screws by first placing 0.062 K-wires in the proposed paths of fixation and check under fluoroscopy.
- Place bone graft in burr holes of all the fusion sites after confirming good compression and fixation of the fusions.

Reference

1. Jeng CL, Vora AM, Myerson MS. The medial approach to triple arthrodesis. Indications and technique for management of rigid valgus deformities in high-risk patients. *Foot Ankle Clin.* 2005;10:515-521.

Section 4
Cavovarus Foot Deformity

Chapter 7
Forefoot-Driven Cavovarus Deformity

MACALUS HOGAN

Forefoot Deformity

Preoperative Evaluation

- Neurologic assessment
- Coleman block testing determines forefoot versus hindfoot deformity.
  - Failure to achieve deformity correction on x-ray when positioning lateral foot/hindfoot on 1-cm block suggests fixed deformity (Figure 7-1).
- Assess muscle imbalance that may contribute to recurrence.

Surgical Planning and Sterile Instruments/ Equipment

- Thigh tourniquet
- Overholt clamp
- Langenback retractors
- Small Hohmann retractors
- Sagittal saw
- Sutures (1-0 Vicryl, 2-0 Vicryl, 3-0 nylon, 3-0 Ticron, 3-0 Prolene)
- Forceps
- Scalpel
- Implants
  - 3.5-mm fully threaded screws
  - 4.0-mm partially threaded screws
- Small burr

Positioning

- Supine on the table with heel near the end of the table
- Hip bump placed under the ipsilateral side with foot perpendicular to the floor
- Thigh tourniquet with padding to prevent skin breakdown/injury
- Bone foam or sterile bump (optional, but may permit improved exposure of the medial aspect of the foot)

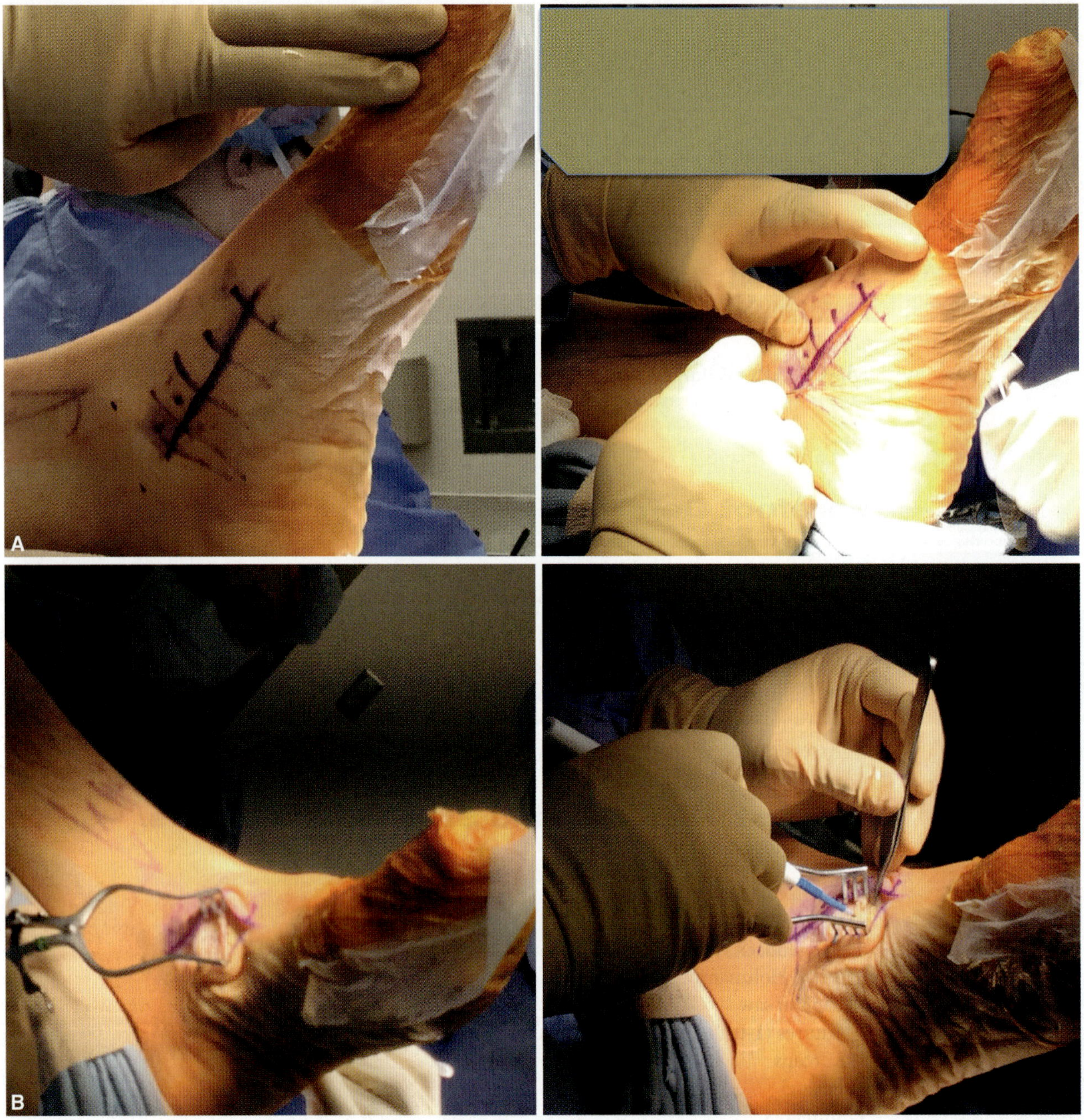

Figure 7-1. A, Create a 3- to 4-cm incision over the insertion of the posterior tibial tendon (PTT) on the navicular bone. B, Dissect through subcutaneous tissue to expose the flexor retinaculum and PTT sheath.

Surgical Approach

- Technique No. 1—Posterior tibial tendon (PTT) transfer
  - Create a 3- to 4-cm incision over the insertion of the PTT on the navicular bone.
  - Dissect through subcutaneous tissue.
  - Incise the flexor retinaculum and PTT sheath.
  - With an Overholt clamp, tension the tendon to release from the insertion site with a scalpel as far distal as possible.
  - Incise another 3-cm site at the distal aspect of the medial leg, but three fingerbreadths above the ankle.
  - Dissect through the subcutaneous tissue.
  - Incise the fascia and retract with Langenback retractors.

- Identify the flexor hallux longus (FHL) and retract the tendon to visualize the PTT just deep to the FHL tendon.
- Pull the PTT tendon into view to bisect the tendon.
- Tag both halves with 1-0 Vicryl sutures.
- A third incision is made on the lateral side of the shank at the height ventral to the fibular bone.
- Dissect through subcutaneous tissue to retract the fascia.
- Insert narrow forceps through the interosseous membrane from the medial incision site to the lateral incision.
- Grab a single thread with forceps and pull through the medial wound.
- Grab the two tag sutures placed on each half of the PTT.
- Transfer the split PTT to the lateral wound pulling the end of the thread.
- Expose the anterior tibial tendon (ATT) with a 2- to 3-cm incision.
- Dissect through subcutaneous tissue.
- Incise the ATT sheath and insert forceps through the sheath to the extensor compartment to visualize the PTT halves.
- Grab the tagged suture of one-half of the PTT and transfer it distally.
- Expose the extensor digitorum longus (EDL) tendon with a dorsal incision and incise the EDL tendon sheath.
- Transfer the other half of the PTT using the tagged suture.
- Secure the tendon transfer by suturing the medial half of the PTT to the ATT and the lateral half of the PTT to the peroneus brevis tendon.
- Place the ankle in neutral to tension the tendon transfer.
- Correct hindfoot equinus, if present, so the foot rests in the corrected position after suturing the transfers.

- Technique No. 2—First metatarsal (MT) dorsiflexion osteotomy
  - A dorsal incision is made over the proximal first MT.
  - Dissect down to extensor tendons and retract laterally.
  - Continue to dissect down to bone.
  - Dissect subperiosteum.
  - Mark a line transverse on the bone, 1 cm from joint for the bone cut.
  - Place small Hohmann retractors around bone to protect soft tissues.
  - Perform dorsal closing wedge osteotomy with a sagittal saw.
  - The first cut is perpendicular to the diaphysis and 90° through the bone.
  - The second cut is 2 to 3 mm distal and angled back toward the plantar endpoint of the first cut.
  - Complete the first cut and remove the bone wedge.
  - Restore the anatomic alignment of the talus and the first MT on a lateral radiograph (~0°).
  - Make a small shallow hole with a small burr in the dorsal aspect of the bone to recess the screw head.
  - Reduce the first MT and insert a 3.5-mm lag screw from the burr hole through osteotomy.
- Technique No. 3—Jones procedure
  - Utilizes both tendon force balancing (extensor hallucis longus transfer) and correction of first MT bony deformity.[1]
  - Create transverse incision over interphalangeal (IP) joint of great toe and cut the extensor hallu-ces.
  - Create a joint arthrotomy large enough to visualize the collateral ligaments and articular carti-lage, using blunt and sharp dissection to mobilize the joint.
  - Demur the cartilage from the proximal and distal aspects of the IP joint.
  - In an antegrade/retrograde manner, insert a Kirschner wire (K-wire) through the distal articular surface out beneath the nail. Then, from the distal aspect retract the same wire and reinsert it through the joint.
  - Following sharp dissection to the K-wire surface distally, drill a hole adequate to permit the insertion of a 4-mm cannulated partially threaded screw.
  - Locate the distal extensor hallucis longus and bring it into a longitudinal dorsal incision over the first MT neck. Using a 4-mm drill hole, create medial and lateral (complete using blunt dissec-tion to avoid an iatrogenic fracture) aspects of the MT neck.
  - Pass the tendon lateral to medial, then suture the distal end back onto the proximal tendon using a nonabsorbable Ticron or Prolene suture.

Dangers

- Care of the superficial peroneal nerve with interosseous membrane preparation
- Avoid over- or undercorrection of the foot while tensioning the tendon transfers.
- Avoid the tendency to take too little of a dorsal wedge, which leaves the first MT plantarflexed and makes the patient susceptible to recurrence.
- Avoid the first tarsometatarsal joint when inserting the lag screw.
- May consider plantar fascia release if midfoot flexion remains prominent after first MT osteotomy

Complications

- Infection
- Recurrence (more common with too little of dorsal wedge)
- Residual dorsiflexion when first MT not corrected (Jones alone)[2]
- Hardware irritation
- Wound dehiscence
- Nonunion
- Claw toes
    - Secondary to intrinsic foot muscle contracture
    - In those cases where claw toes are already associated with a cavovarus foot, correction of tarsal deformity may lead to claw toe resolution.

Postoperative Care

- Posterior splint with sidebar stirrups in the immediate postoperative period with ankle in neutral dorsiflexion
- Skin staples/sutures removed 3 to 4 weeks into the postoperative period
- Transition to short leg boot for a total of 6 to 8 weeks.[3]
- Non–weight-bearing for 8 weeks
- Once osseous healing has occurred, transition to supportive shoes and start physical therapy for gait training, strengthening, and stretching.

References

1. Giannini S, Girolami M, Ceccarelli F, Maffei G. Modified Jones operation in the treatment of pes cavovarus. *Ital J Orthop Traumatol.* 1985;11:165-170.
2. de Palma L, Colonna E, Travasi M. The modified Jones procedure for pes cavovarus with claw hallux. *J Foot Ankle Surg.* 1997;36:279-283.
3. Ortiz C, Wagner E. Tendon transfers in cavovarus foot. *Foot Ankle Clin.* 2014;19:49-58.

Chapter 8
Hindfoot-Driven Cavovarus Deformity

MACALUS HOGAN

Hindfoot Deformity

Preoperative Evaluation

- Patient history and physical
  - In cases of a tight Achilles tendon, a lengthening procedure or gastrocnemius recession should be performed before any osteotomy procedure.
  - This will reduce deforming forces on the heel.
- Preoperative radiographic analysis critical to surgical indication and determination (Figure 8-1)
- Visual inspection and gait analysis
- Motor and neurologic assessment
- Compare to contralateral extremity
- Perform Coleman block testing: determine the presence of fixed hindfoot deformity, thereby warranting additional surgical correction[1] (Figure 8-2).
  - Place patient's heel and lateral foot onto a 2.5-cm block, permitting the first to fourth metatarsals (MTs) to fall into pronation.
  - Block size may be increased to reduce weight-bearing impact of first MT.
  - Obtain anteroposterior (AP) and lateral x-rays to document deformity changes with block.
- Document and prioritize muscle imbalances that contribute to deformity recurrence.

Surgical Planning and Sterile Instruments/ Equipment

- Radiolucent operating room table
- C-arm flouroscopy
- Thigh tourniquet

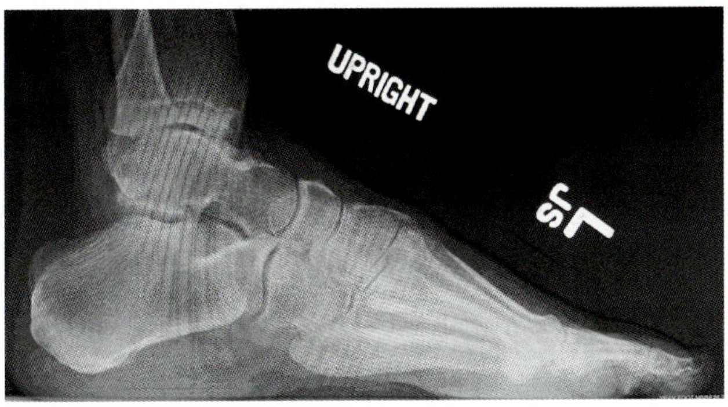

Figure 8-1. Preoperative lateral radiograph demonstrates moderate cavovarus deformity with early degenerative changes.

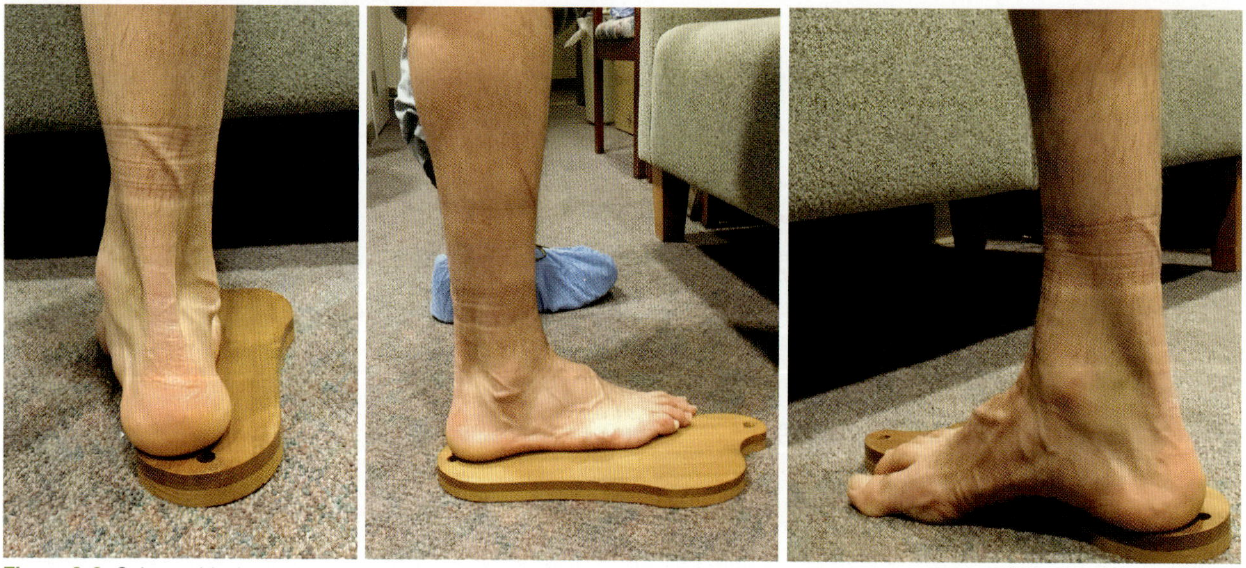

Figure 8-2. Coleman block testing used to determine the presence of flexible versus fixed hindfoot deformity.

- #15 blade
- Small Hohmann retractors
- Narrow sagittal saw
- Kirschner wires (1.6- or 2.0-mm K-wires)
- Implants
  - 6.5- or 6.7-mm partially threaded cancellous screws
- Rasp
- Smooth-toothed calcaneal laminar spreader
- Joker and/or Freer elevator
- Sutures (nonabsorbable)

Positioning/Prep

- Visually inspect surgical leg in preoperative area.
  - Confirm there are no active ulcers/infections.
  - Mark the operative extremity.
  - Preoperative ankle block with 1% lidocaine and 0.5% bupivacaine typically adequate for hindfoot procedure
- Position patient supine on the table.
  - Heel should be positioned near the end of the table.
  - Place a bump (centered at the level of anterior superior iliac spine [ASIS]) under the hip of the operative leg to increase foot internal rotation.
  - May use either bone foam or sterile bump (surgeon preference) to improve access to the medial and lateral aspects of the foot
- Well-padded calf tourniquet
- Use a plastic shield barrier or foam tape to prevent skin breakdown secondary to retained operative prep.

Surgical Approach

- Gastrocnemius recession—if tight Achilles tendon
  - Create a 3-cm longitudinal incision on medial aspect of leg, distal and overlying the myotendinous junction of the gastrocnemius, advancing your incision down to through the fascia in the same manner.
  - Isolate the gastrocnemius from the underlying soleus, using a malleable to separate this structure from the underlying tissue.
  - Make a transverse cut through the gastrocnemius fascia.

- Close wound with a 2-0 or 3-0 Vicryl/braided absorbable sutures.
- Layered dermal and superficial closure with a 3-0 Vicryl followed by a 4-0 absorbable monofilament
- Lateral calcaneal valgus producing osteotomy with peroneal longus to brevis transfer
  - Palpate and mark the distal fibula and fifth MT.
  - Template an L-shaped incision for an extensile lateral approach with the top aspect of the vertical limb beginning at the level of and one fingerbreadth (1 cm) posterior and inferior to the lateral malleolus (Figure 8-3A-D).
    - This permits an exposure 1 cm anterior to the Achilles tendon.

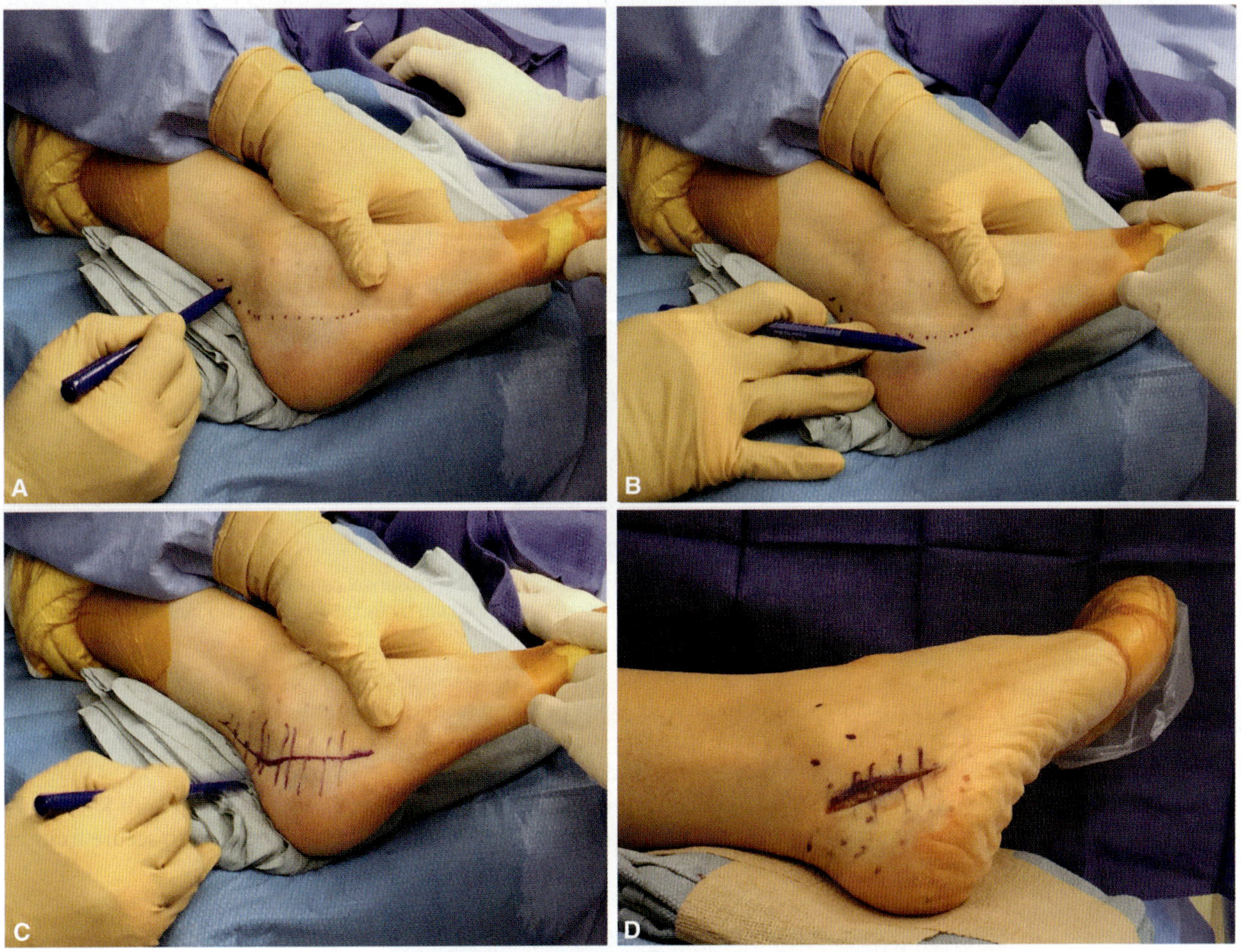

Figure 8-3. Palpate and mark the distal fibula (A) and fifth metatarsal (B). Template an L-shaped incision for an extensile lateral approach, with the top aspect of the vertical limb beginning at the level of and one fingerbreadth (1 cm) posterior and inferior to the lateral malleolus (C). D, Incision placement for isolated calcaneal osteotomy.

  - Extend the incision inferior and parallel to the peroneus longus until the peroneal tendons are identified.
  - Incise the peroneal tendon sheath over the extent of the superficial incision while maintaining the integrity of the superior peroneal retinaculum.
  - Excise a portion of the peroneal longus and Z-lengthen the peroneal brevis with a nonabsorbable suture.
  - Continue to dissect inferiorly, carefully identifying and retracting the sural nerve to avoid injury.
  - Dissect down to the calcaneus, and extend inferiorly via subperiosteal dissection.
  - Osteotomy and deformity correction
    - Use small Hohmann retractors to protect your surgical field during saw use, placing them superiorly to protect the Achilles tendon insertion, and anteriorly to preserve the plantar fascia origin.
    - Make a calcaneal osteotomy perpendicular to the calcaneal inclination axis with a sagittal saw.

- Decrease the calcaneal pitch.
- Move the free piece 8 to 10 mm laterally to achieve hindfoot valgus position of 5°.
- Make a midline longitudinal incision adjacent to the posterior plantar heel pad and continue through the subcutaneous fat to bone.
- Maintain the corrected position of the heel with K-wires (Figure 8-4A).
- Insert two 6.5-mm partially threaded cancellous screws via lag by technique, ensuring that the subtalar joint is not penetrated via multiview fluoroscopy (Figure 8-4B).
    - Use a rasp to smoothen any prominent lateral bone after the heel is properly shifted and positioned.

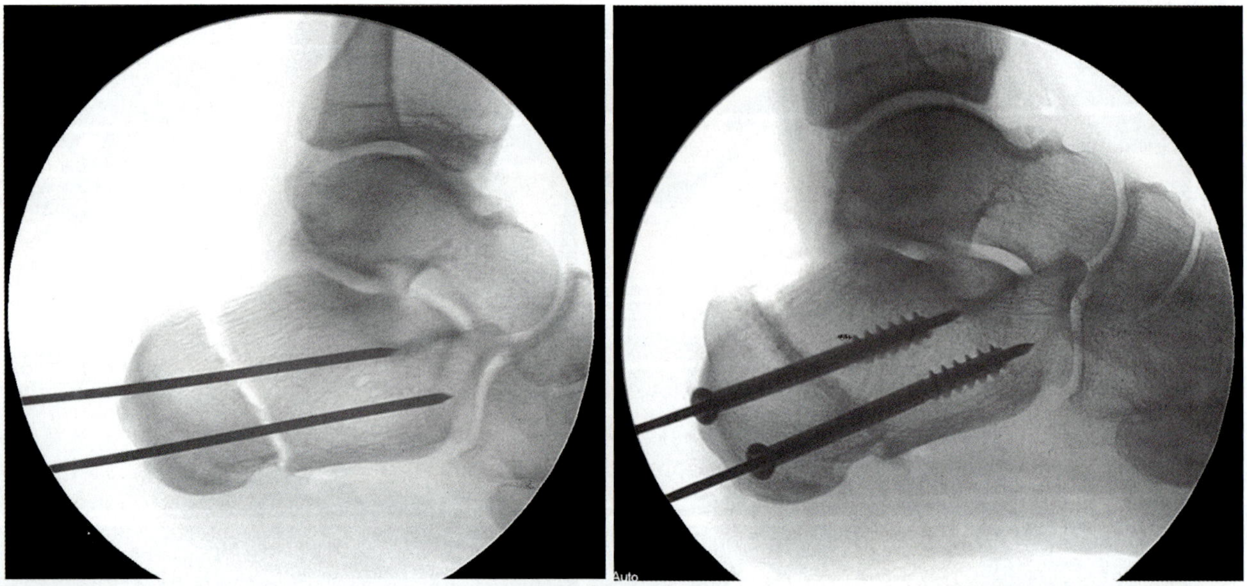

Figure 8-4. A, Placement of Kirschner wires to maintain corrected position following calcaneal osteotomy perpendicular to the calcaneal inclination axis. B, Insertion of two 6.5-mm partially threaded cancellous screws via lag by technique, ensuring that the subtalar joint is not penetrated.

- Alternative osteotomy technique: Dwyer closing wedge osteotomy
    - As an alternative to the straight perpendicular cut utilized in the lateral displacement osteotomy, a wedge of bone may be removed.
    - Dorsiflex the foot to complete the closing wedge before provisional fixation with K-wires.
    - Cannulated 6.5-mm partially threaded cancellous screws can still be used to secure fixation (Figure 8-5).

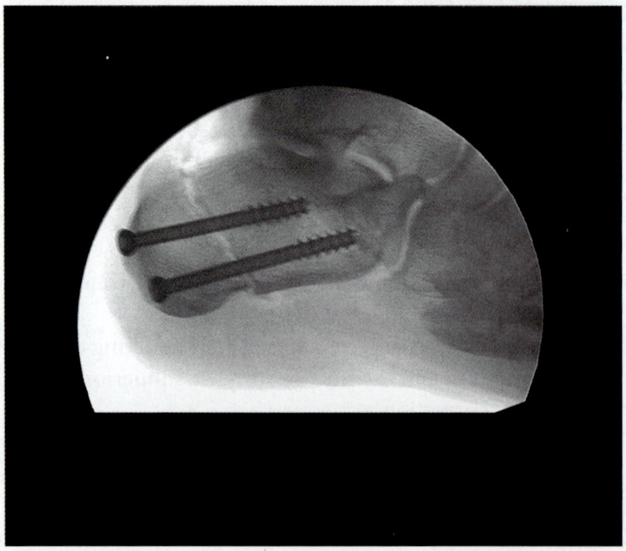

Figure 8-5. Intraoperative images of cannulated 6.5-mm partially threaded cancellous screws used to secure fixation.

- First MT dorsiflexion osteotomy
  - Although sentinel literature originally recommended deferring forefoot correction until the full effects of hindfoot surgery could be measured,[2] simultaneous forefoot osteotomies have been associated with improved patient-reported outcomes and functional scores.[3]
  - This may be performed in a manner similar to that described in Chapter 7.

Closure

- Irrigate wound with normal saline.
- Close deep/fascial layers with 2-0 braided Vicryl sutures.
- Close dermal layer with a 3-0 Maxon or an equivalent absorbable suture, followed by a 3-0 nylon suture for superficial closure.
- Place Steri-Strips loosely over the incision.
- Cover with Betadine-soaked Adaptic and sterile 4 × 4 gauze pads.
- Wrap with sterile Webril.
- Place patient in a posterior splint with sidebar stirrups to ensure a neutral/slightly dorsiflexed position without valgus/varus toggle.

Dangers

- Ensure screws are not placed too far lateral.
- Care of the sural nerve during dissection down to calcaneus and during gastrocnemius recession
- Additional dangers related to first MT osteotomy as described in Chapter 7

Complications

- Infection
- Sural nerve entrapment
- Diffuse heel pain
- Recurrence
- Hardware irritation
- Wound dehiscence
- Delayed union or nonunion

Postoperative Care

- Posterior splint with side bar stirrups in the immediate postoperative period (2 weeks) with ankle in neutral dorsiflexion
- Skin staples/sutures removed 3 to 4 weeks into the postoperative period
- Transition to short leg boot for a total of 6 to 8 weeks.
- Non–weight-bearing for 8 weeks
- Once osseous healing has occurred, transition to supportive shoes and start physical therapy for gait training, strengthening, and stretching.

References

1. Coleman SS, Chesnut WJ. A simple test for hindfoot flexibility in the cavovarus foot. *Clin Orthop Relat Res.* 1977;(123):60-62.
2. Dwyer FC. The present status of the problem of pes cavus. *Clin Orthop Relat Res.* 1975;(106):254-275.
3. Sammarco GJ, Taylor R. Cavovarus foot treated with combined calcaneus and metatarsal osteotomies. *Foot Ankle Int.* 2001;22:19-30.

Section 5
Ankle Arthritis

Chapter 9
Tibiotalar Arthrodesis: Anterior Approach

MACKENZIE T. JONES
SCOTT ELLIS

Introduction

Ankle arthrodesis has been the treatment of choice for end-stage ankle arthritis. Even with the availability of total ankle arthroplasty, a fusion still has many advantages such as less need for revision,[1] consistent results with regard to patient pain relief,[2] low cost of initial surgery,[3] and success in young active patients who would not be good candidates for arthroplasty.[4]

There are multiple approaches available for an ankle arthrodesis including arthroscopic, lateral, posterior, and anterior. The anterior approach provides good exposure, making it easier for the surgeon to achieve the correct position of the heel in the coronal plane.[5] In addition, it is often preferred for patients with post-traumatic arthritis because the anterior approach will avoid any prior lateral incisions. Another advantage is that the anterior approach allows the fibula to be spared so that the joint can potentially be converted into arthroplasty in the future using the same incision.[6]

Sterile Instruments/Equipment

- Tourniquet
- Headlight
- Esmarch bandage
- Trocar for iliac crest aspiration
- #15 blade
- Dissecting scissors
- Langenbeck retractor
- Army/navy retractor
- Deep Gelpi
- Reciprocating saw
- Curved Lambotte osteotome
- Straight curette
- Curved curette
- Microsagittal saw
- Burr
- 2.5-mm drill
- Wire driver
- 0.062 Kirschner wires (K-wires)
- Implants:
  - Anterolateral plate
  - Additional anteromedial plate for double-plating technique

  - 3.5-mm locking screws
  - 4.0-mm cortical screw
  - 7.5-mm headless partially threaded variable pitch compression screw
- 0-Vicryl, 2-0 Vicryl, 3-0 Vicryl, and 3-0 nylon sutures

Positioning

- The patient is placed in the supine position.
  - Support the ipsilateral pelvis to control external rotation of the leg. The patella should be directed upward to facilitate surgical approach and operation.
  - Pad all bony prominences to protect nerves.
- Place a nonsterile tourniquet on the operative thigh. Prep and drape the lower extremity in a sterile manner.
- Exsanguinate the lower extremity using an Esmarch bandage and inflate the tourniquet 250 to 300 mm Hg.

Iliac Crest Aspiration

Although there is no data to support the idea that an iliac crest aspiration promotes bone fusion, the procedure has low morbidity, with a chance of reducing the risk of nonunion.[7]

- Introduce the trocar into the iliac crest, proximal to the anterior superior iliac spine.
- Advance the trocar into the bone, taking care not to violate the cortex of the crest.
- Remove 60 mL to be processed.
- Remove the trocar and place Steri-strips over the small poke hole followed by a clean, sterile dressing.
- Concentrate aspirate with one of a number of commercially available systems.

Surgical Approach

- Perform an anterior approach to the ankle centered between the medial and lateral malleoli (Figure 9-1). Make an incision through the skin using a #15 blade that is long enough to insert the plate but just distal to the talonavicular joint to expose the talar neck in its entirety.

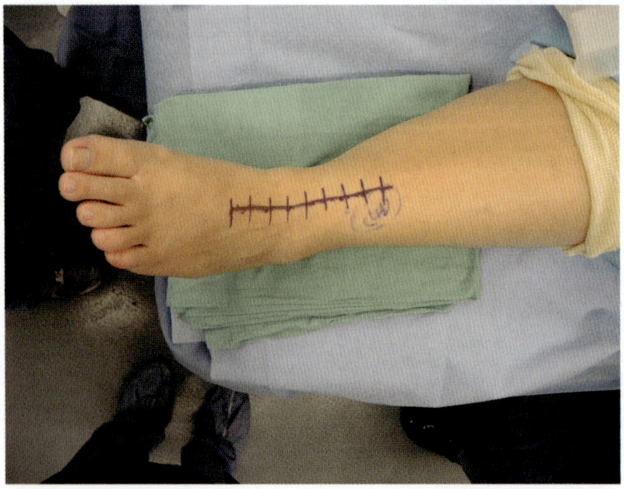

Figure 9-1. The skin incision is drawn over the anterior ankle.

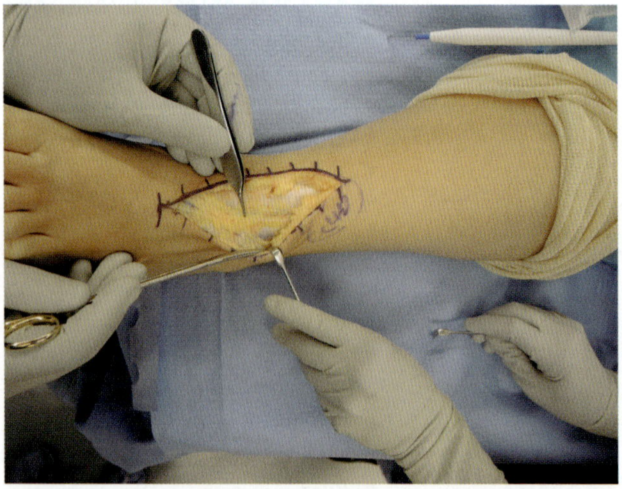

Figure 9-2. The superficial peroneal nerve is identified.

- Carefully dissect the subcutaneous tissue using dissecting scissors.
- Identify the superficial peroneal nerve and retract it laterally (Figures 9-2 and 9-3).
- Divide the extensor retinaculum longitudinally.
- Retract the tibialis anterior tendon medially and the extensor hallucis longus laterally using a Langenbeck retractor (Figure 9-4).
- Perform a longitudinal capsulotomy.

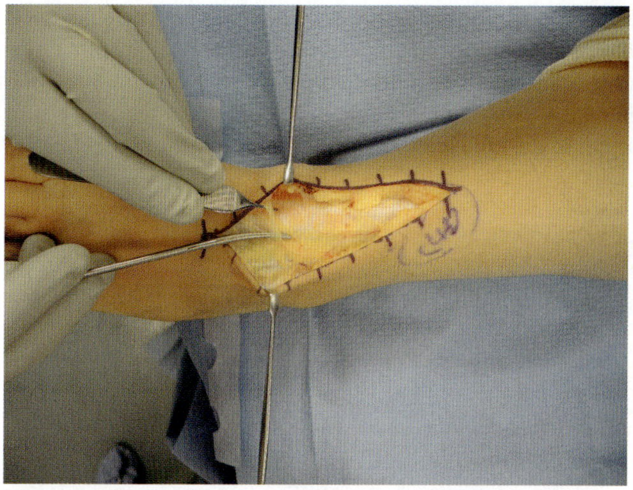

Figure 9-3. The medial branch of the superficial peroneal nerve is identified and must be cut.

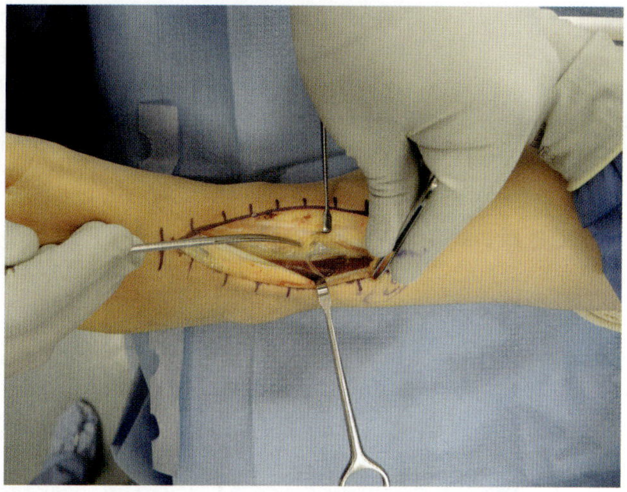

Figure 9-4. The deep bundle anterior tibial artery and deep peroneal nerve are visible beneath the retracted tendons.

- Elevate the capsule both medially and laterally to expose the joint.
- Place the deep Gelpi retractor below the capsule (Figure 9-5).
- Remove any osteophytes at the anterior aspect of the ankle using a reciprocating saw, first at the tibia and then at the talus (Figures 9-6 and 9-7).

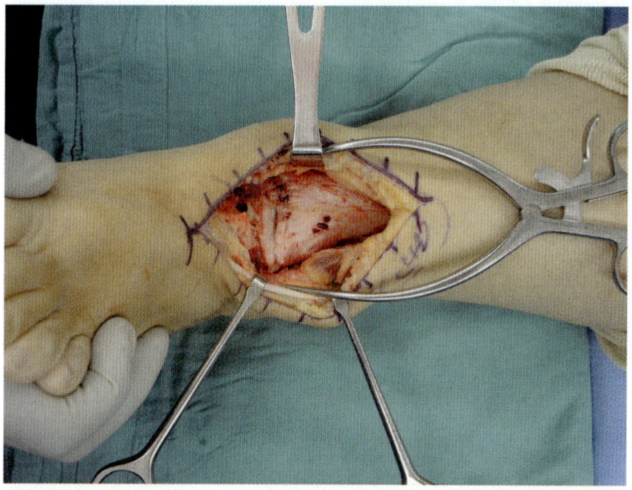

Figure 9-5. Use the army/navy, Langenbeck, and deep Gelpi retractors to expose the joint under the capsule.

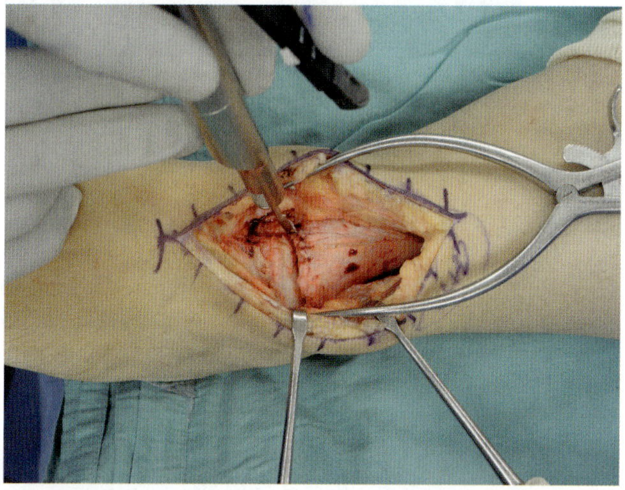

Figure 9-6. A reciprocating saw is used to make a cut in the tibia that is in line with the gutters to gauge the amount of anterior bone spur to remove.

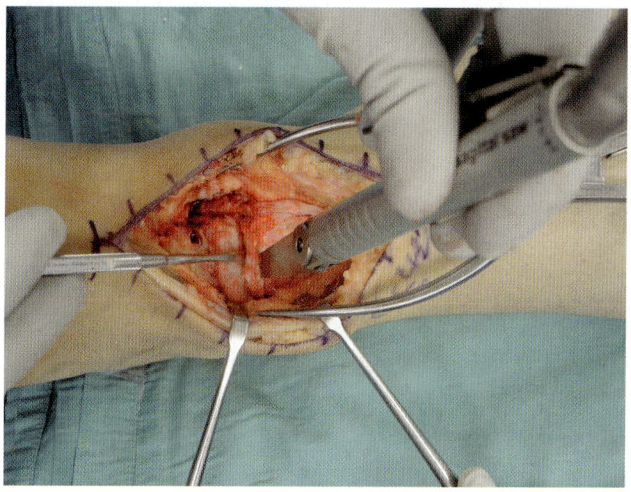

Figure 9-7. A microsagittal saw is used to remove bone spur from the tibial side of the joint.

- Prepare the joint from anterior to posterior. Use a smooth laminar spreader to aid in visualization of the joint (Figure 9-8), alternating between medial and lateral positions, and scrape any remaining cartilage from the tibia and talus using a combination of an osteotome, a microsagittal saw, and straight and curved curettes (Figure 9-9).
  - Take care to preserve the anatomic shape of the bones.

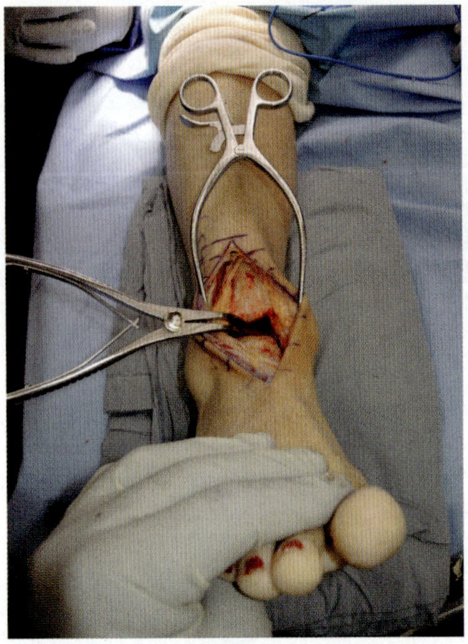

Figure 9-8. A smooth laminar spreader is inserted between the tibia and talus to expose the joint.

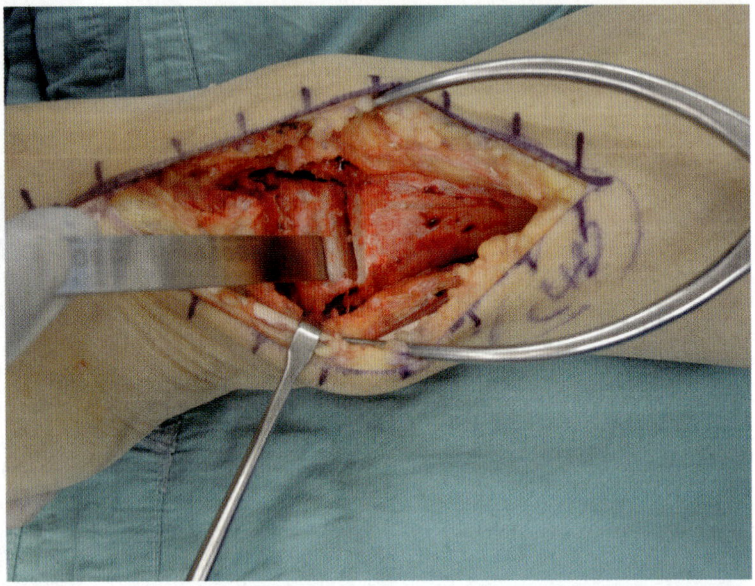

Figure 9-9. An osteotome is used to scrape cartilage from the talar side of the joint.

- Once all of the cartilage is removed, prepare the subchondral bone by creating multiple drill holes using a 2.5-mm drill and then fenestrate those holes using a curved osteotome (Figure 9-10).
  - Take care to prepare the joint far posteriorly as well.
- Bone graft the joint using a mixture of autograft, allograft, or biologic adjunct at the surgeon's discretion. Bone marrow aspirate can be used at this stage as well.

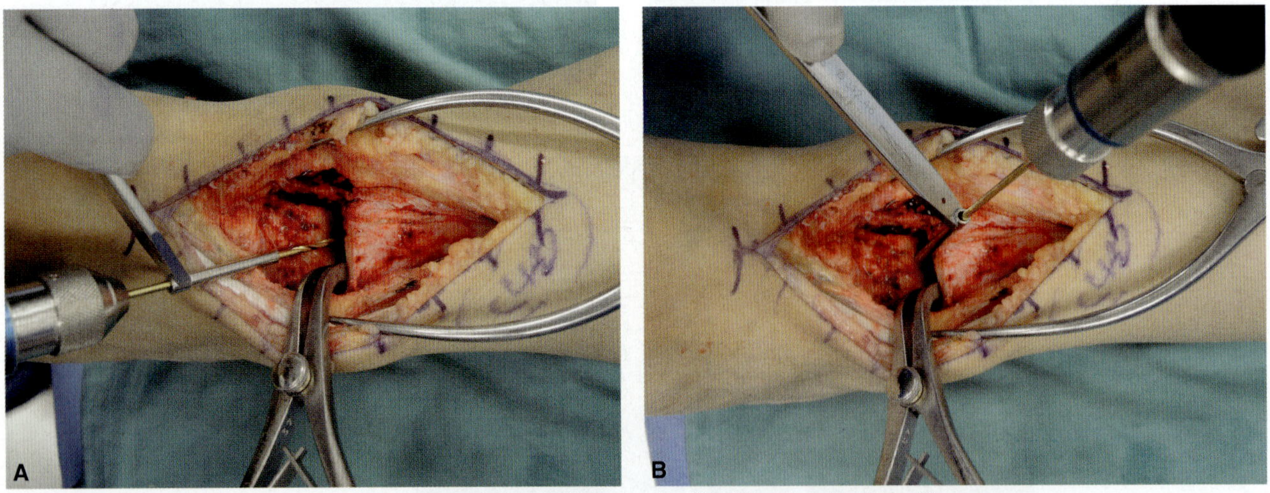

Figure 9-10. A 2.5-mm drill is used to prepare the subchondral bone on the tibia (A) and on the talus (B).

Reduction and Fixation Technique

For fixation, a headless compression screw can be used to prevent symptomatic hardware.[8]

- Reduce and pin the joint using 0.062 K-wires.
  - Take care to align the hindfoot to ensure that the ankle is in the optimum position.[9]
    - Ankle should be in a neutral position with respect to dorsiflexion and plantarflexion.
    - Joint should have 0° to 5° of slight valgus angulation.
    - Achieve approximately 5° to 10° of external rotation.
- Use intraoperative fluoroscopy with anteroposterior (AP) and lateral views to confirm provisional fixation and appropriate alignment of the joint (Figure 9-11).

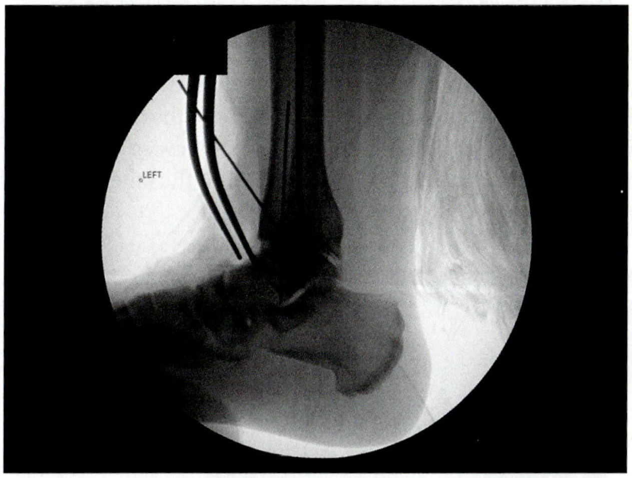

Figure 9-11. An intraoperative radiograph shows the ankle reduced and pinned. The anteroposterior view is not shown, but subsequent figures show the relative position after hardware placement.

- Position a guidewire for the 7.5-mm headless partially threaded variable pitch compression screw from the medial aspect of the tibia into the center portion of the talus. Take care not to disturb the subtalar joint space. In general, this should be directed posteriorly so as to make room for the anterior plate and screws to be placed.
- Place the screw to achieve compression across the joint.
- Use intraoperative fluoroscopy with AP and lateral views to confirm placement of the screw (Figure 9-12).

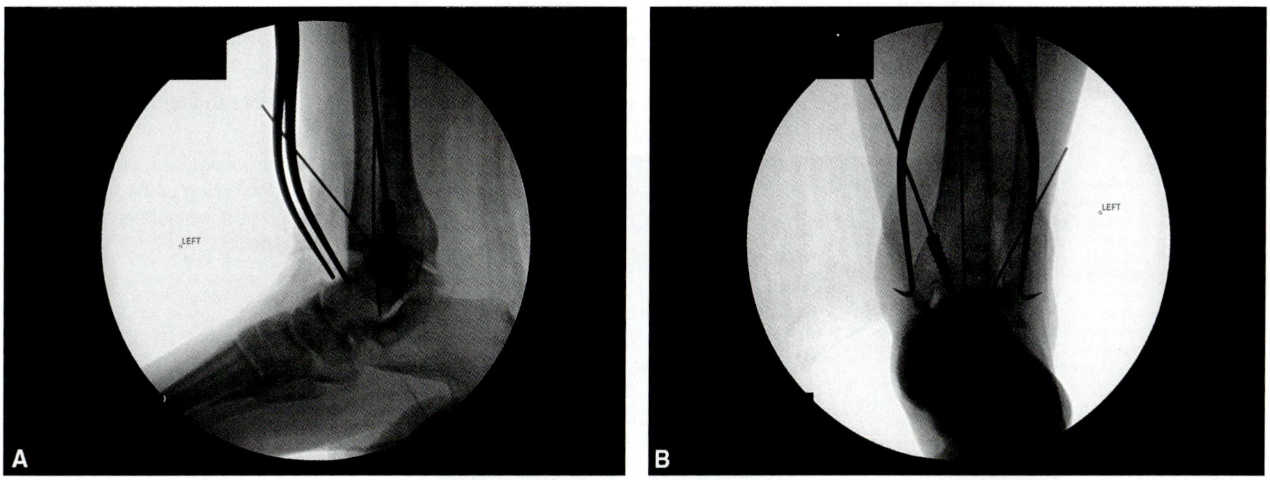

Figure 9-12. Lateral (A) and anteroposterior (B) intraoperative radiographs confirm the placement of the variable pitch compression screw.

Anterior Plating

Anterior fusion can be fixed with either a single anterior plate or a double-plating technique. Supplementation with anterior plating is ideal for patients with post-traumatic bone defects or poor bone quality following a long period of immobilization because they will require more rigid fixation. Because a major stressor on the fused ankle is dorsiflexion during gait, an anterior plate can provide more rigid fixation.[10] Anterior plating has been found to increase construct rigidity and decrease micromotion at the site of ankle fusion compared to screw fixation alone. In patients with minimal bony resection, an additional advantage of anterior plating is that the potentially deforming force of the Achilles tendon acts instead as an effective posterior tension plate, compressing the ankle joint and preventing overcorrection and dorsiflexion.[11]

Technique No 1: Anterior Single Plate

- Place the anterolateral plate onto the ankle.
  - Take care to ensure that the plate does not impinge on the talonavicular joint.
- Position appropriate length screws into the talus as well as into the tibia to secure the plate onto the bone.
  - Be very careful when assessing screw length on lateral view so as not to violate subtalar joint.
- The first 3.5-mm locking screw should be at the bottom of the anterolateral plate and connected to the talus (Figure 9-13).

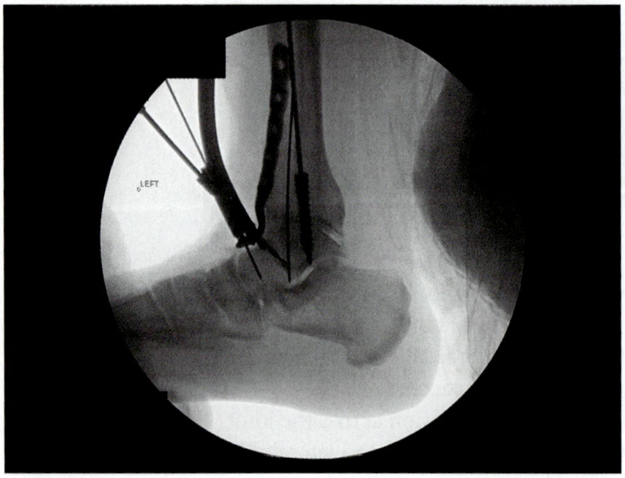

Figure 9-13. This intraoperative radiograph shows the first screw placed in the anterolateral plate, which goes through the talus.

  - Place locking cap over each before placing the next screw to secure the construct and prevent misalignment.
- The next 3.5-mm locking screw will connect the anterolateral plate to the tibia, establishing compression at the joint.
- The final screw will be a 4.0-mm cortical screw that is placed through both the tibia and talus (Figure 9-14).

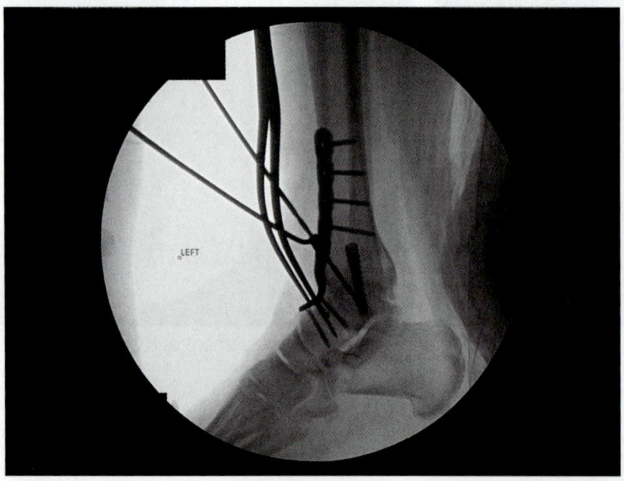

Figure 9-14. Intraoperative radiograph is taken to show the drilling of the "home run screw," which provides stabilization across the tibiotalar joint.

- Use intraoperative fluoroscopy with AP and lateral views to confirm placement of the plate and screws (Figures 9-15 and 9-16).
  - Note that screw length may be difficult to interpret in the lateral view, especially for those in the talar neck directed toward the subtalar joint.

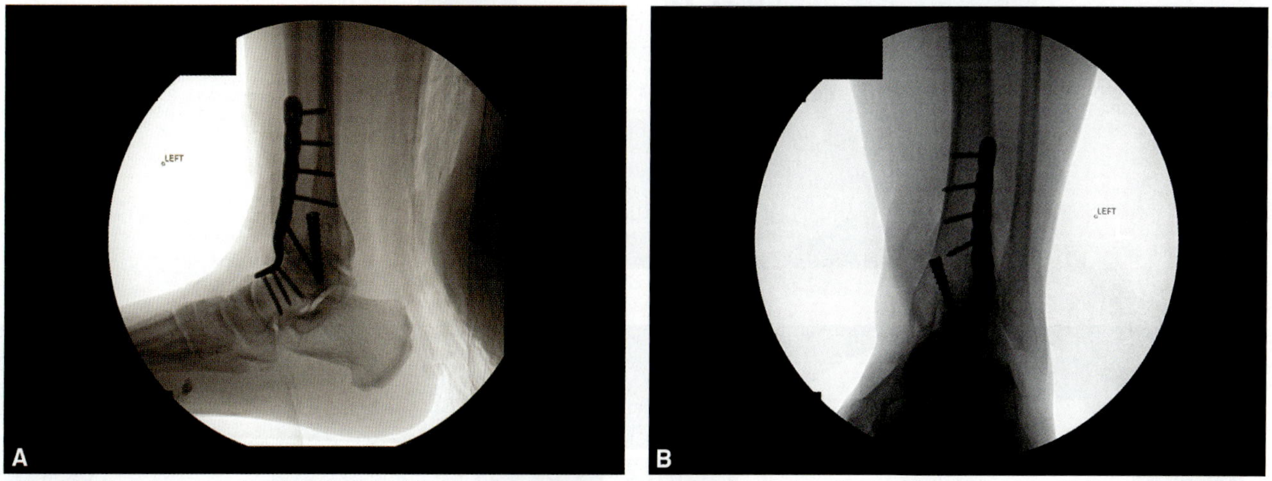

Figure 9-15. Anteroposterior (A) and lateral (B) intraoperative radiographs show the final positioning of the anterolateral plate and screws.

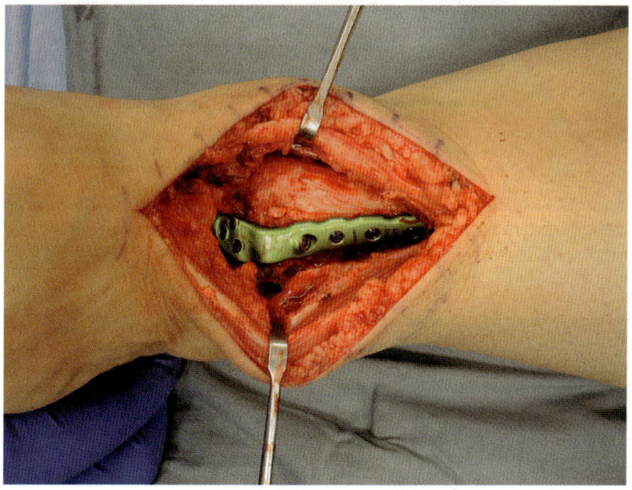

Figure 9-16. Photograph shows a final view of the anterior plate positioning before closing.

Technique No 2: Anterior Double Plate

This alternative technique, anterior double plating, has been shown to help achieve a solid arthrodesis despite difficult bone quality and/or comorbidities for bone healing by improving fixation of the talus and increasing compression of the talus and tibia.[12]

- Position the anterolateral plate onto the bone (Figure 9-17).
  - Follow Technique No. 1, but be sure to leave space for the expected second plate.
- Position the anteromedial plate onto the talus.
- Secure the plate distally through the talus and then proximally at the tibia using 3.5-mm locking screws.
- Position the 4.0-mm cortical screw through the plate and tibia into the posterior portion of the talar dome.
  - Take care not to violate the subtalar joint with any of the screws.
- Use intraoperative fluoroscopy with AP and lateral views to confirm placement of the plate and screws (Figures 9-18 and 9-19).

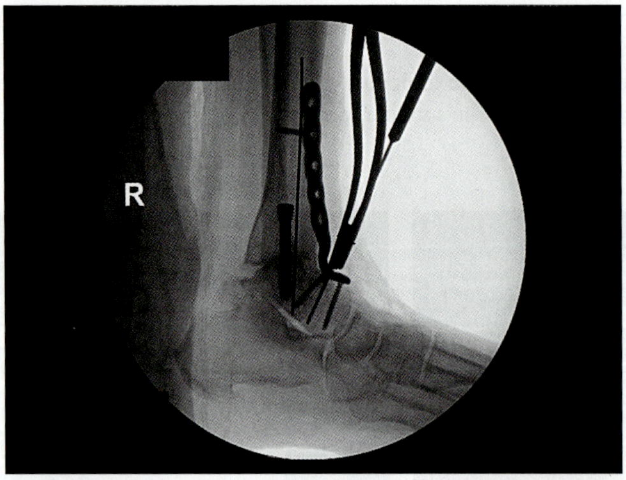

Figure 9-17. This lateral intraoperative radiograph confirms the placement of screws through the anterolateral plate and into the talus.

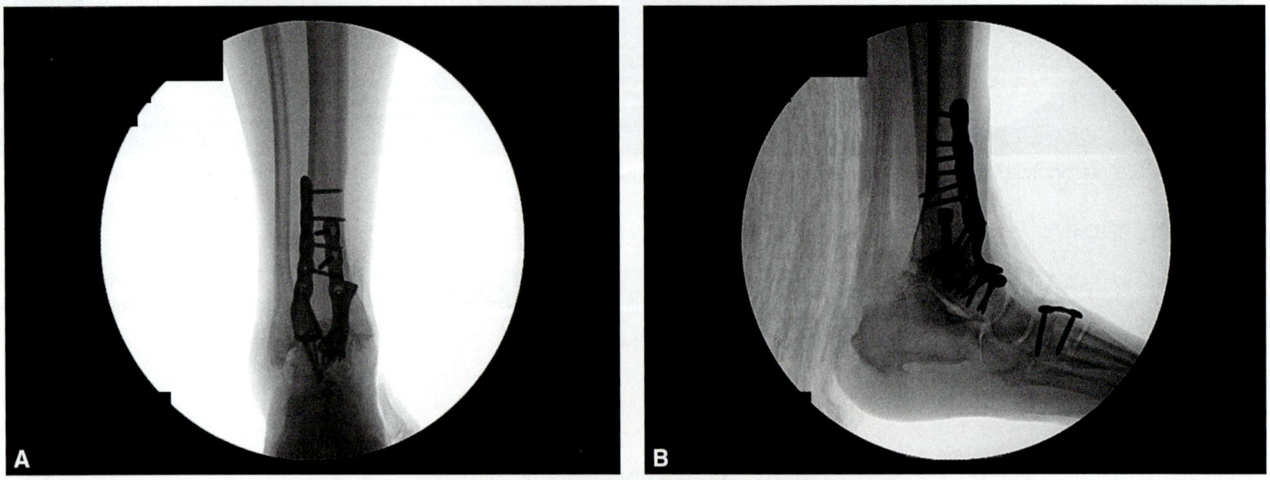

Figure 9-18. Anteroposterior (A) and lateral (B) intraoperative radiographs show the final placement of the two anterior plates. Note that a plate is also placed over the medial cuneiform to fix a Cotton osteotomy that was performed to increase the arch of the foot separate from the ankle fusion.

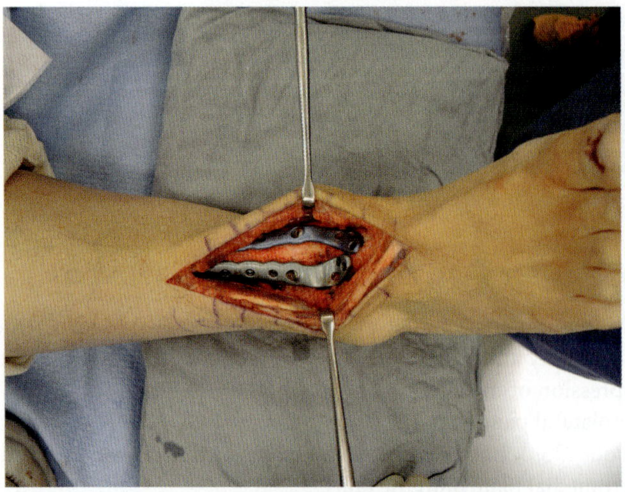

Figure 9-19. Photograph shows a final view of the anterior double plates before closing.

Closing

- Irrigate, clean, and dry the wound.
- Let down the tourniquet and confirm hemostasis.
- Close the capsule with a 0-Vicryl suture (Figure 9-20). Sometimes the capsule is difficult to close over the anterior plates and can be left.
- Close the extensor retinaculum with a 2-0 Vicryl suture (Figure 9-21).

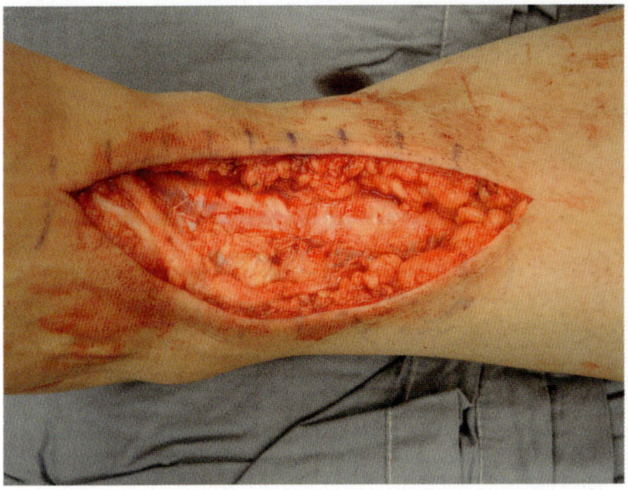

Figure 9-21. Photograph shows the closed extensor retinaculum.

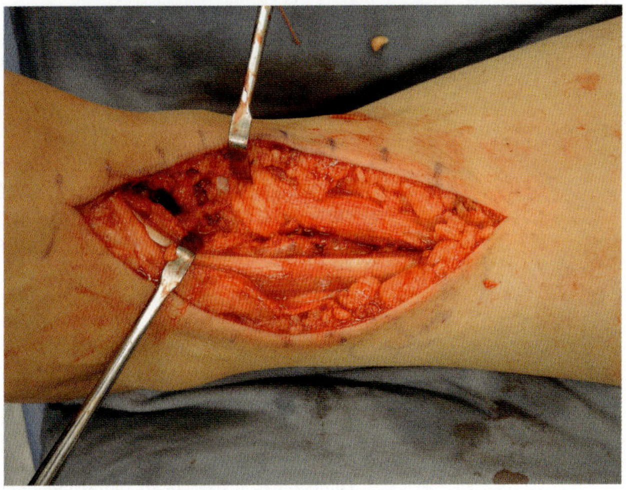

Figure 9-20. Photograph shows the closed capsule between the anterior tibial tendon and extensor hallucis longus tendon.

- Close subcutaneous tissue with a 3-0 Vicryl suture.
- Close the skin with a 3-0 nylon suture placed in a horizontal mattress pattern and in an interrupted manner (Figure 9-22).
- Place Xeroform over the incision, followed by a clean sterile dressing, followed by a well-padded posterior U-splint.

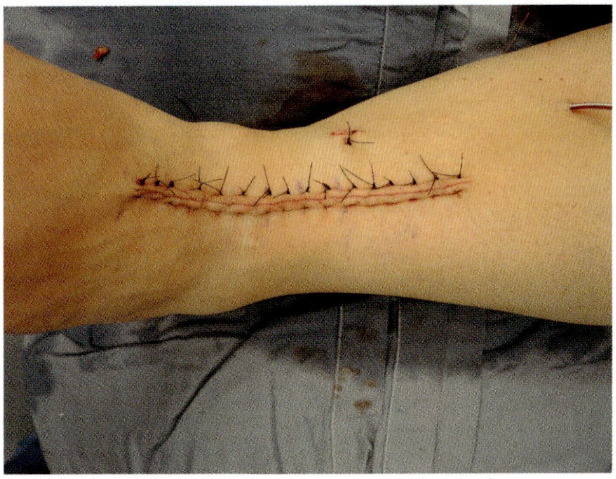

Figure 9-22. Photograph shows the closed incision with sutures in a horizontal mattress pattern.

References

1. Daniels TR, Younger ASE, Penner M, et al. Intermediate-term results of total ankle replacement and ankle arthrodesis. *J Bone Joint Surg Am.* 2014;96(2):135-142.
2. Lynch AF, Bourne RB, Rorabeck CH. The long-term results of ankle arthrodesis. *J Bone Joint Surg Br.* 1988;70(1):113-116.
3. Nwachukwu BU, McLawhorn AS, Simon MS, et al. Management of end-stage ankle arthritis: cost-utility analysis using direct and indirect costs. *J Bone Joint Surg Am.* 2015;97(14):1159-1172.
4. McGuire MR, Kyle RF, Gustilo RB, Premer RF. Comparative analysis of ankle arthroplasty versus ankle arthrodesis. *Clin Orthop Relat Res.* 1988;(226):174-181.
5. Helm R. The results of ankle arthrodesis. *J Bone Joint Surg Br.* 1990;72(1):141-143.
6. Ahmad J, Raikin SM. Ankle arthrodesis: the simple and the complex. *Foot Ankle Clin.* 2008;13(3):381-400.
7. Sen MK, Mclau T. Autologous iliac crest bone graft: should it still be the gold standard for treating nonunions? *Injury.* 2007;38(1):S75-S80.
8. Odutola AA, Sheridan BD, Kelly AJ. Headless compression screw fixation prevents symptomatic metalwork in arthroscopic ankle arthrodesis. *Foot Ankle Surg.* 2012;18(2):111-113.
9. Buck P, Morrey BF, Chao EY. The optimum position of arthrodesis of the ankle. A gait study of the knee and ankle. *J Bone Joint Surg Am.* 1987;69(7):1052-1062.
10. Guo C, Yan Z, Barfield WR, Hartsock LA. Ankle arthrodesis using anatomically contoured anterior plate. *Foot Ankle Int.* 1991;268:70-77.
11. Mears DC, Gordon RG, Kann SE, Kann JN. Ankle arthrodesis with an anterior tension plate. *Clin Orthop Relat Res.* 1991;268:70-77.
12. Plaass C, Knupp M, Barg A, Hintermann B. Anterior double plating for rigid fixation of isolated tibiotalar arthrodesis. *Foot Ankle Int.* 2009;30(7):631-639.

Suggested Readings

1. Brodsky JW, Kane JM, Coleman S, Bariteau J, Tenenbaum S. Abnormalities of gait caused by ankle arthritis are improved by ankle arthrodesis. *Bone Joint J*. 2016;98(10):1369-1375.
2. Chalayon O, Wang B, Blankenhorn B, et al. Factors affecting the outcomes of uncomplicated primary open ankle arthrodesis. *Foot Ankle Int*. 2015;36(10):1170-1179.
3. Coester LM, Saltzman CL, Leupold J, Pontarelli W. Long-term results following ankle arthrodesis for post-traumatic arthritis. *J Bone Joint Surg Am*. 2001;83(2):219-228.
4. DiGiovanni CW, Lin SS, Daniels TR, et al. The importance of sufficient graft material in achieving foot or ankle fusion. *J Bone Joint Surg Am*. 2016;98(15):1260-1267.
5. Haddad SL, Coetzee JC, Estok R, Fahrbach K, Banel D, Nalysnyk L. Intermediate and long-term outcomes of total ankle arthroplasty and ankle arthrodesis. *J Bone Joint Surg Am*. 2007;89(9):1899-1905.
6. Haskell A, Dedini R, Dini M. Safe zone for placement of talar screws when fusing the ankle with an anterior plating system. *Foot Ankle Int*. 2015;36(6):730-735.
7. Jones CP, Cohen B, Lewis J, Davis WH. CT scan outcomes of ankle arthrodesis with anterior plating. *Foot Ankle Orthop*. 2016;1(1). doi:10.1177/2473011416S00045.
8. Muir DC, Amendola A, Saltzman CL. Long-term outcome of ankle arthrodesis. *Foot Ankle Clin*. 2002;4:703-708.
9. Pedowitz DI, Kane JM, Smith GM, Saffel HL, Comer C, Raikin SM. Total ankle arthroplasty versus ankle arthrodesis: a comparative analysis of arc of movement and functional outcomes. *Bone Joint J*. 2016;98(5):634-640.
10. Sinclair V, O'Leary E, Pentlow A, Hepple S, Harries B, Winson I. The long-term outcomes of arthroscopic ankle arthrodesis and the prevalence of adjacent degenerative joint disease. *J Bone Joint Surg Br*. 2017;98:S19.

Chapter 10

Total Ankle Arthroplasty With Prophecy® Infinity® Surgical Technique (Wright Medical, Memphis TN)

AUSTIN E. SANDERS
CONSTANTINE A. DEMETRACOPOULOS

Sterile Instruments/Equipment

- Tourniquet
- Headlight
- Retractors
  - Skin hooks
  - Ragnell retractors
  - Langenbeck retractors
  - Gelpi retractor
- Metzenbaum scissors
- Reciprocating saw
- Microsagittal and large oscillating saw
- Pituitary rongeurs
- Long straight and angled curettes
- 2.4-mm Steinnman pins
- Implants
  - Talar dome
  - Tibial tray
  - Polyethylene insert
- Bone cement

Preoperative Planning

- Indications: end-stage ankle arthritis
- Contraindications: an active infection or a history of one, peripheral vascular disease, osteomyelitis, a current infection or a history of one, inadequate neuromuscular status, sepsis, skeletal immaturity, neuropathy, severe ankle instability or severe malalignment that cannot be corrected, insufficient bone stock, excessive loads due to patient weight or activity, pregnancy, uncooperative patient or neurologic disorders resulting in noncompliance, and osteonecrosis of the talus.
- Physical examination
  - Assess motion of the ankle and hindfoot.
  - Assess stability of the ankle.
  - Assess for malalignment of the limb beginning proximally and extending to the hindfoot. Include any associated foot deformity such as a flatfoot or cavus deformity.
  - Determine neurovascular status; include assessment for subtle neuropathy utilizing a 5.07 Semmes–Weinstein monofilament examination.

- Radiographs:
  - Obtain standardized weight-bearing radiographs of the ankle and foot, including a hindfoot alignment view.
  - Include hip-to-ankle alignment views if physical examination suggests deformity more proximally.
  - The anterior tibial distal angle can be measured to determine the presence of a recurvatum deformity (>83°) in the tibia.
  - The lateral distal tibial angle (LDTA) (normal = 89° ± 3°) can be measured to determine coronal plane deformity. An LDTA <86° indicates a valgus deformity.
  - A tibial talar angle >10° represents an incongruent deformity.
  - If there is significant proximal deformity, realignment with osteotomy or arthroplasty may be indicated depending on the patient's clinical presentation.
  - The hindfoot alignment view may not only demonstrate hindfoot malalignment but also suggest possible compensatory deformity in the subtalar joint, which, if present, may be revealed once tibiotalar deformity is corrected.

Positioning

- The patient is supine on the operating room table with all extremities well padded.
- A bump is placed underneath the ipsilateral hip to bring the foot into a neutral position or into slight internal rotation.
- A nonsterile tourniquet should be placed on the operative thigh.
- The lower extremity is prepped and draped in a normal sterile manner.
- Exsanguinate the lower extremity using an Esmarch bandage and inflate the tourniquet.

Surgical Technique

- The incision is made one fingerbreadth lateral to the tibial crest and extends distally to the level of the talonavicular joint (Figure 10-1).
- Dissect through the subcutaneous tissue to identify the superficial peroneal nerve. Often, a medial branch of the nerve at the level of the tibiotalar joint may need to be sacrificed to sufficiently mobilize the nerve to protect it throughout the remainder of the case.
- The extensor retinaculum is incised over the extensor hallucis longus tendon (Figure 10-2).
- The deep neurovascular bundle is mobilized and retracted laterally, and the tibialis anterior is retracted medially. Make every attempt to preserve the tibialis anterior into its own sheath to prevent postoperative adhesions (Figure 10-3).
- A midline capsulotomy is performed to protect the neurovascular bundle. Once distal to the tibiotalar joint, the capsulotomy may be angled slightly medially to avoid the deep bundle (Figure 10-4).
- Excess soft tissue is removed from the anterior aspect of the distal tibia. Any loose osteophytes may be removed as indicated by the preoperative plan. Stable osteophytes must be preserved to ensure proper fit of the tibial cutting guide.
- The alignment guide is placed against the anterior aspect of the distal tibia. The fit of the alignment guide with respect to the patient's tibia may be compared to that of the preprinted distal tibial model to ensure that the guide is positioned correctly in the patient. The guide is pinned to the tibia (Figures 10-5 and 10-6).
- Confirm correct positioning of the alignment guide with an anteroposterior (AP) fluoroscopic imagine (Figure 10-7).

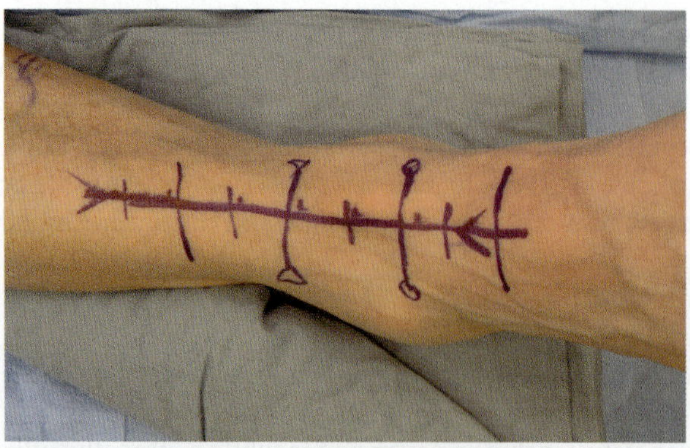

Figure 10-1. Marked midline incision centered on the joint.

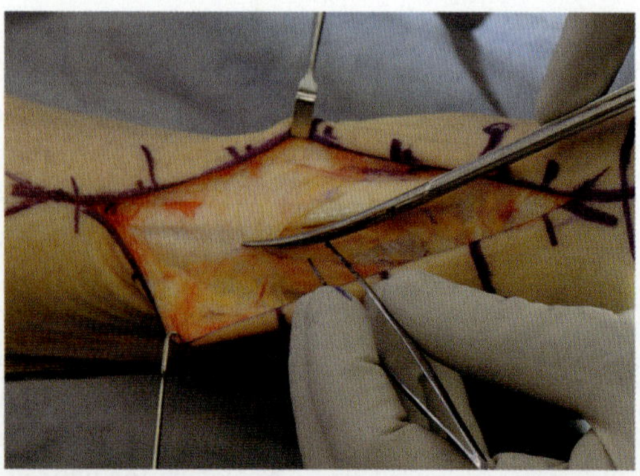

Figure 10-2. The extensor retinaculum is incised over the extensor hallucis longus tendon.

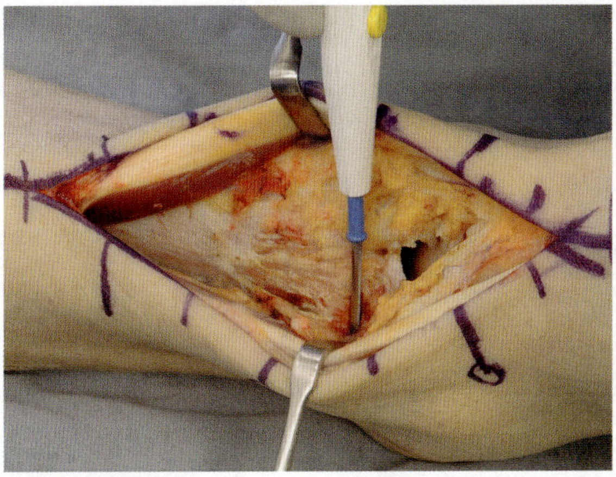

Figure 10-3. The capsule is elevated both medially and laterally, either with sharp dissection or with Bovie electrocautery.

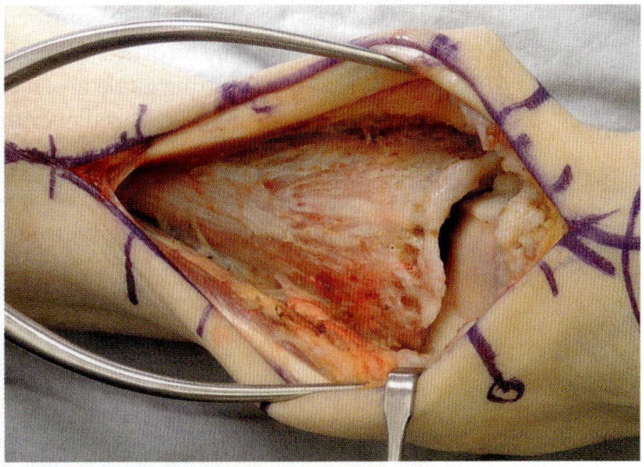

Figure 10-4. Exposed tibiotalar joint.

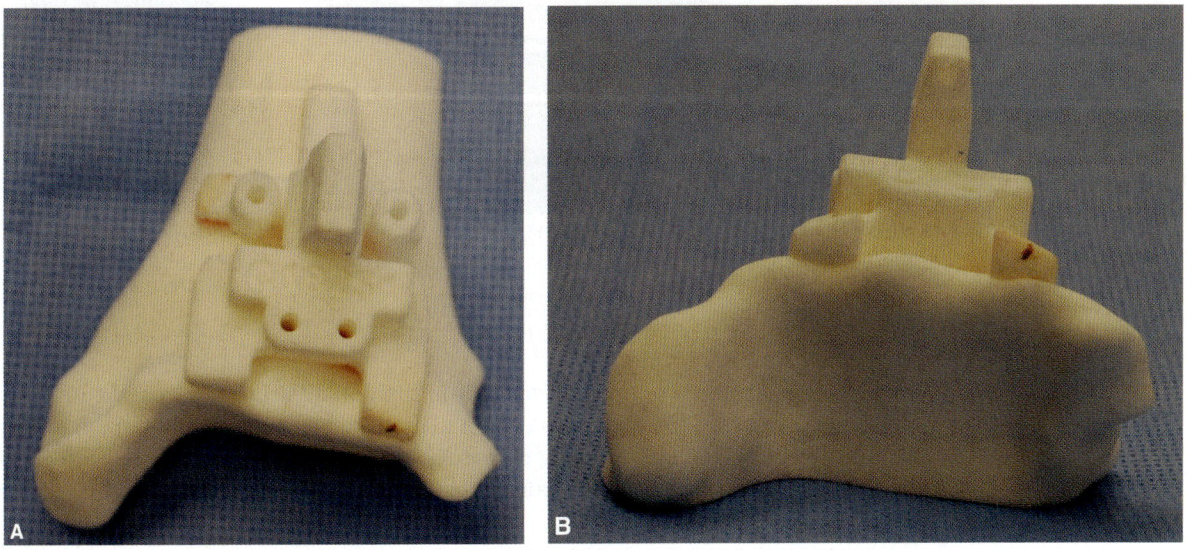

Figure 10-5. Tibial alignment guides. Note the fit of the guides in the coronal (A) and axial (B) planes.

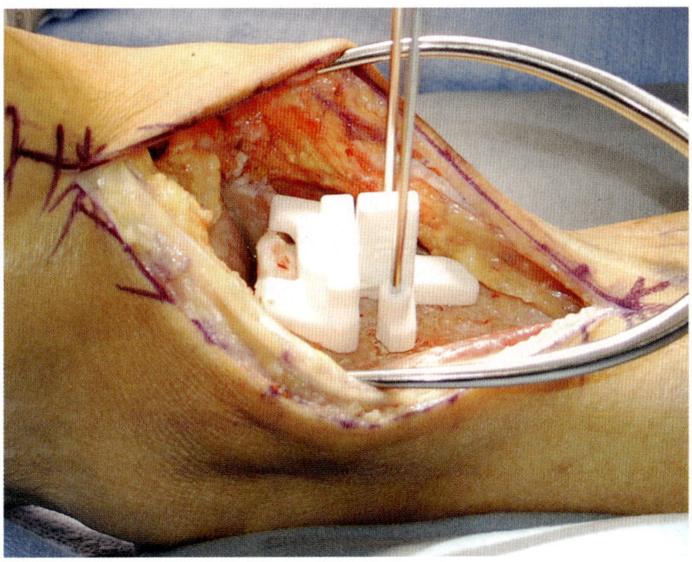

Figure 10-6. Tibial guide with two Steinnman pins.

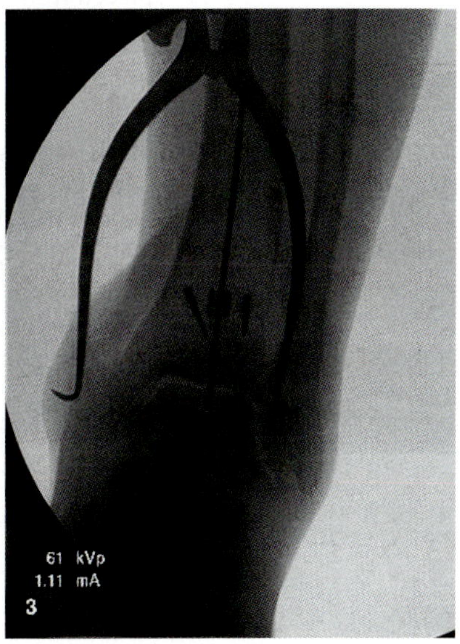

Figure 10-7. Intraoperative fluoroscopic image demonstrating the tibial alignment guide is correctly positioned in the coronal plane.

- Once the alignment is confirmed, two additional pins are placed through the alignment guide. All pins should be bicortical to ensure proper fixation.
- The coronal sizing guide is placed over the pins and secured to the distal tibia (Figure 10-8).
- The sizing guide is placed over the pins and secured to the tibia (Figure 10-9).

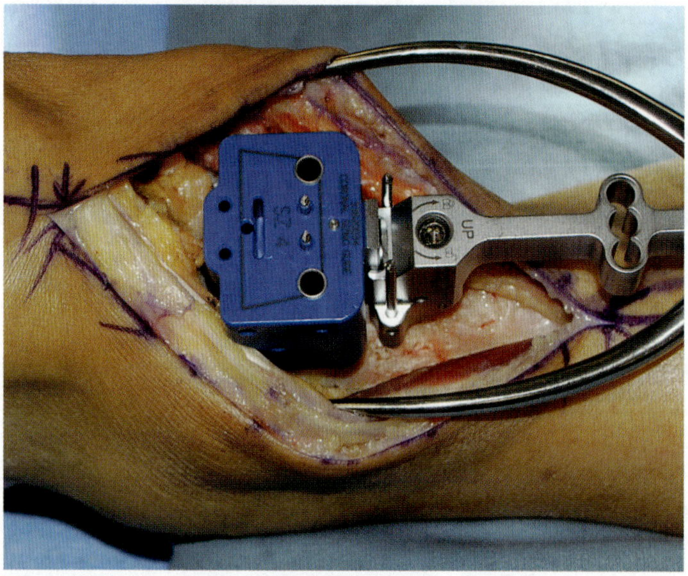

Figure 10-8. The coronal sizing guide flush against the tibia.

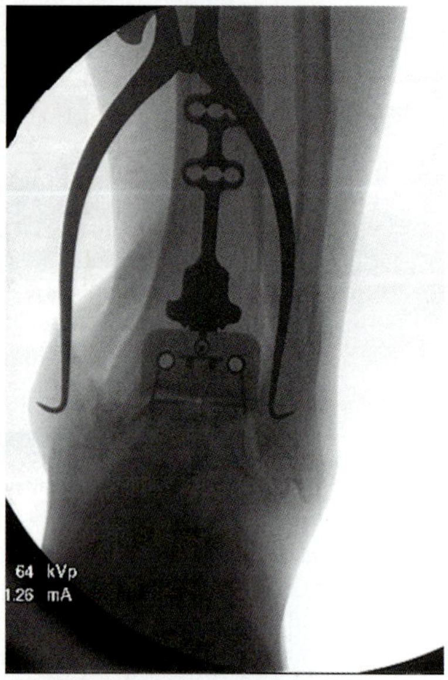

Figure 10-9. Intraoperative fluoroscopy confirming the appropriate size of the coronal sizing guide for the tibial cut.

- Intraoperative fluoroscopy is utilized to confirm appropriate sizing of the tibial cut, as well as correct position of the cut guide with respect to its medial/lateral position. Care must be taken not to oversize the component because of concern about violating the malleoli. The corners of the tibial cut should match the medial and lateral gutters. In addition, the implant should be centered with respect to the distal tibia.
- Once the correct position is confirmed, the corners of the tibial cut are reamed (Figure 10-10).
- Remove the coronal sizing guide and replace with the resection guide by sliding it over the two distal pins. Additional fixation can be achieved with a more central pin through the cutting guide, placed from medial to lateral to avoid the neurovascular bundle posterior to the medial malleolus.
- The tibial cut is performed with a large oscillating saw through the cut slots (Figure 10-11).

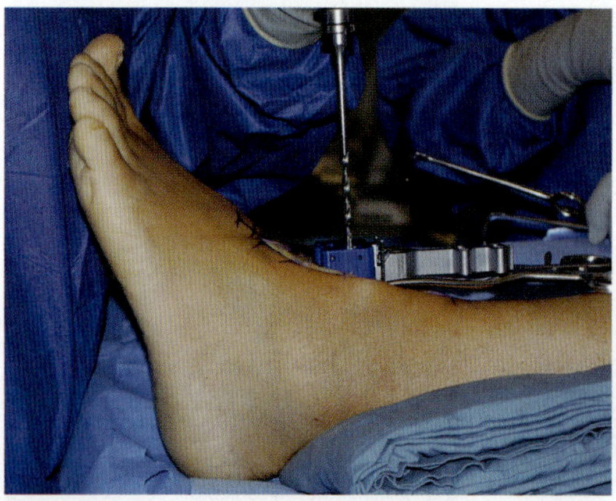

Figure 10-10. Corner reaming is performed in preparation for the tibial cut.

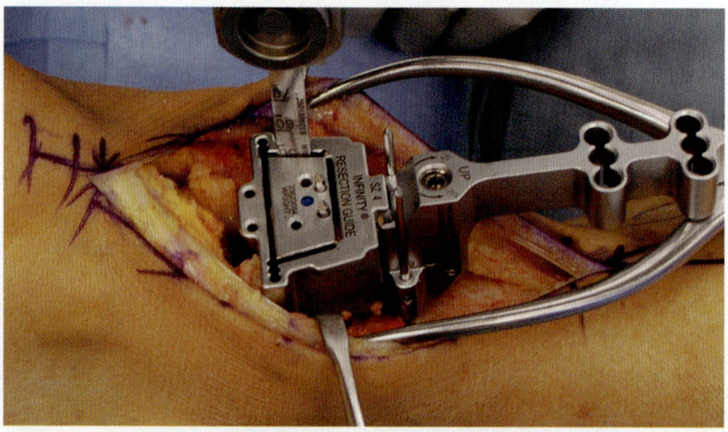

Figure 10-11. The tibial cut is performed.

- The corner cutter can be used to ensure that the cut is completed all the way posteriorly. The osteotome has hash marks indicating the appropriate depth that the instrument should be advanced depending on the expected size of the tibial implant (Figure 10-12).

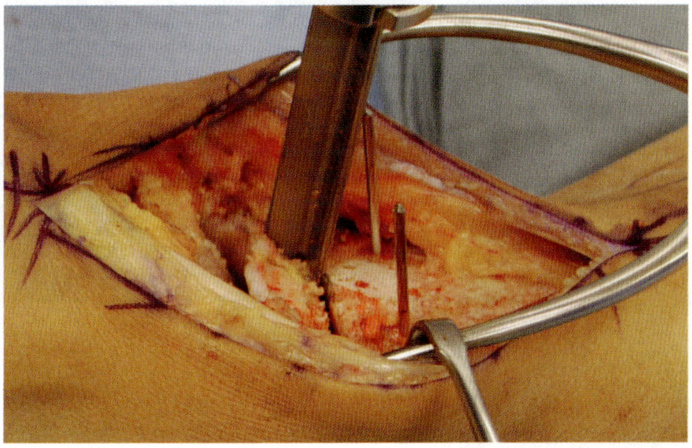

Figure 10-12. The corner osteotome is used to free the tibial cut.

- The tibial bone is removed. A pituitary rongeur, as well as long and straight curettes, may be necessary to remove all bone from the posterior aspect of the joint (Figures 10-13 and 10-14).
- Place the foot into plantar flexion and then place the talar alignment guide in the best fit location. Utilize the provided model of the talus to assure proper fit. Often, the guide will sit distal on the talar neck and head, just proximal to the talonavicular joint (Figure 10-15).
- Secure with one Steinnman pin through the top of the guide and place the other into one of the anterior pin holes, taking care to retract the deep neurovascular bundle (Figure 10-16).
- Once the alignment has been confirmed, remove the alignment guide and replace it with the appropriately sized resection guide. Be sure to check the sizing of the talar component in the preoperative plan. The cutting guide for the talus may be a size smaller than the one used for the tibia.

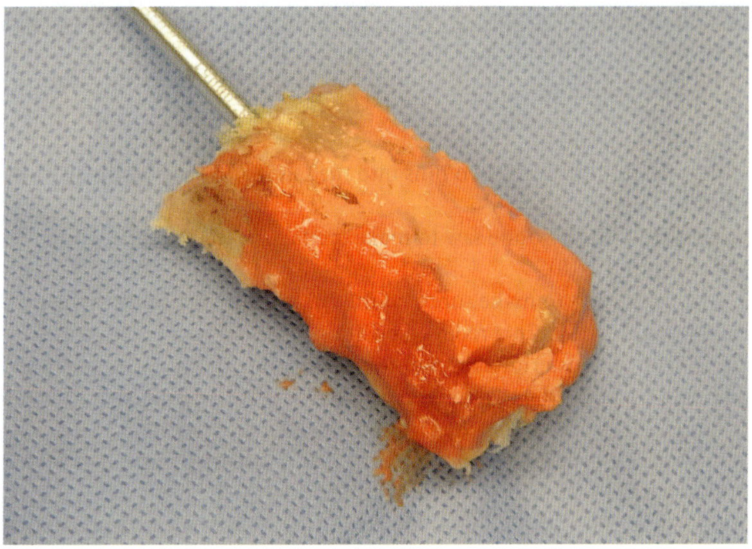

Figure 10-13. The distal tibial cut is removed.

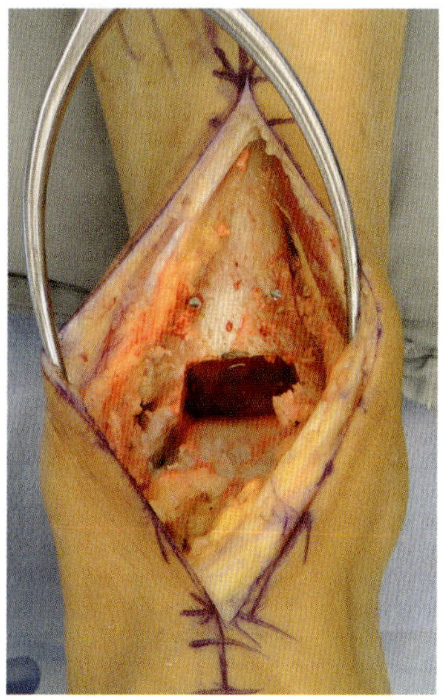

Figure 10-14. Tibial resection is removed.

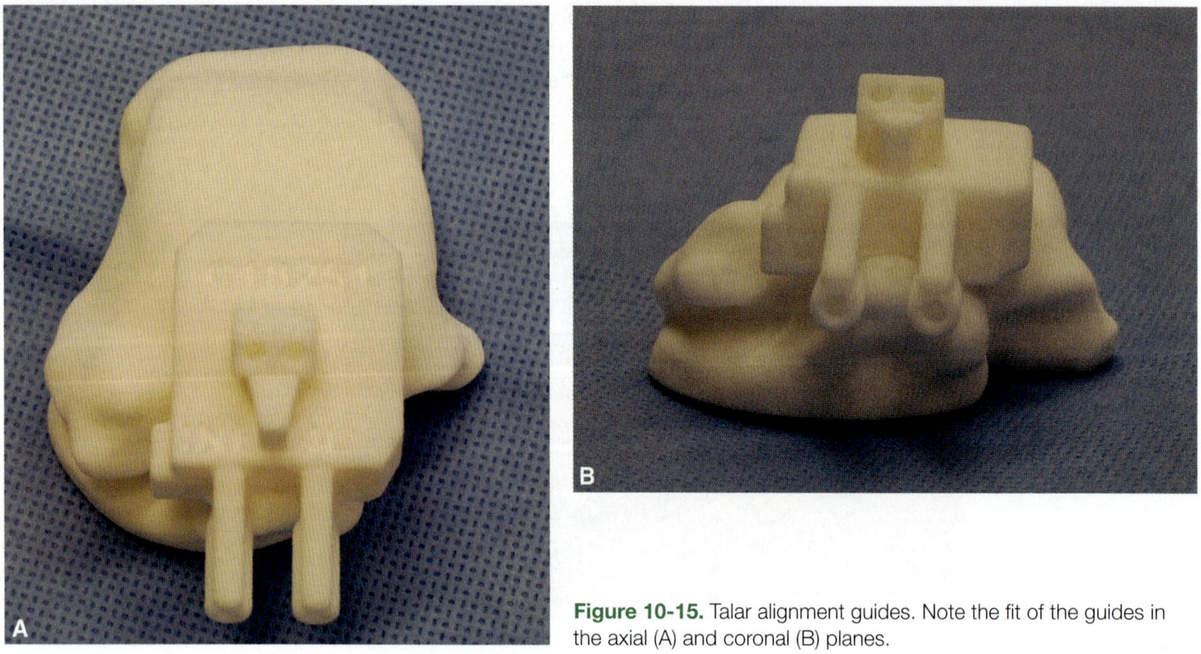

Figure 10-15. Talar alignment guides. Note the fit of the guides in the axial (A) and coronal (B) planes.

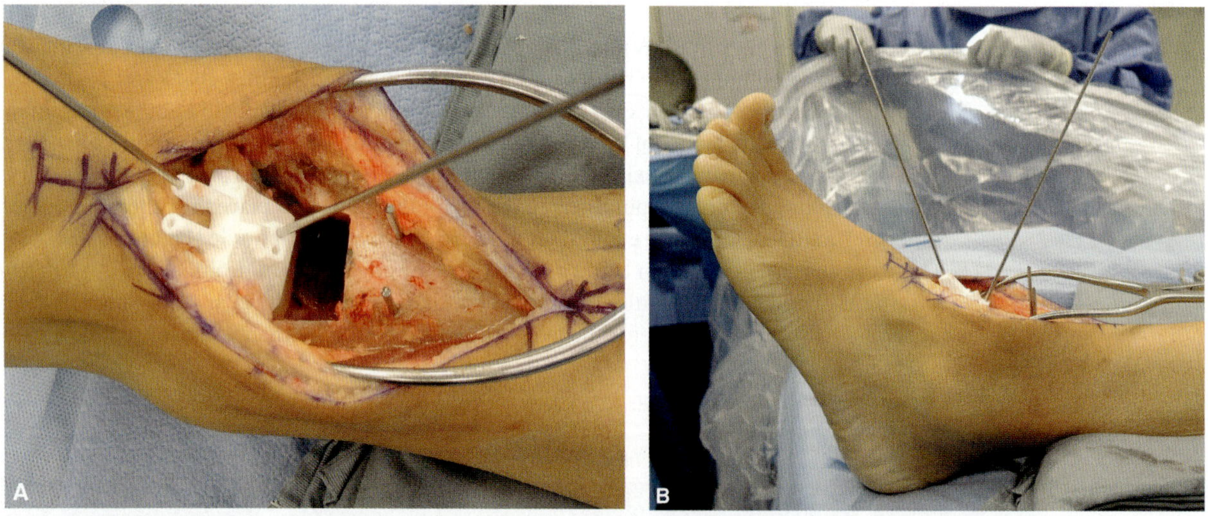

Figure 10-16. The talar guide is pinned onto the talus. View from top (A); view from the side (B).

- Secure the tibial cutting guide with two pins into the talus, and pins for the medial and lateral gutter (Figure 10-17).
- Use the appropriate oscillating bone saw to make the talar resection through the distal slot of the resection guide (Figure 10-18).
- Remove the talar cut. Check to make sure that the cut is flat and parallel to the tibial cut when holding the ankle and hindfoot in a reduced position. This is a good opportunity to remove any remaining bone from the posterior aspect of the ankle joint.
- Place the tibial tray trial over the two tibial pins into the resected joint space flush with the tibia. Ensure the trial is flush to the tibia using laminar spreaders (Figure 10-19).
- The amount of posterior overhang may be adjusted by translating the tibial trial anteriorly a maximum of 3 mm utilizing the black handle screwdriver.
- Use the intraoperative fluoroscopic image (Figure 10-20) to size the tibial component. The notch posteriorly indicates a standard tibial size, and the end of the trial indicates a size long tibial component (Figure 10-20).

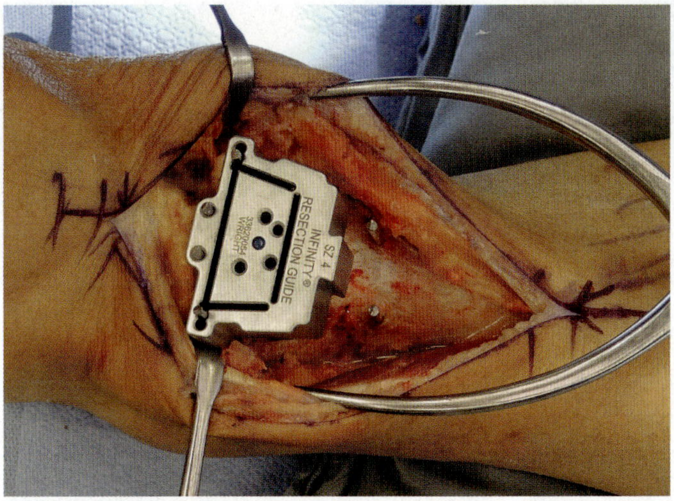

Figure 10-17. Talar cutting guide is pinned in preparation for the tibial cut.

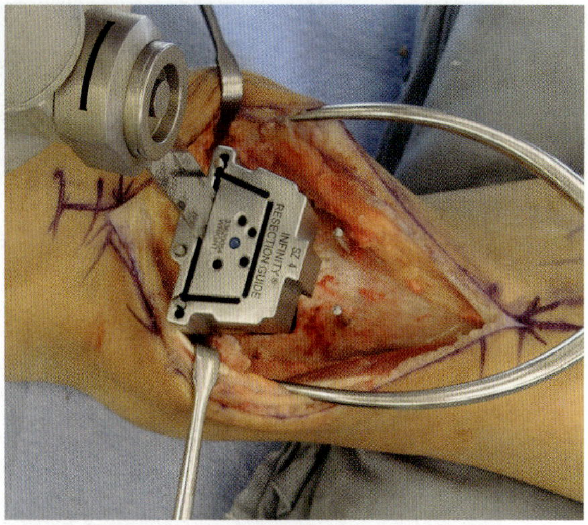

Figure 10-18. Talar cut is performed.

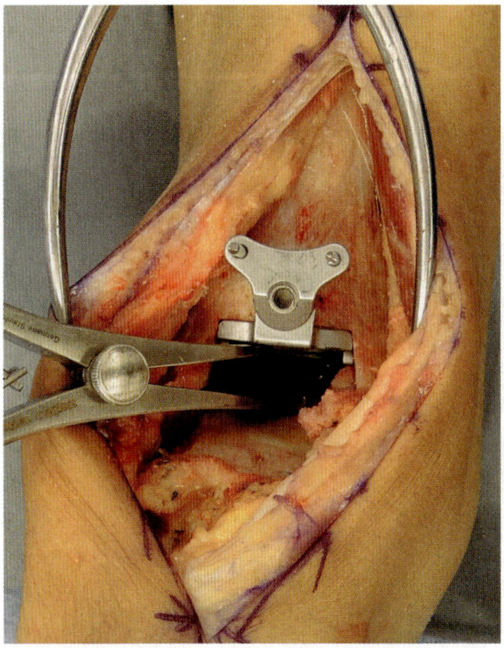

Figure 10-19. The tibial trial is secured against the tibial cut, and a laminar spreader is utilized to confirm that there is no liftoff of the trial.

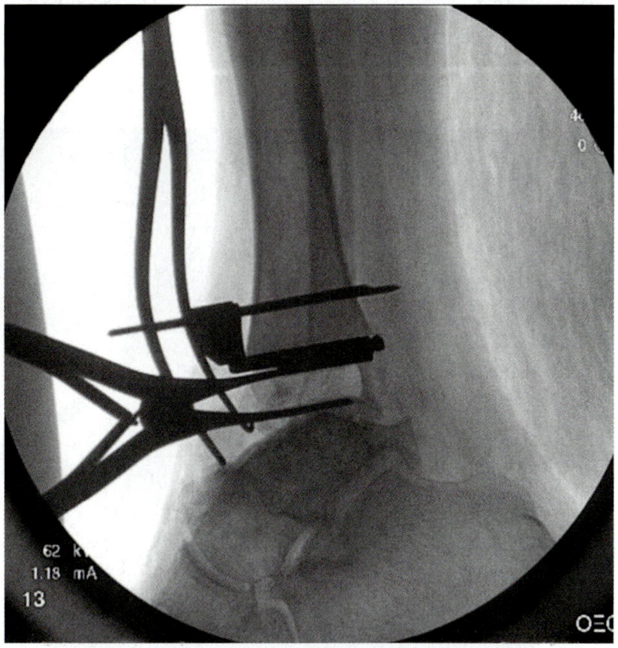

Figure 10-20. Intraoperative fluoroscopy confirms the trial is flush against the tibial cut.

- Use the broaches to prepare the tibia for the posterior and anterior pegs. The posterior peg is broached first, and the broach is left in place to secure the trial to the tibia (Figure 10-21).
- Insert a trial polyethylene insert and the talar chamfer reference guide into the ankle. A final decision on the size of the talus must be made before the anterior and posterior chamfers are performed (Figures 10-22 and 10-23).
- Take the ankle through its range of motion to allow the talar trial to achieve its correct rotation. Rotation of the talus is referenced off the rotation of the tibial component. Intraoperative fluoroscopy is utilized to confirm size, and that the referencing guide is in line with the posterior margin of the talar cut.
- The talar chamfer referencing guide is pinned and the anterior and posterior chamfer cutting guide is placed over the pins.
- Place two temporary fixation screws through the talar chamfer resection guide into the talus (Figure 10-24).

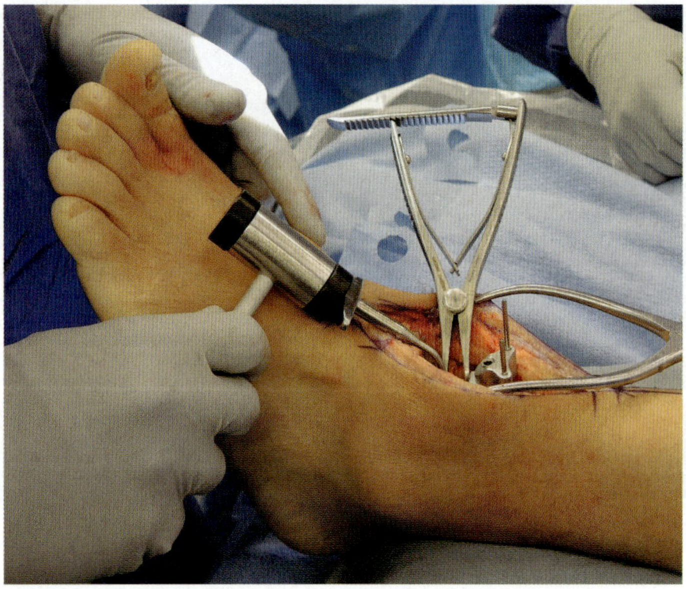

Figure 10-21. The tibia is broached for the posterior peg.

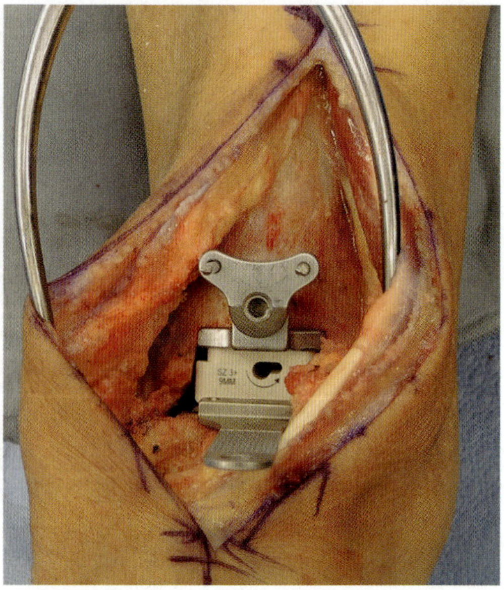

Figure 10-22. The tibial trial, polyethylene trial, and talar chamfer referencing guide are inserted into the ankle.

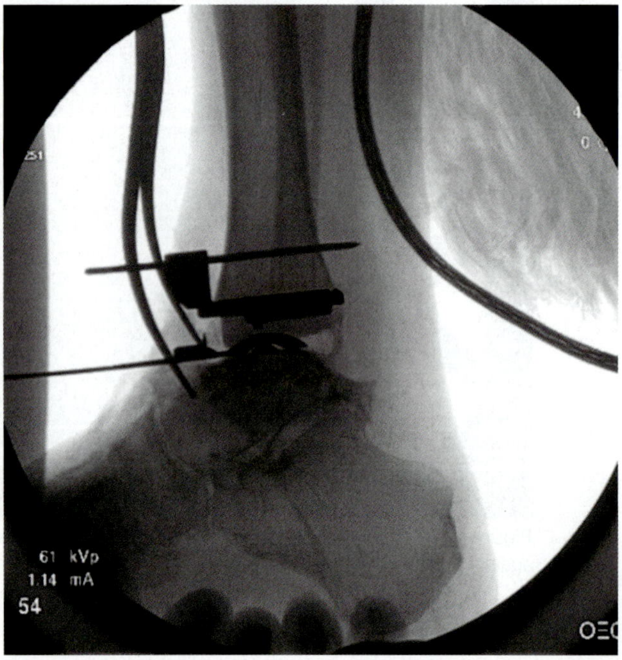

Figure 10-23. Lateral fluoroscopic view demonstrating the talar chamfer referencing guide is in line with the posterior margin of the talar cut.

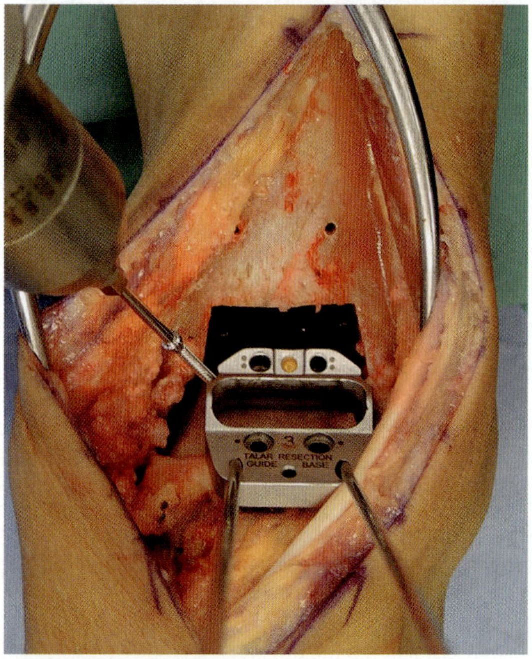

Figure 10-24. Temporary fixation screws are placed into the talar chamfer cutting guide.

- Perform the posterior talar chamfer resection through the opening in the talar resection guide base (Figure 10-25).
- After assembling the anterior talar pilot guide onto the anterior face of the talar resection guide base, ream through all four holes of the pilot guide using the talar reamer.
- Replace the pilot guide with the anterior talar finish guide and slide the talar reamer medial to lateral to finish the cut.
- Reassemble the pilot guide onto the talar resection guide base rotated 180° from the previous positioning and repeat plunge cutting the four holes and finish the cut by sliding the talar reamer guided by the finish guide (Figure 10-26).

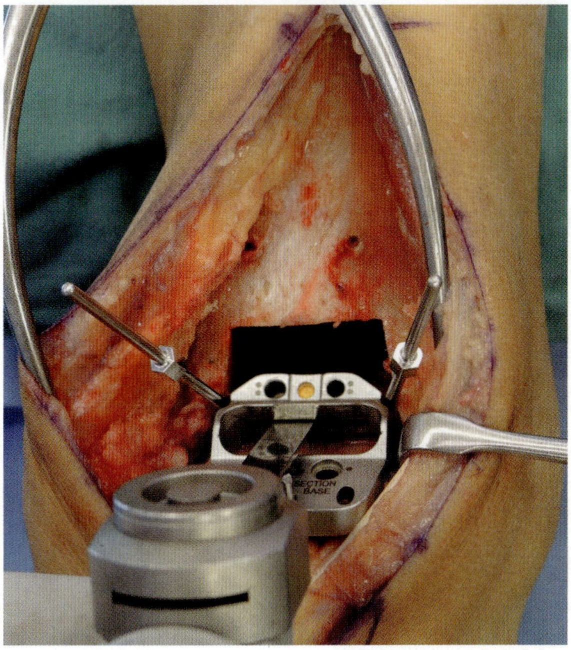

Figure 10-25. Posterior chamfer of the talus is performed.

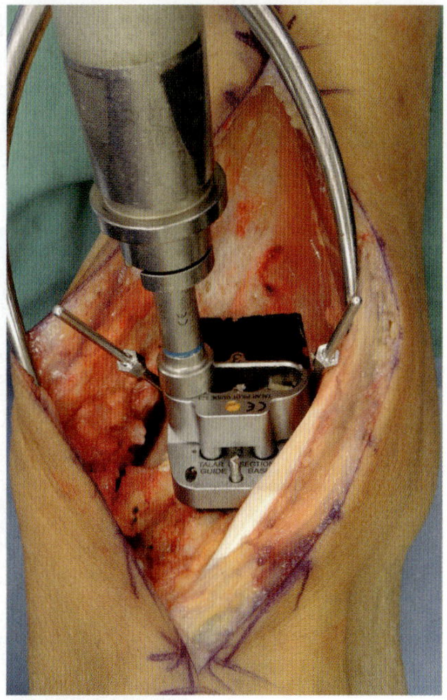

Figure 10-26. The anterior chamfer is prepared utilizing the talar reamer.

- Remove the talar chamfer cutting guide from the talar and replace it with the talar peg drill guide. Insert the tibial trial with a polyethylene trial into the ankle as well. Check, both with direct visualization and with intraoperative fluoroscopy, the medial to lateral position of the talar peg drill guide. Also, check with a lateral fluoroscopic image that the talar peg drill guide is flush against the bone.
- Using the 4-mm anterior peg drill, prepare the talus for the medial and lateral pegs (Figure 10-27).
- All trial components are removed. The ankle should be thoroughly irrigated, cleaned, and dried. Confirm that all bone has been removed from the posterior aspect of the joint. Also confirm that the medial and lateral gutters have been cleared.

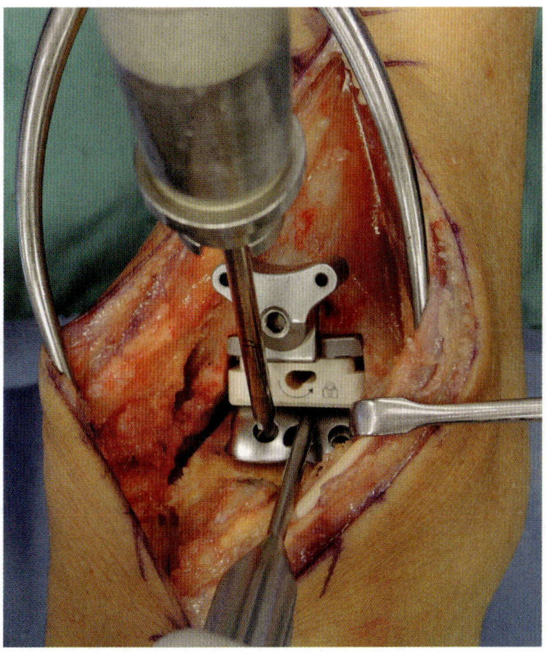

Figure 10-27. The anterior pegs for the talar component are prepared.

- The tibial component is inserted first. Line up the pegs of the tibial component with the prepared holes in the tibia. Start with the indirect impactor, and begin by impacting the tibial component posteriorly. Place gentle pressure against the handle anteriorly. Alternate impaction between the anterior and posterior slot with the indirect impactor. Final impaction can be performed with the direct tibial impactor, although great care must be taken to avoid translating the tibial component posteriorly (Figure 10-28).

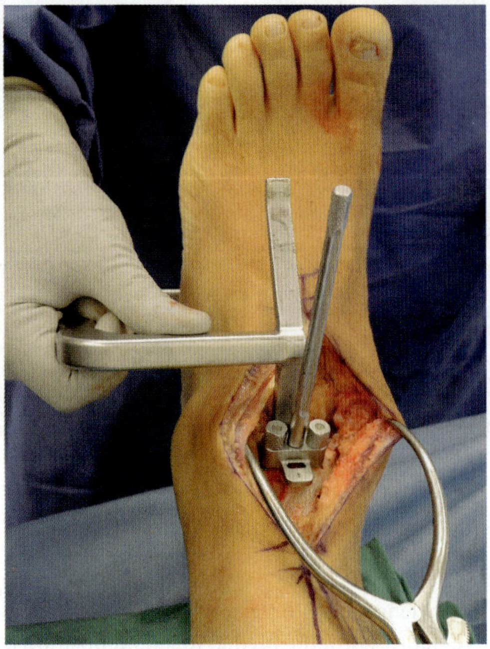

Figure 10-28. The tibial component is impacted into the tibial with the indirect impactor.

- You may insert the tibial tray protector to avoid scratching the tibial component while you prepare to insert the talus. The protector must be removed before impacting the talus into position.
- The talar component is impacted next. Align the pegs of the component with the prepared holes in the talus. Begin impaction posteriorly, and then complete impaction anteriorly (Figures 10-29 and 10-30).

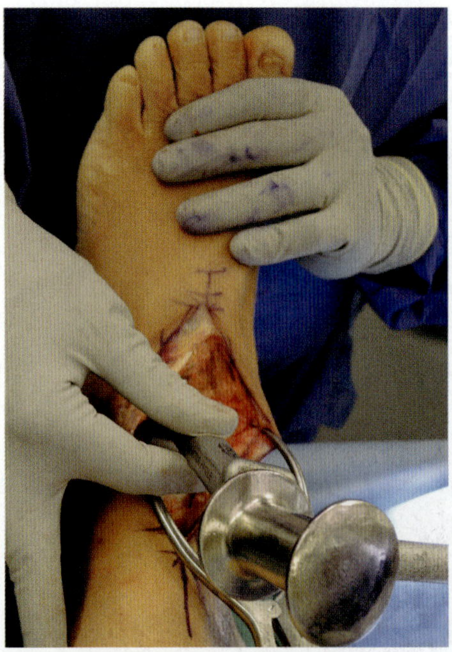

Figure 10-29. The talus is impacted into position.

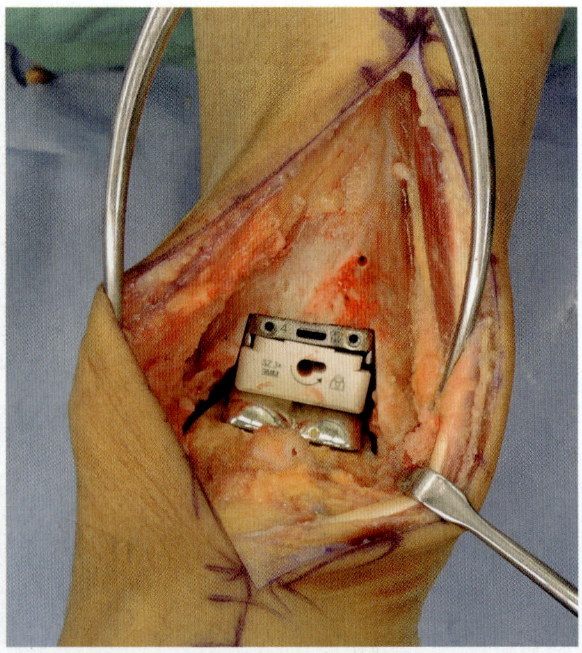

Figure 10-30. Image demonstrating the final implants positioned inside the ankle with a trial polyethylene insert.

- Assess range of motion and stability of the ankle. Perform additional procedures to balance the ligaments and provide a plantigrade, well-aligned foot. Also assess for the need for a gastrocnemius recession or tendoachilles lengthening if there is limitation on dorsiflexion.
- Assess polyethylene trials to determine the best size that will provide stability to the joint without sacrificing motion.
- Position the two posts on the tibial components, and place the polyethylene with the insert over the posts. Secure the two screws at the top of the posts. Use the inserter to place the polyethylene into the tibial component. Final impaction can be performed with the impactor. Utilize the posts to provide counterpressure to ensure that the tibial component is not translated posterior when impacting the polyethylene into position (Figure 10-31).
- Final impaction of the polyethylene insert can be performed with the direct impactor while holding counterpressure with the posts (Figures 10-32 and 10-33).

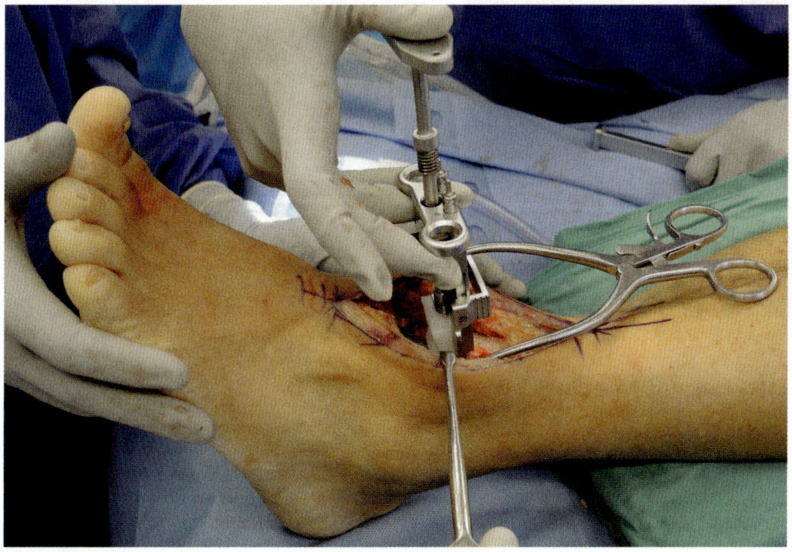

Figure 10-31. The polyethylene is inserted into the tibial component.

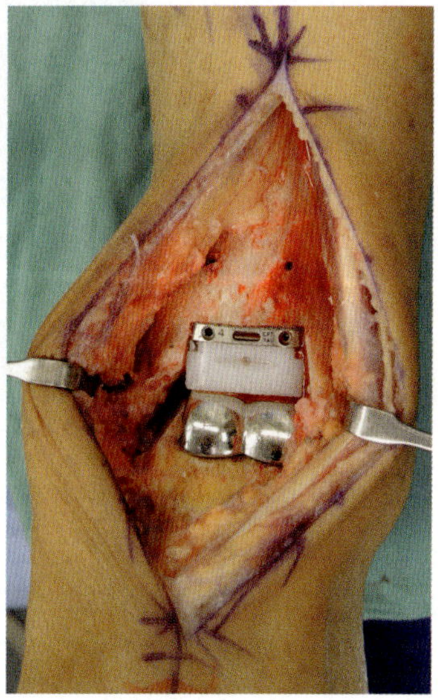

Figure 10-32. Image showing the final implants in the ankle joint.

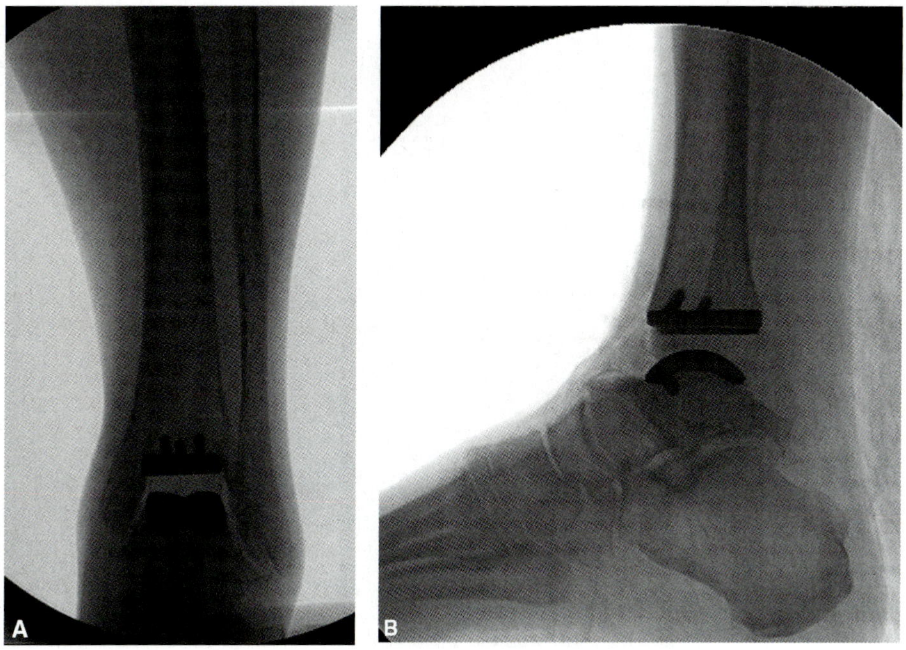

Figure 10-33. Final AP (A) and lateral (B) intraoperative fluoroscopic images demonstrating positioning of the implants.

- A 0-Vicryl is used to close the capsule (Figure 10-34).
- A drain is placed deep to the extensor retinaculum.

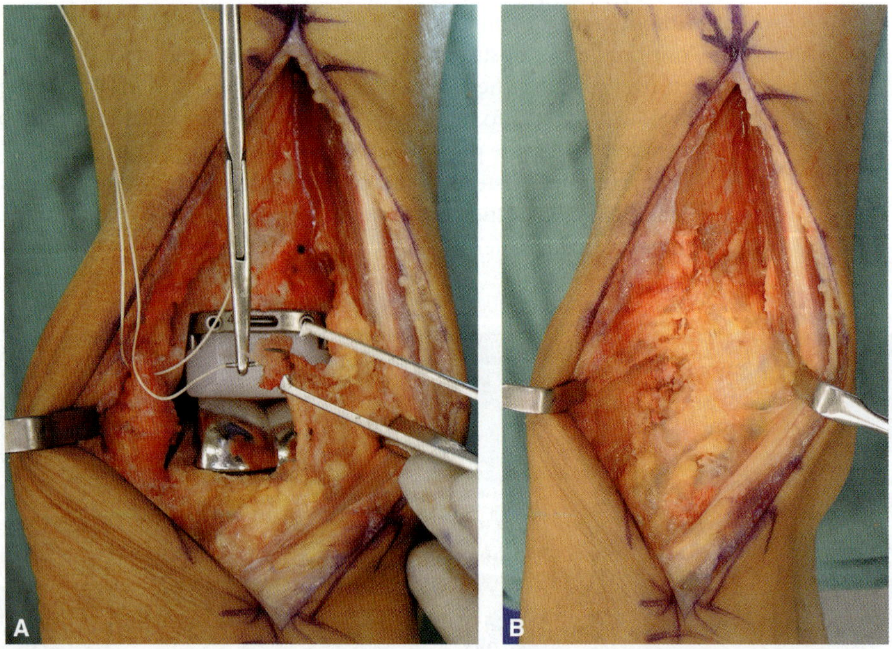

Figure 10-34. A, The capsule is closed over the implant. B, A meticulous and complete capsular closure is important for minimizing wound complications that track into the joint and provides added soft-tissue stability around the implant.

- A 2-0 Vicryl is used to close the extensor retinaculum (Figures 10-35 and 10-36).
- The subcutaneous tissue is closed with a 3-0 Vicryl suture and the skin is closed with a 3-0 nylon suture.
- Place Xeroform over the incision followed by a clean sterile dressing, followed by a well-padded posterior U-splint (Figure 10-37).

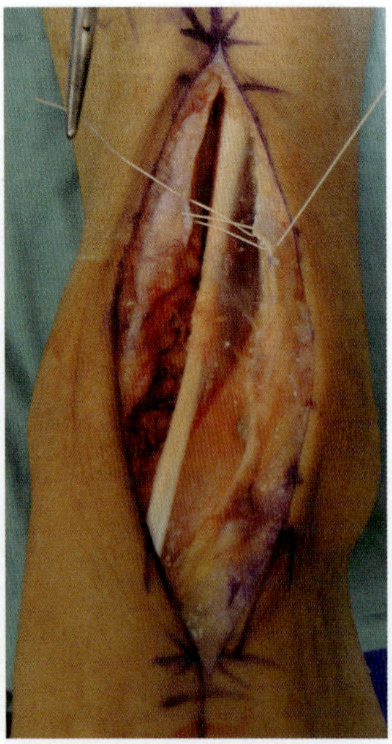

Figure 10-35. The retinaculum is closed with a 2-0 Vicryl suture.

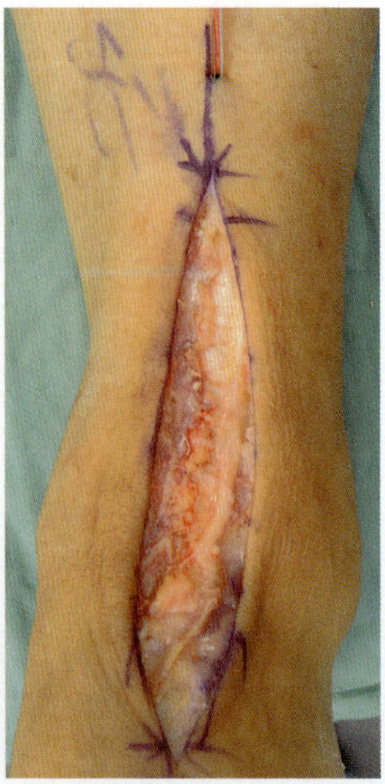

Figure 10-36. Closure of the extensor retinaculum.

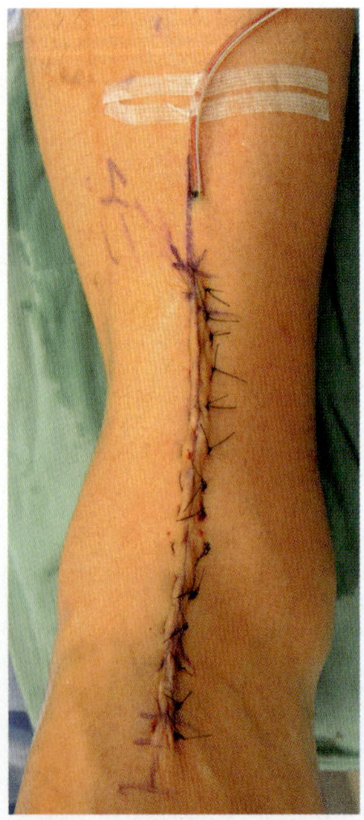

Figure 10-37. Closure of the skin.

Section 6
Tendon Disorders

Chapter 11
Hamstring Harvest and Principles of Autograft Reconstruction

SYDNEY C. KARNOVSKY
MARK C. DRAKOS

Sterile Instruments/Equipment

- Tourniquet
- Linvatec tendon stripper
- Graft Master
- 0-Vicryl, 3-0 Vicryl, 3-0 nylon sutures
- #15 blade knife
- Metzenbaum scissors
- Penrose drain
- Right-angle clamp

Positioning (Supine or Prone)

- Place the patient in a supine or prone position, depending on what position is needed for the rest of the case.
- Place a nonsterile tourniquet on the operative thigh. Prep and drape the lower extremity in a sterile manner.
- Exsanguinate the lower extremity and inflate the tourniquet 250 mm Hg.

Surgical Approach

- Perform a medial approach to the tibia. Make a 3-cm incision at the midway point between the top of the tibial tubercle and the posteromedial border of the tibia using a #15 blade knife (Figures 11-1 and 11-2).
- Use a knife and a 90° right-angle clamp to expose the site of interest and divide the sartorial fascia in line with its fibers, exposing both the gracilis and semitendinosus. This is oblique to your prior incision (Figure 11-3).
- Identify the gracilis and semitendinosus between the sartorial fascia and the superficial medial collateral ligament. They are in between layer 1 and layer 2 (Figure 11-4).
- Identify the gracilis and/or semitendinosus and then place a Penrose around each tendon (Figures 11-5 to 11-7).
- The tendon will be held in place with multiple adhesions to the medial head of the gastrocnemius.
  - Remove those adhesions using the Metzenbaum scissors.

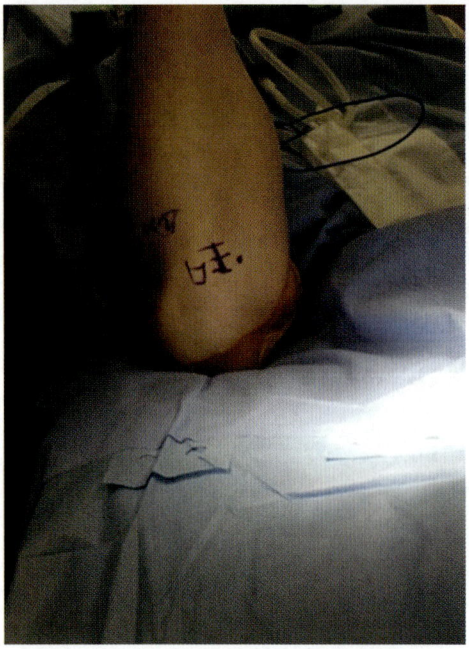

Figure 11-1. The incision will be at the dashed line, between the tibial tubercle (the box) and the posteromedial border of the tibia (the dot). The patient is in a prone position.

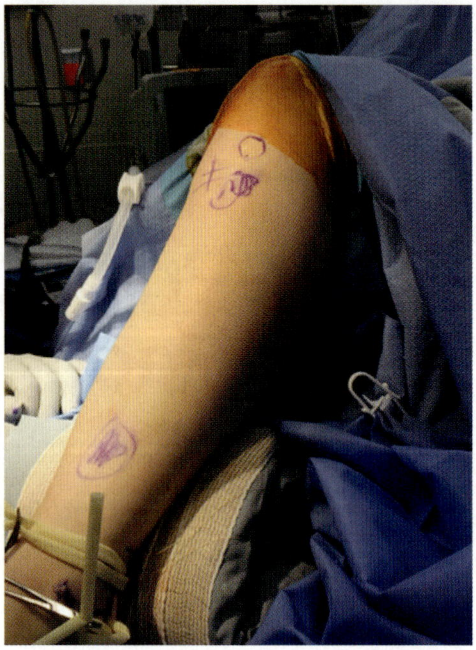

Figure 11-2. The incision will be at the dashed line, between the tibial tubercle (the circle) and the posteromedial border of the tibia. The patient is in a supine position.

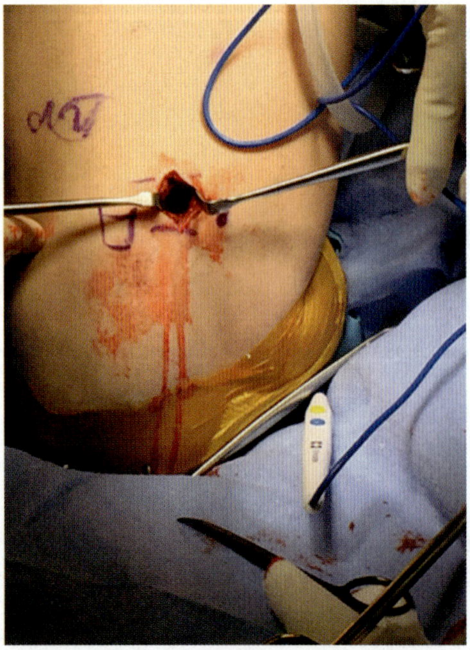

Figure 11-3. An incision is made on the superior border of the sartorial fascia (with the patient in a prone position).

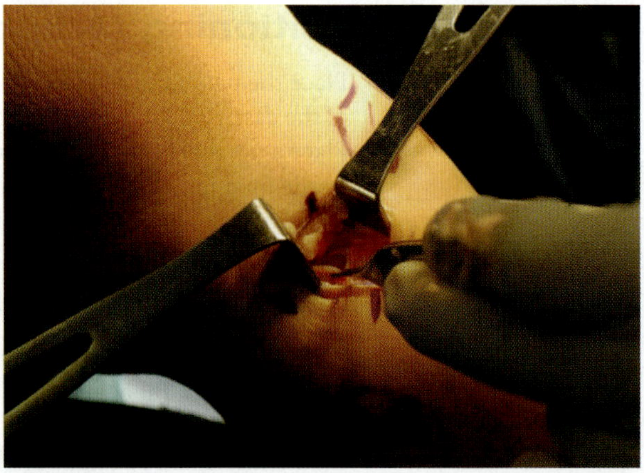

Figure 11-4. The hamstring tendons are identified between the sartorial fascia and medial collateral ligament.

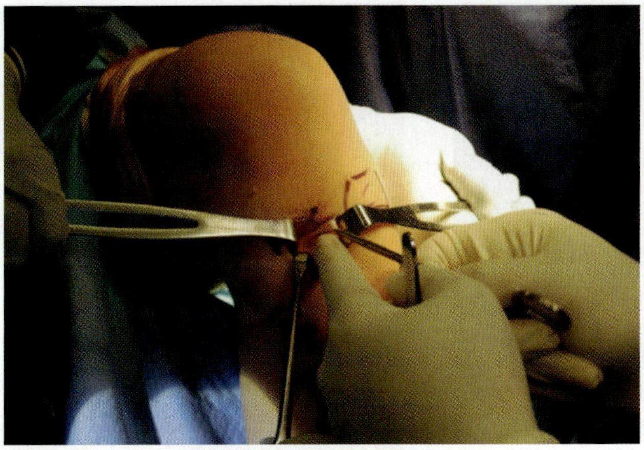

Figure 11-5. Layer 1 and layer 2 are identified (with the patient in a supine position).

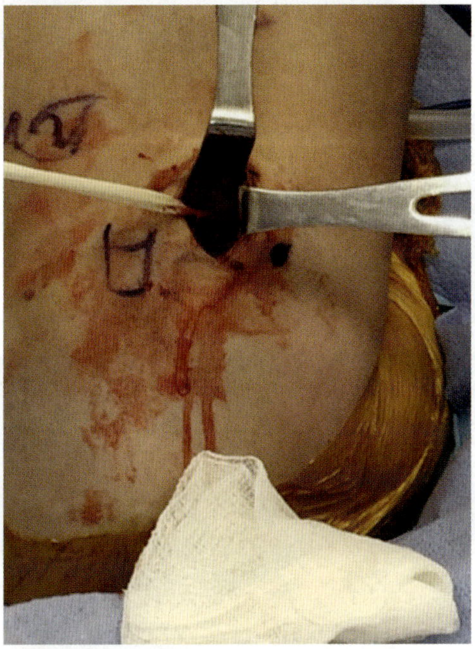

Figure 11-6. The gracilis is mobilized (with the patient in a prone position).

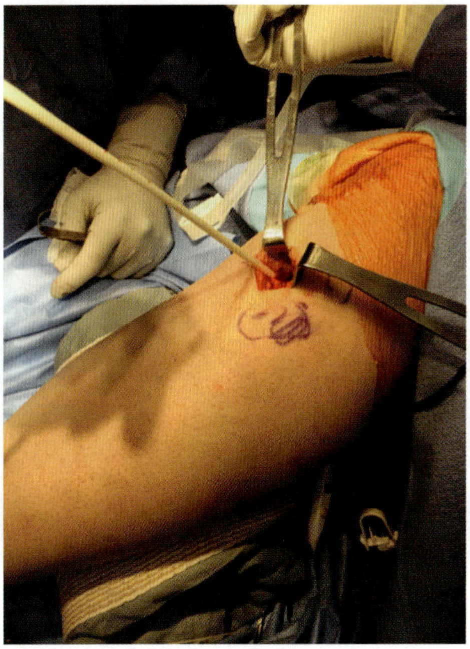

Figure 11-7. The gracilis is mobilized (with the patient in a supine position).

- Harvest both tendons using a Linvatec tendon stripper. The knee should be placed as shown in the position in Figure 11-4 to increase visualization and facilitate passage of the tendon stripper. The knee should be in a flex position as well (Figures 11-8 to 11-12).
- Bring the harvested tendon(s) to a separate table to prepare them (Figure 11-13).
  - First, remove any remnants of muscle from the tendon(s) using a ruler (Figure 11-14).
  - Attach the tendons to the Graft Master. The average gracilis will have a diameter between 3.5 and 4.3 mm and a length between 22 and 28 cm (Figure 11-15).
  - The average semitendinosus will have a diameter between 4 and 5 mm and a length between 23 and 30 cm.
  - If using only the gracilis, and the diameter is <5 mm, fold the tendon back on itself to increase the diameter. Depending on the defect the tendon will be filling, you can fold over the tendons to create a double or quadruple bundle graft.
    - Note that double bundling the graft increases diameter by 1 to 1.5 mm.

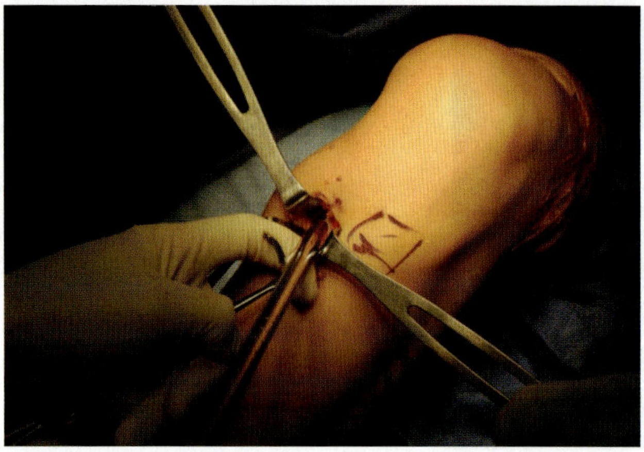

Figure 11-8. The knee is in the position as shown in Figure 11-4. The Linvatec tendon stripper is placed at the site of the incision.

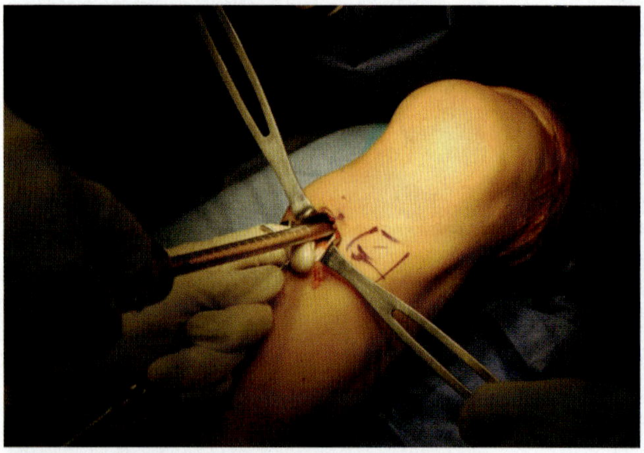

Figure 11-9. The tendon stripper is used to harvest the tendon.

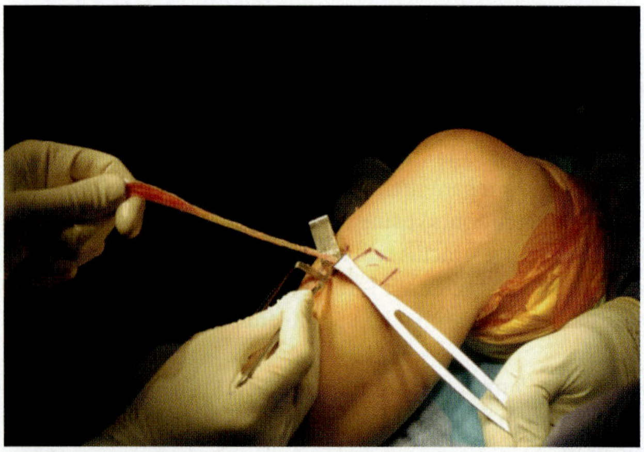

Figure 11-10. The gracilis is harvested (with the patient in a supine position). The site remains open to identify the semitendinosus.

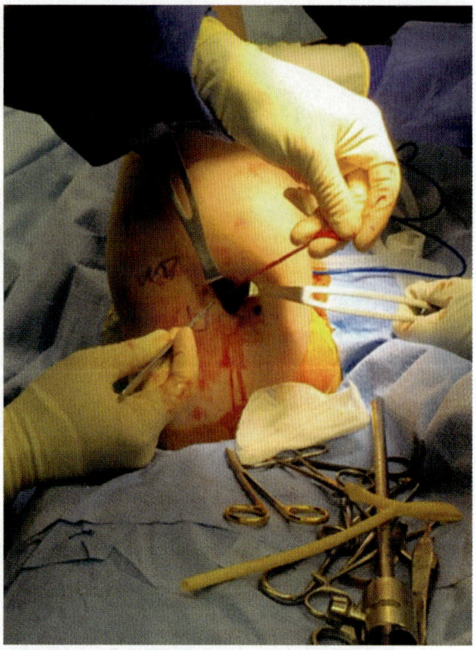

Figure 11-11. The gracilis is harvested (with the patient in a prone position).

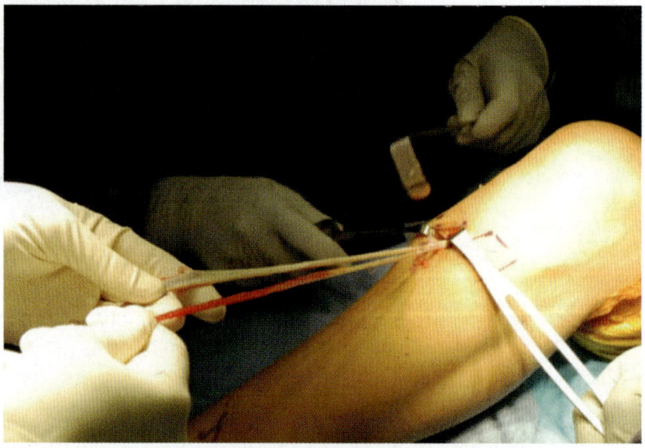

Figure 11-12. The gracilis and semitendinosus are both harvested.

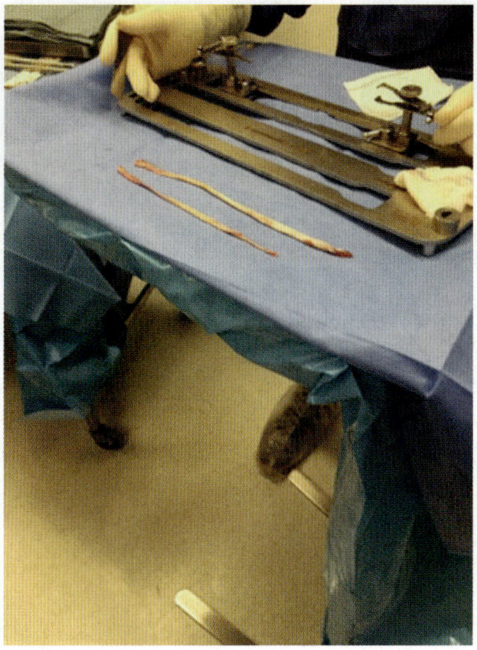

Figure 11-13. The tendons are brought to a side table to be prepared to use as an autograft.

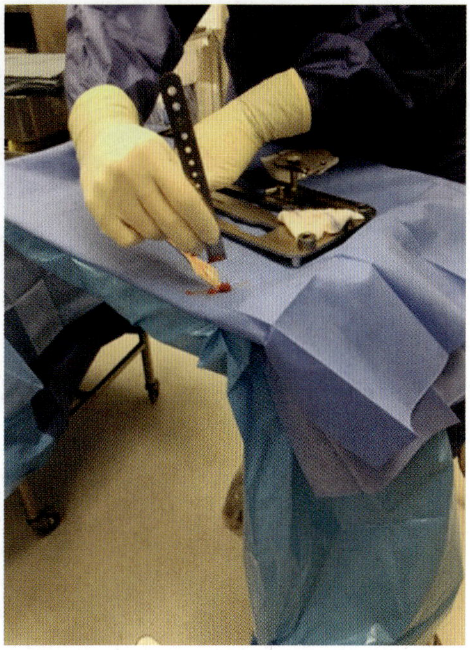

Figure 11-14. Muscle remnants are removed from the tendons using a ruler.

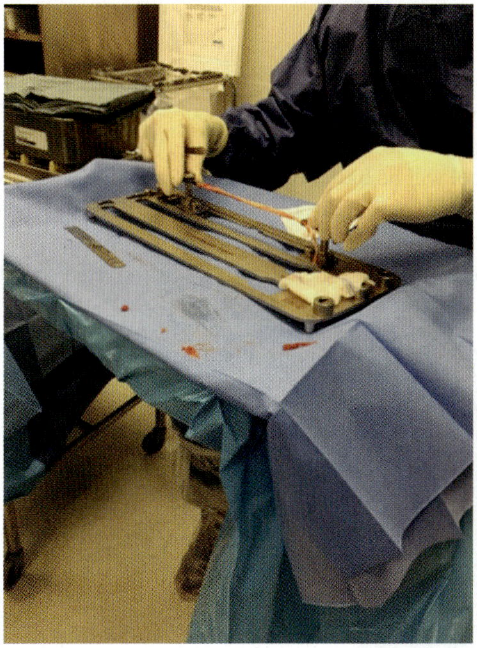

Figure 11-15. The tendons are attached to the Graft Master.

- Using a 0-Vicryl suture, tubularize the tendon(s) with a modified Krakow stitch (Figures 11-16 and 11-17).
- Measure the length and diameter of the new tendon.

Note: In a prone position, the tendons can be more difficult to feel because the tension is released with the knee flexed. To help feel the tendons, you can extend the knee to feel the superior border of the tendons and the sartorial fascia. However, the tendons should be harvested with the knee in the flexed position.

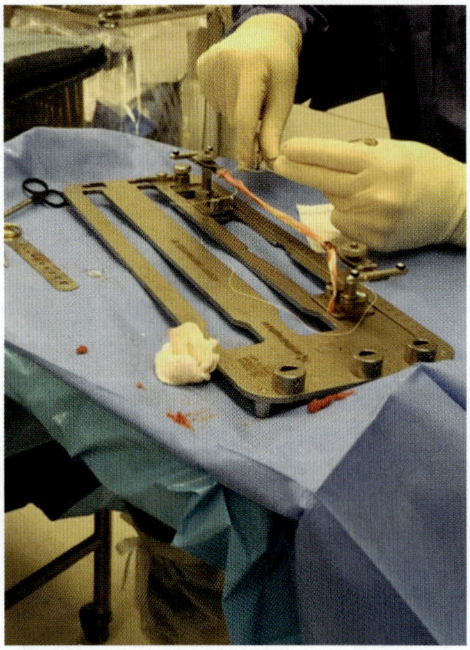

Figure 11-16. The tendons are secured to each other at the ends.

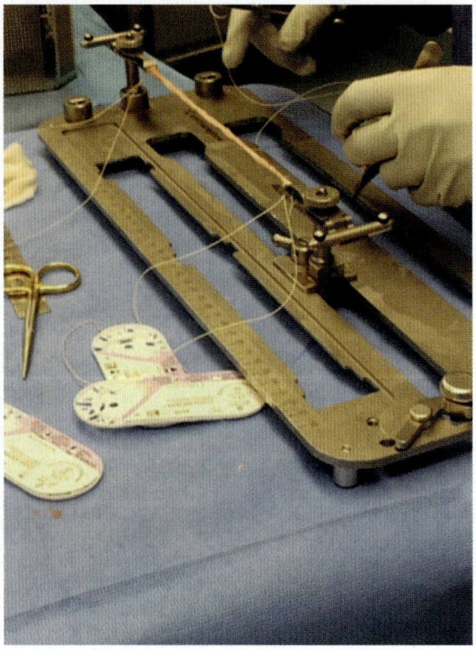

Figure 11-17. The tendons are tubularized.

Closing

- Thoroughly irrigate the wound.
- Close the sartorial fascia using a 3-0 Vicryl.
- Close the skin using a 3-0 nylon (Figure 11-18).
- Apply Steri-strips and sterile dressing to the wound.
- Often, the postoperative protocol will be based on the concomitant pathology and site of the donor tendons. The hamstring harvest part of this can be weight-bearing as tolerated post procedure, encouraging early knee range of motion to minimize stiffness.
- Other than range of motion, there is no specific rehabilitation required specifically for the knee.

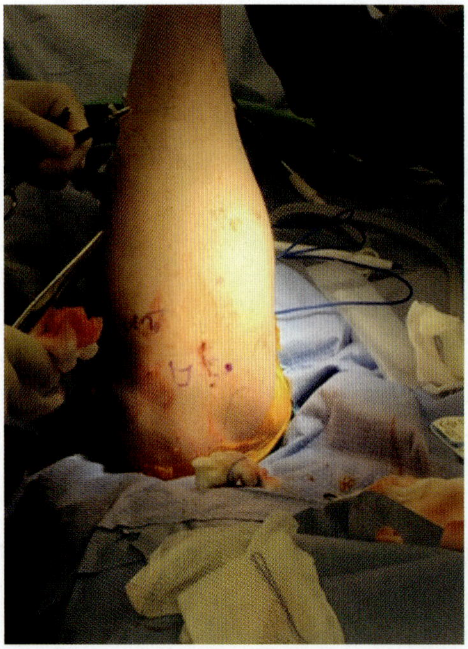

Figure 11-18. The site of incision is closed.

Chapter 12
Achilles Tendinopathy

SYDNEY C. KARNOVSKY
MARK C. DRAKOS

Sterile Instruments/Equipment

- Tourniquet
- #2 Orthocord
- 0-Vicryl, 3-0 nylon sutures
- Saw
- Oscillating rasp
- G4 anchor
- Arthrex Bio-Tenodesis screw
- Linvatec tendon stripper
- Tendon weaver

Positioning

- Place the patient in a prone position.
- Place a nonsterile tourniquet on the operative thigh. Prep and drape the lower extremity in a sterile manner.
- Exsanguinate the lower extremity and inflate the tourniquet 250 mm Hg.

Surgical Approach

- Identify the Achilles, and make an incision over the tendon (Figures 12-1 to 12-3).
  - Cheat medial to midline because of improved vascular supply.

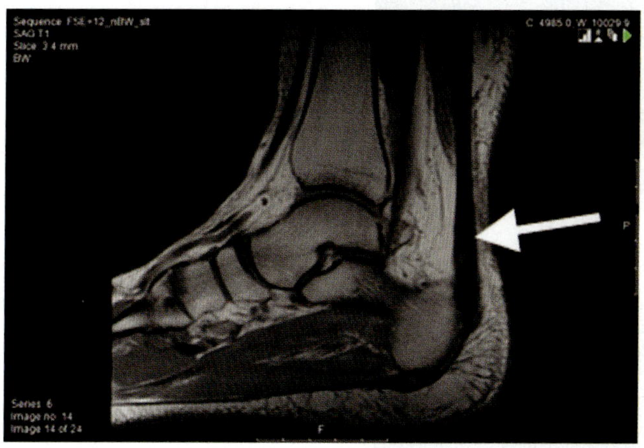

Figure 12-1. The patient's area of tendinopathy is identified on the magnetic resonance imaging (arrow indicating area of tendinopathy). This is a patient with mid-substance tendinosis.

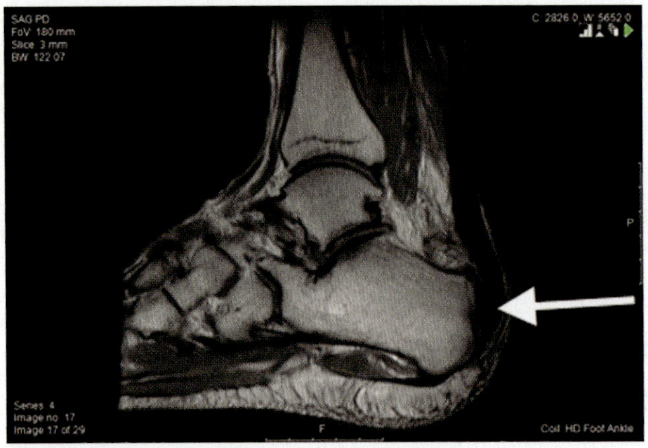

Figure 12-2. The patient's area of tendinopathy is identified on the magnetic resonance imaging (arrow indicating area of tendinopathy). This is a patient with insertional tendinosis.

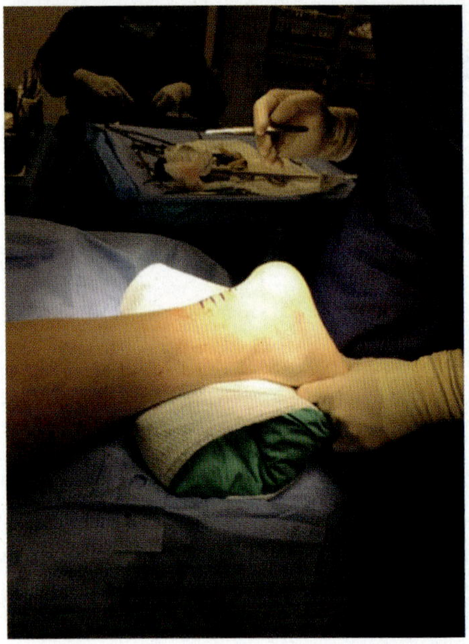

Figure 12-3. The site of the incision is identified and marked on the patient's leg in a prone position.

- Base the size and location of the incision on the degree and location (either mid-substance or insertional) of tendinosis.
  Dissect the incised area to the level of the Achilles tendon (Figure 12-4).

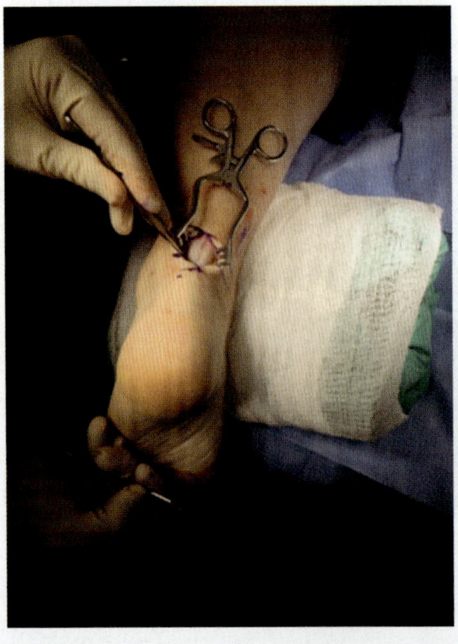

Figure 12-4. An incision is made over the Achilles tendon and the paratenon layer is incised.

- Incise the paratenon sharply in line with its fibers.
- Identify the area of tendinosis. Look for small tears, tissue integrity, and tissue quality. Determine whether any tissue looks salvageable (Figure 12-5).

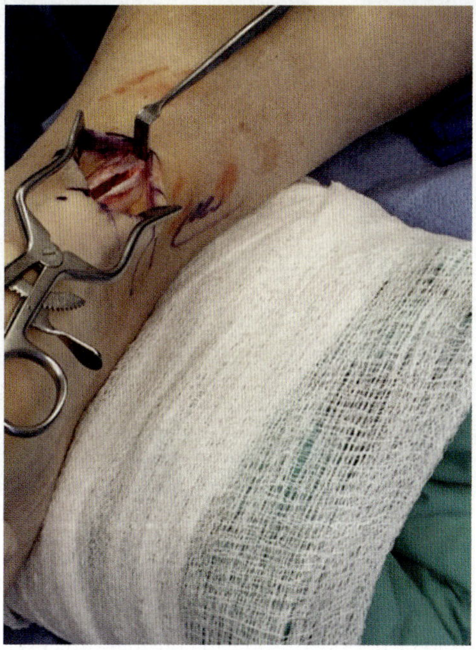

Figure 12-5. The area of tendinosis is exposed.

- Proceed to debride the area of tendinosis and remove the parts of the tendon that have significant degeneration within them (Figures 12-6 to 12-9).

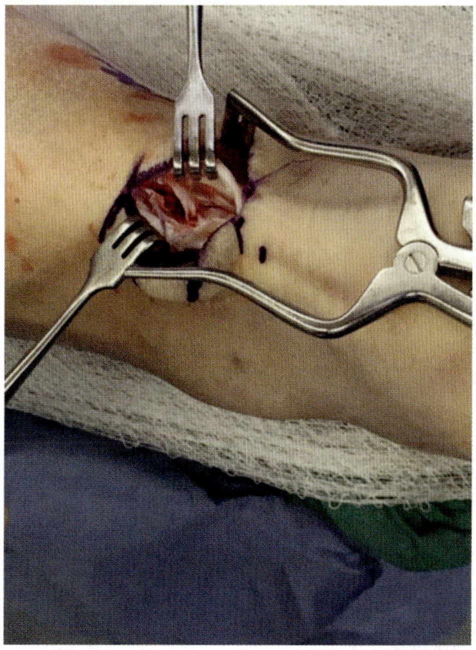

Figure 12-6. Degenerated and unhealthy tendon is removed.

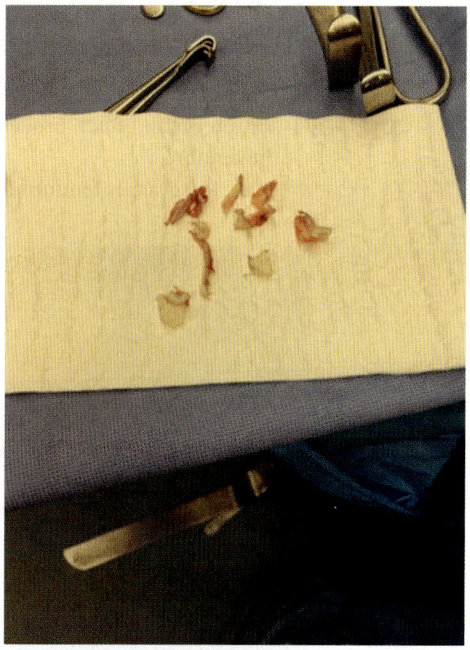

Figure 12-7. The removed tissue from a patient with mid-substance tendinopathy.

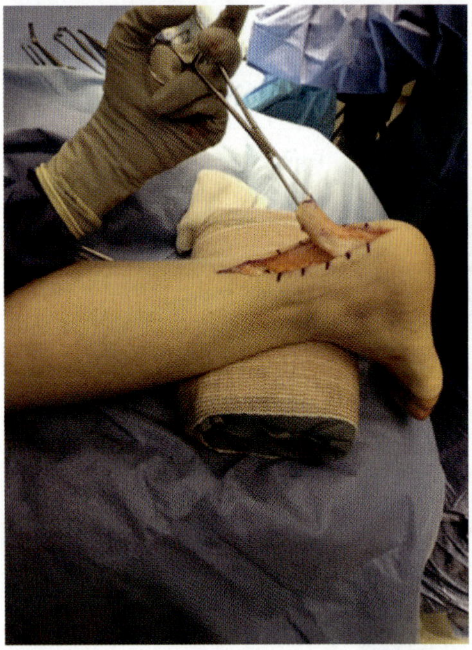

Figure 12-8. The area of tendinopathy in the stump of a tendon of a patient with insertional tendonitis.

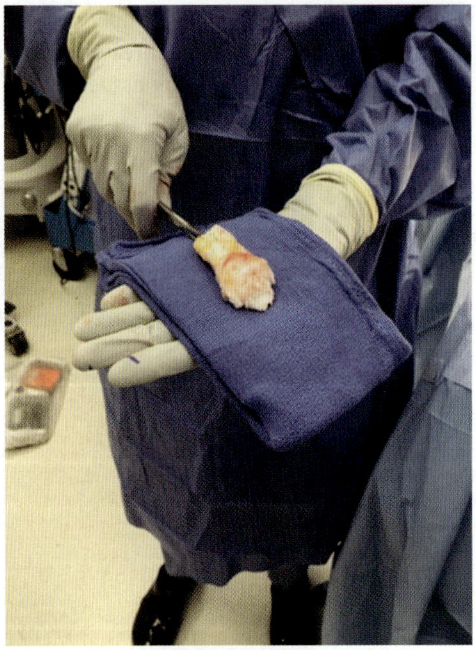

Figure 12-9. The removed tissue from a patient with insertional tendinopathy.

- Use a midline-splitting-type approach.
  - If <50% of the tissue needs to be debrided, you can consider direct repair of the remaining tendon if the tendon appears to be of good quality.
  - If >50% of the tendon is unhealthy and needs to be removed, consider augmentation with a hamstring autograft.
    - In this case, harvest a gracilis to use as an autograft (see Chapter 11).

The Repair Will Vary Depending on the Area of Tendinosis

Mid-Substance Tendinosis

- If the patient has mid-substance tendinosis and after removal of the damaged tendon the site of insertion is still intact, proceed to use a prepared hamstring autograft (see Chapter 11) to reconstruct the tendon.
- Dock the gracilis tendon in the distal Achilles stump (Figure 12-10).

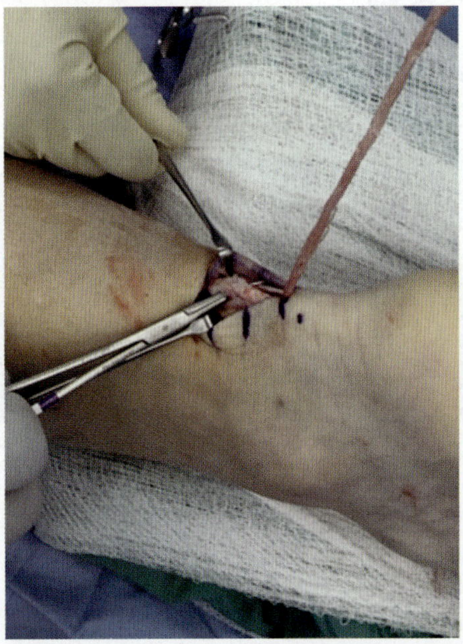

Figure 12-10. The gracilis and semitendinosus are docked into the distal Achilles stump.

- Weave it in a proximal distal manner in the defect of the Achilles. Depending on the extent of tendinosis, you will usually be able to get at least four to six passes of the gracilis (Figure 12-11).
  - Tension the new tendon with approximately 10° to 15° of plantar flexion.
- Repair the Achilles over the top with a #2 orthocord (Figure 12-12).

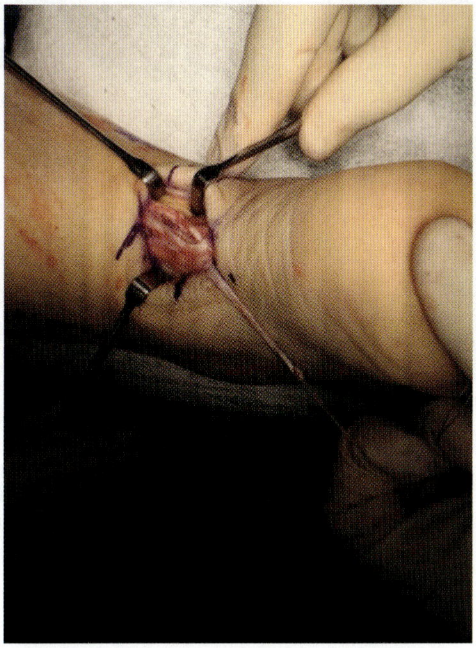

Figure 12-11. The gracilis and semitendinosus are woven up and down to reconstruct the Achilles defect.

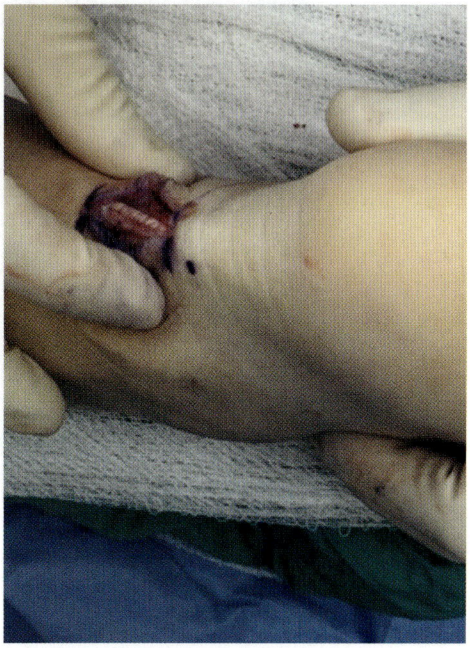

Figure 12-12. The Achilles (with the gracilis and semitendinosus graft) is repaired with #2 orthocord.

Insertional Tendinosis

- For patients with insertional tendinosis, the incision should be made on the lateral aspect of the calcaneus and Achilles insertion. The incision should be 3 to 4 cm.
- Patients with insertional tendinosis usually have a Haglund deformity, which should be removed with a saw.
- Use an oscillating rasp to contour the posterior calcaneus to make it smooth.
- Insert a G4 anchor (four sutures).
- The Achilles should be repaired using a modified Mason–Allen-type stitch. The areas of tendinosis are debrided and repaired, and the Achilles is repaired down into bone.
- If >50% of the tendon involved has extensive Achilles tendinopathy with a large insertional deficit such that the tendon would have to be detached, consider augmenting with a hamstring autograft.
  - In this case, you should use both the gracilis and semitendinosus (see Chapter 11 for harvesting these tendons).
- Drill a tunnel in the base of the calcaneus, the same diameter as the prepared hamstring autograft (usually about 6 mm) (Figure 12-13).
- Bring the graft through the tunnel (Figure 12-14).
- Fix the graft in place with an Arthrex Bio-Tenodesis screw (Figure 12-15).
  - The screw should be the same size as the tunnel or within 0.25 mm to encourage a strong bite.
- Bring the graft proximally (Figure 12-16).
- Tension it with 10° to 15° of plantar flexion (Figure 12-17).
- Use a Pulvertaft maneuver to bring the graft through the healthy proximal portion of the Achilles (Figure 12-18).

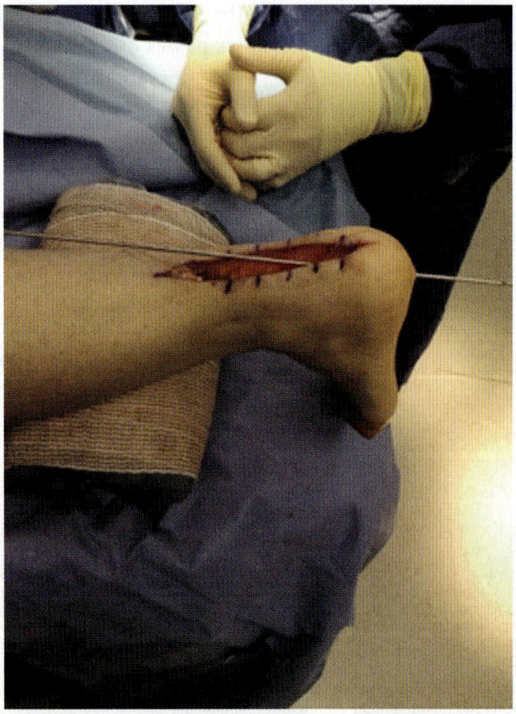

Figure 12-13. A tunnel is made in the calcaneus.

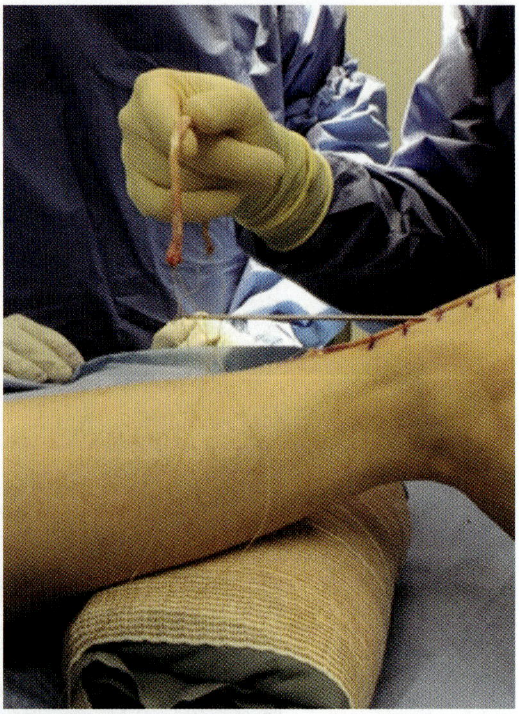

Figure 12-14. The graft is brought through the bone tunnel.

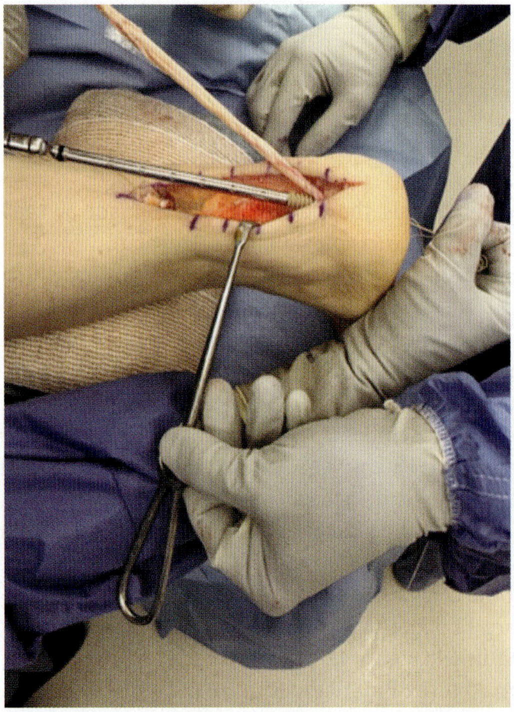

Figure 12-15. The graft is secured in place with an Arthrex Bio-Tenodesis screw.

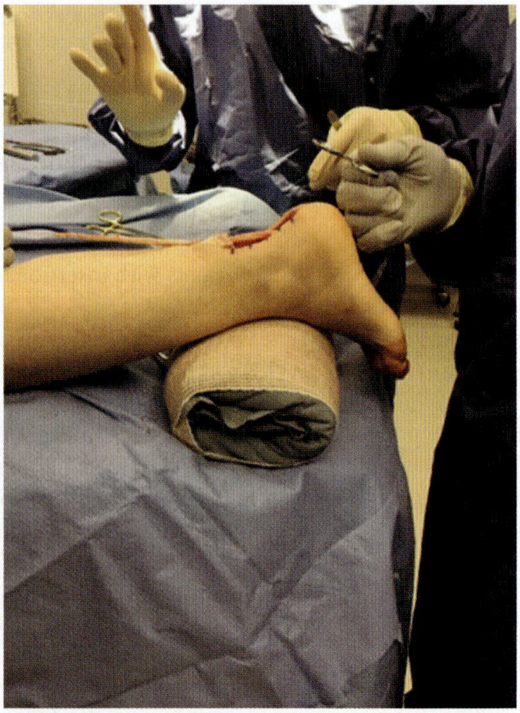

Figure 12-16. The graft is brought through the proximal Achilles stump in a Pulvertaft-type manner and then with #2 orthocord.

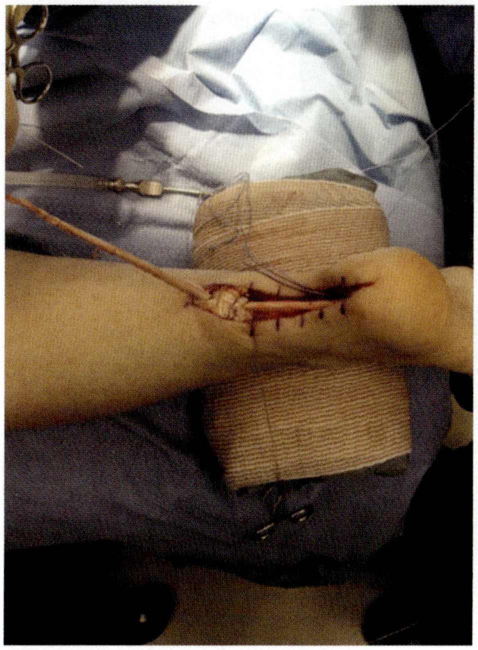

Figure 12-17. The graft is tensioned with the ankle in 10° to 15° of plantar flexion.

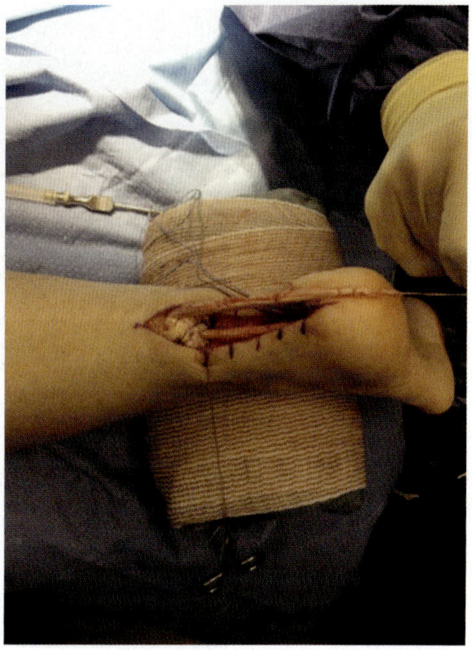

Figure 12-18. The graft is brought back through the distal Achilles insertion with an anchor or suture from the Bio-Tenodesis screw.

- Bring the graft back down and tie it to the stitches out of the Bio-Tenodesis screw and any remaining tendon distally (Figure 12-19).
- A negative Thompson test is confirmed and the patient's foot is held at neutral to confirm it can get to neutral with the grafted tendon secured in place (Figures 12-20 and 12-21).

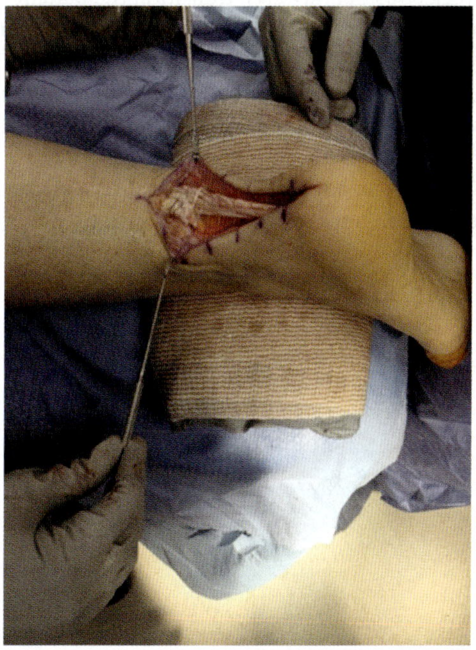

Figure 12-19. The graft is woven in a proximal distal manner and secured in place.

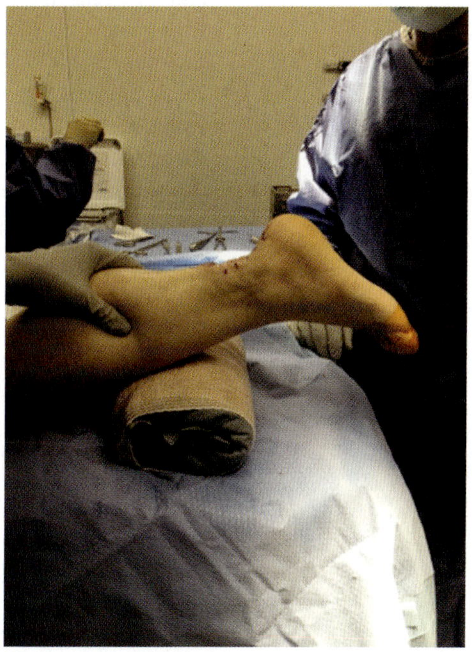

Figure 12-20. The Thompson test result is negative.

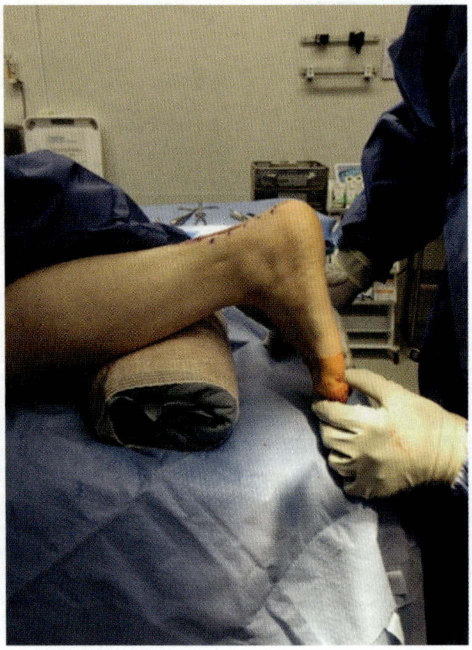

Figure 12-21. The patient's foot can be dorsiflexed to neutral.

Closing

- Thoroughly irrigate the wound with normal sterile saline solution.
- Repair the subcutaneous tissues with a 0-Vicryl.
- Close the skin using a 3-0 nylon.
- Apply Steri-strips and sterile dressing to the wound.
- Place the patient in a non-weight-bearing splint for 2 weeks.
- After the split is removed, transition the patient to a cast and have the patient remain non-weight-bearing for 2 more weeks.
- After 2 weeks in a cast (4 weeks postoperatively), transition the patient into a CAM walker boot with a heel lift and allow partial weight-bearing with active range of motion with dorsiflexion to neutral.
- Begin physical therapy at 6 weeks postoperatively and progress from partial to full weight-bearing. Allow the patient to start with 50 lb and advance 25 to 50 lb per week, as guided by the physical therapist.
- Transition to sneakers at 3 months postoperatively and continue physical therapy.
- By 6 months postoperatively, patients should be able to return to most, if not all, activities.

Chapter 13
Acute Achilles Rupture

SYDNEY C. KARNOVSKY
MARK C. DRAKOS

Sterile Instruments/Equipment

- Tourniquet
- #2 Orthocord
- 0-Vicryl, 3-0 nylon sutures
- PARS device
- Periosteal elevator
- Tissue weaver

Positioning

- Place the patient in a prone position.
- Place a nonsterile tourniquet on the operative thigh. Prep and drape the lower extremity in a sterile manner.
- Exsanguinate the lower extremity and inflate the tourniquet 250 mm Hg.

Surgical Approach

- Identify the Achilles, and make an incision over the tendon (Figure 13-1).
  - Cheat medial to midline because of improved vascular supply.

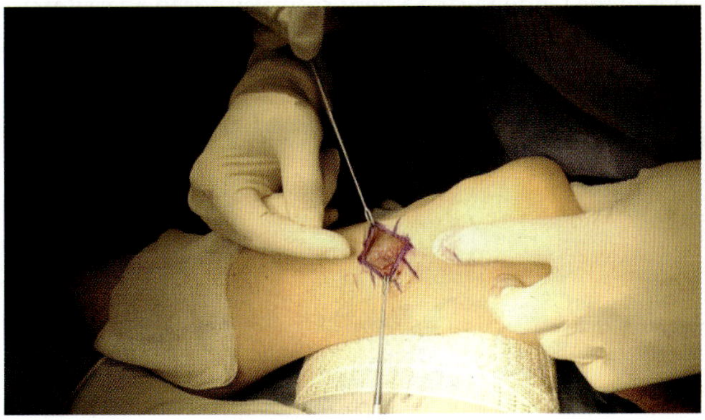

Figure 13-1. The incision over the Achilles tendon has been made, exposing the paratenon.

- Base the size and location of the incision on the location of the rupture.
  - Try to keep incision 2.5 to 3.5 cm or less. Cheat on the higher side of the tear. The inferior Achilles can be delivered into the wound with ankle plantar flexion. If you have a magnetic resonance imaging report to establish the distance of the tear from the Achilles insertion in the calcaneus, this can be helpful for planning. Otherwise, feel for the palpable defect.
- Incise the paratenon sharply in line with its fibers. Evacuate hematoma.
- Dissect the incised area to the level of the Achilles tendon.
- Identify the area of rupture. Identify whether there is associated tendinopathy—look for small tears, tissue integrity, and tissue quality (Figure 13-2).

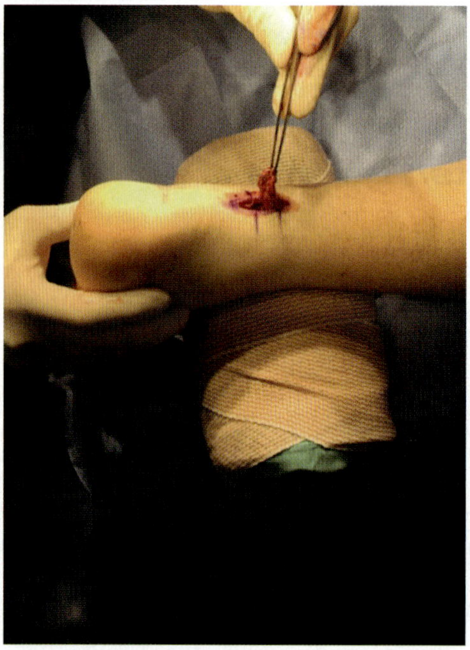

Figure 13-2. The ruptured tendon is identified.

- If there is no degeneration and only an acute rupture, repair the tendon without the use of an additional tendon graft.
  - Mobilize the ends of the tendon using a periosteal elevator to release any adhesions (Figure 13-3).

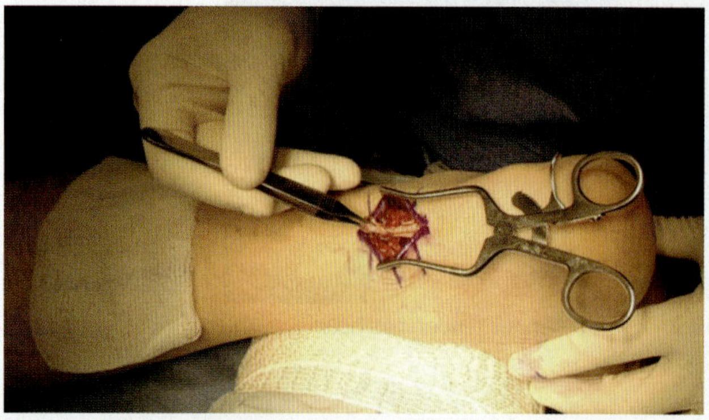

Figure 13-3. The ends of the tendon are mobilized.

- Use a #2 orthocord in a modified Krackow manner to create medial and lateral limbs in the proximal and distal aspect of the tear (Figure 13-4).
  - You can use a PARS device (Arthrex). Using it proximally is not recommended because of the proximity of the sural nerve. However, distally there is usually enough distance between the Achilles and sural nerves, where iatrogenic injury to the nerve is usually less likely. However, if you can mobilize the distal Achilles and get adequate bites of tissue with a Krakow suture, you can eliminate this step (Figure 13-5).
  - If plantaris is present, you can harvest this and incorporate it in the graft (Figure 13-6).

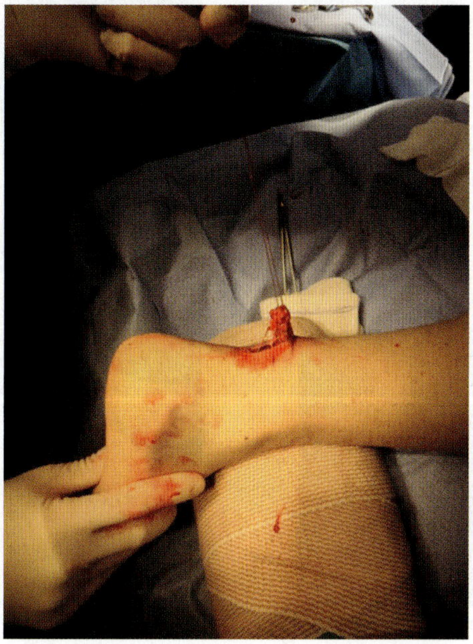

Figure 13-4. A #2 orthocord is used in a modified Krackow manner to repair the medial and lateral limbs of the proximal and distal tear.

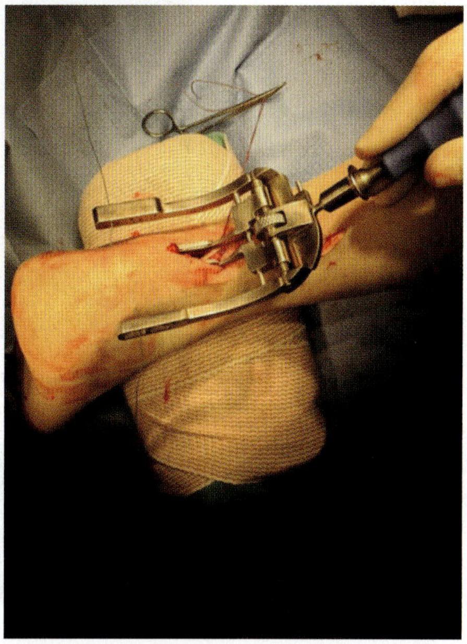

Figure 13-5. A PARS device is used, and the distal tendon is tagged percutaneously.

- Release the posterior compartment of the fascia to take the pressure off of the skin, repair the peritenon superficially, and bring the flexor hallucis longus muscle belly blood supply to the Achilles.
- Place the ankle in maximum plantar flexion and tie down the Krackow sutures (Figures 13-7 and 13-8).

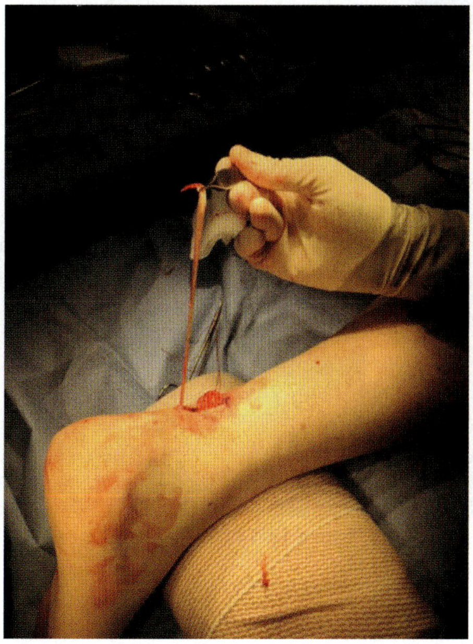

Figure 13-6. The plantaris is harvested, if present.

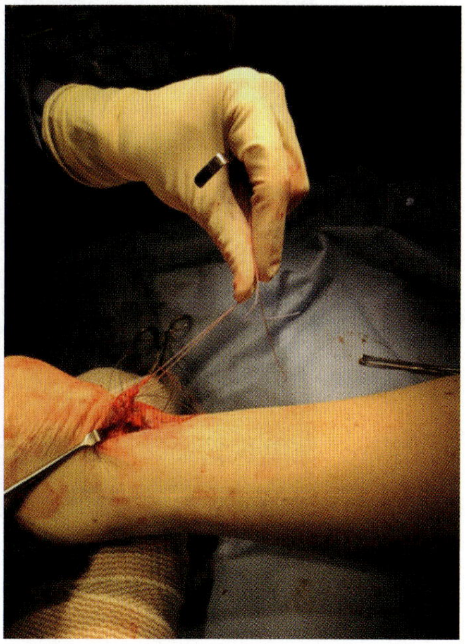

Figure 13-7. The ankle is placed at maximal plantar flexion, and the Krackow sutures are prepared to be tied down.

- Place a modified Bunnell stitch in the distal aspect of the tendon, exiting proximally to further tighter the repair. This should be a #2 orthocord. Ultimately, tendon repair strength is proportional to the number of strands crossing the tear site. Use six half-strands, in this case crossing the repair site to allow for early mobilization (Figures 13-9 to 13-12).

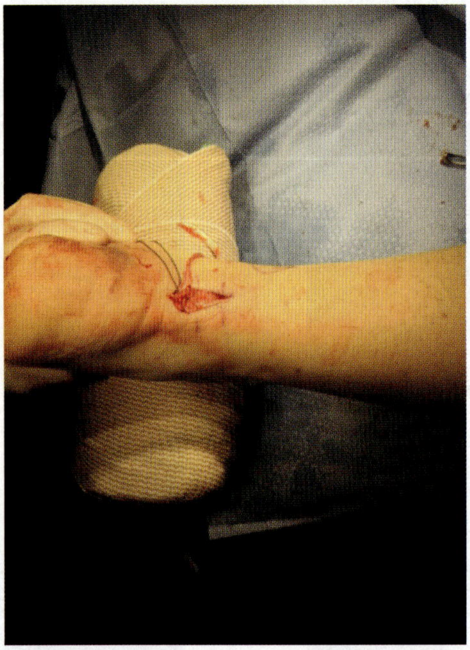

Figure 13-8. The Krackow sutures are tied down.

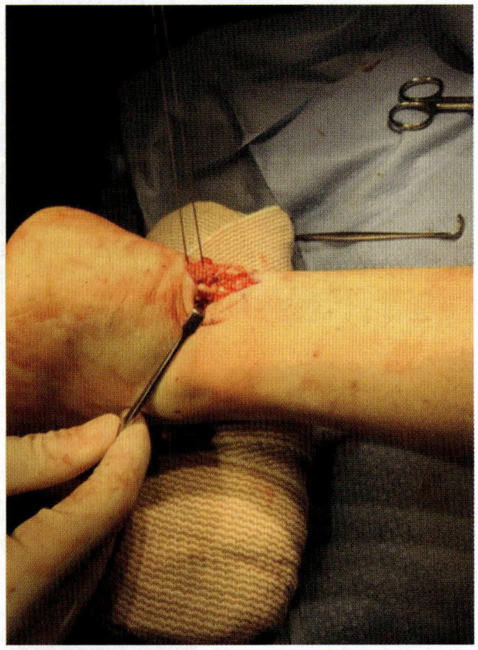

Figure 13-9. A modified Bunnell stitch is placed in the distal aspect of the tendon.

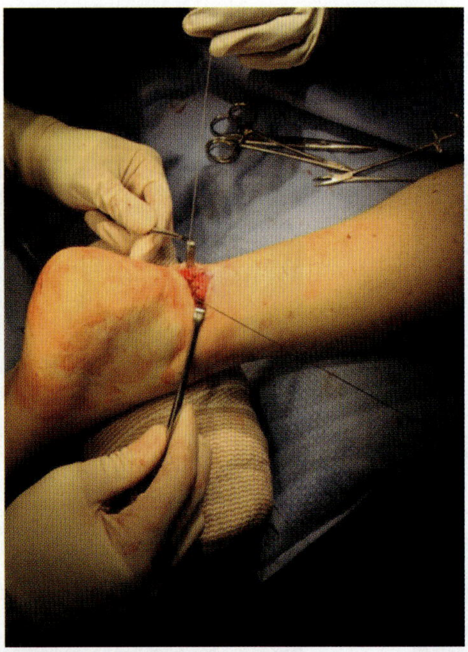

Figure 13-10. A modified Bunnell stitch is used to cross the repair site.

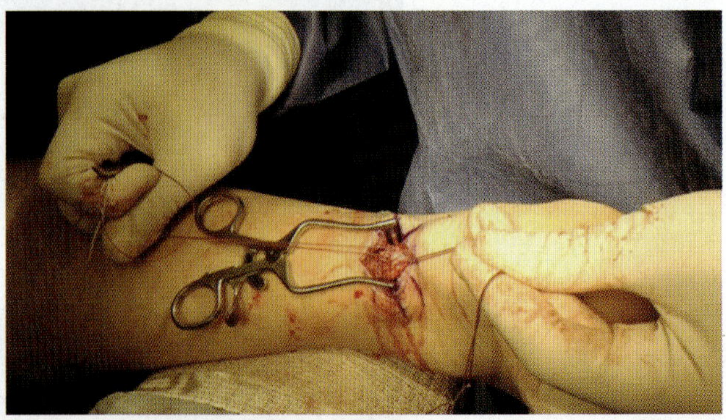

Figure 13-11. A modified Bunnell stitch is used.

- Confirm that tension on the tendon is good and that the Thompson test result is negative.
- Tie down the sutures (Figures 13-13 and 13-14).

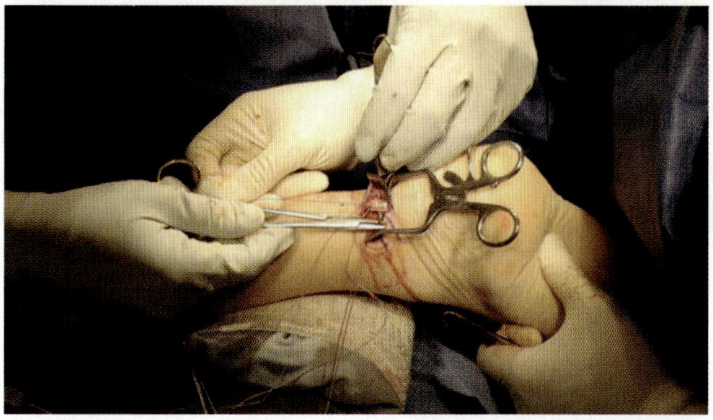

Figure 13-12. A modified Bunnell stitch is brought across the repair site.

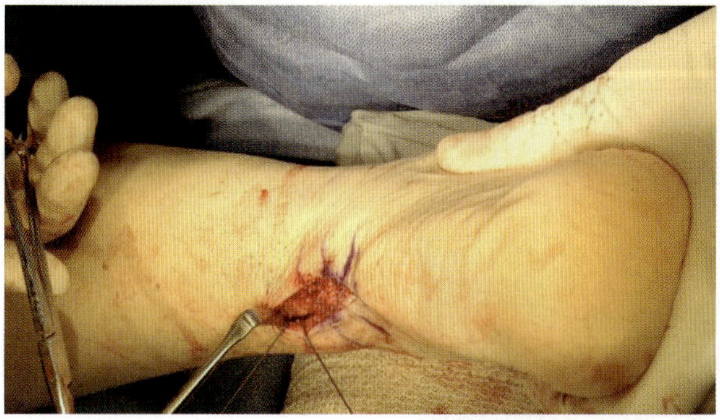

Figure 13-13. The modified Bunnell stitch is tied down.

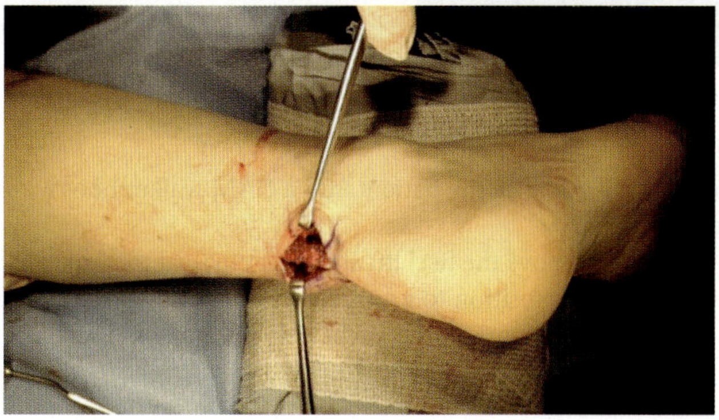

Figure 13-14. The Achilles is now repaired.

Closing

- Thoroughly irrigate the wound with normal sterile saline solution.
- Repair the subcutaneous tissues with a 0-Vicryl (Figure 13-15).
- Close the skin using a 3-0 nylon (Figure 13-16).
- Apply Steri-strips and sterile dressing to the wound.
- Place the patient in a non-weight-bearing splint for 2 weeks.

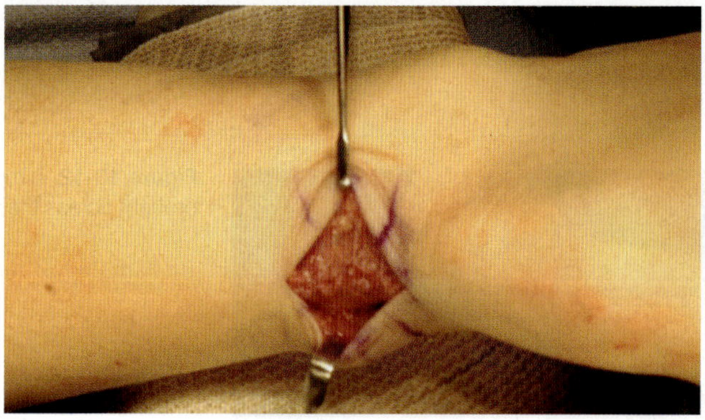

Figure 13-15. The paratenon is repaired.

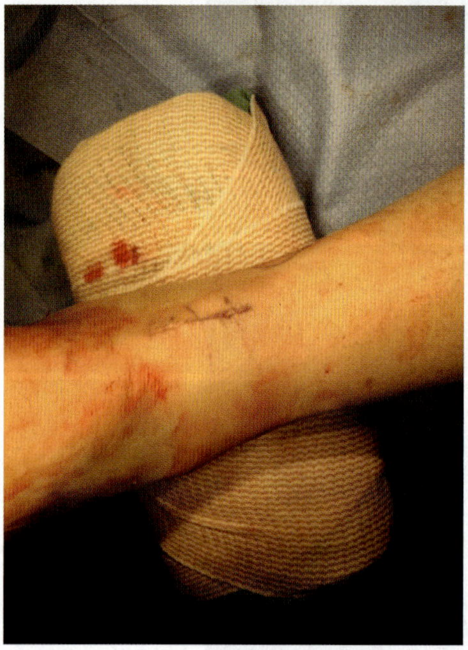

Figure 13-16. The skin is closed.

- At 2 weeks postoperatively, advance the patient into a CAM walker boot with a heel lift and allow partial weight-bearing.
- At 6 weeks postoperatively, remove the heel lift and start physical therapy (in the CAM walker boot).
- At 3 months postoperatively, transition to a sneaker and continue physical therapy.
- At 6 months postoperatively, the patient should be able to return to most, if not all, activities.

Chapter 14
Peroneal Tendinopathy

SYDNEY C. KARNOVSKY
MARK C. DRAKOS

Sterile Instruments/Equipment

- Tourniquet
- #2 orthocord
- 3-0 Vicryl, 3-0 nylon, 0-Vicryl sutures
- Linvatec tendon stripper available
- Bump
- 2-0 drill
- 3-0 Ethibond
- 4-0 burr available
- Rongeur
- G2 anchor

Positioning

- Place the patient in a supine position. Position a large bump under the hip to create a sloppy lateral-type position.
- Place a nonsterile tourniquet on the operative thigh. Prep and drape the lower extremity in a sterile manner.
- Exsanguinate the lower extremity and inflate the tourniquet 250 mm Hg.

Surgical Approach

- Identify the fibula just posterior to bone (Figure 14-1).
- Make a 6-cm incision on the lateral aspect of the patient's fibula.

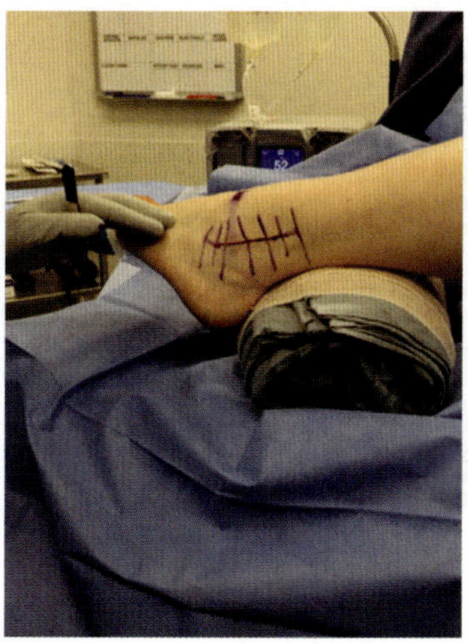

Figure 14-1. The site of the incision is identified and marked on the patient's ankle.

- Incise the peroneal retinaculum. Take care to avoid injury to the sural nerve, which is posterior to the peroneals at this level (Figures 14-2 and 14-3).
- Identify the area of tendinopathy and determine whether there is any dislocation.

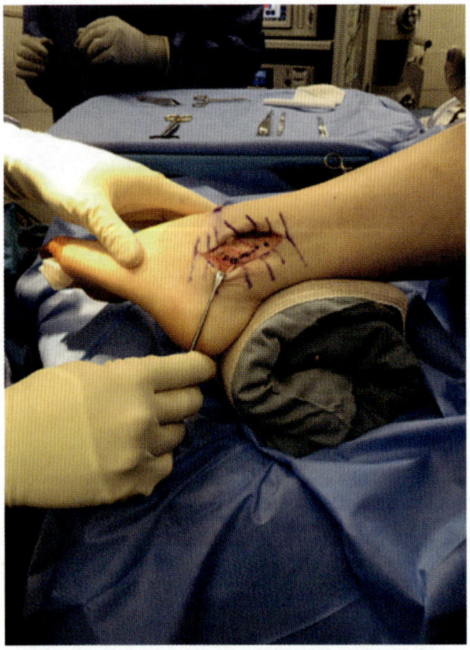

Figure 14-2. The peroneal retinaculum is identified.

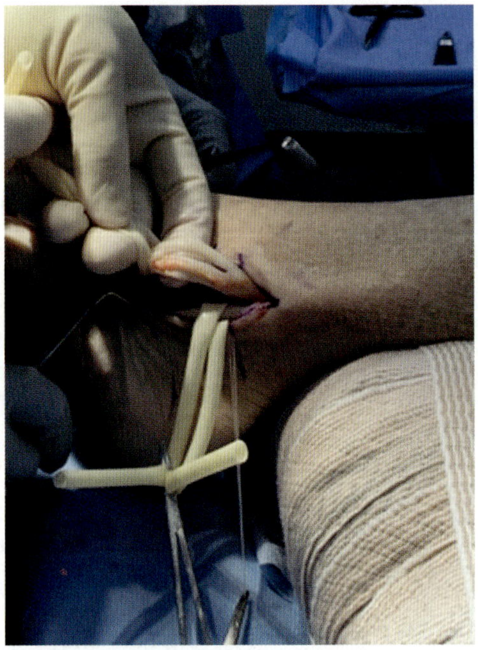

Figure 14-3. The peroneal tendons are identified, and the retinaculum is tagged.

- Determine whether there is any damage to the superior peroneal retinaculum. You should be looking for longitudinal split tears, areas of thickening and tendinopathy, low-lying peroneus brevis muscle belly, and peroneus quartus (Figures 14-4 to 14-6).
- Determine whether the peroneus brevis or longus is damaged and/or torn (Figures 14-7 and 14-8).
- Debride the area of the tendon that is torn. If <50% is torn, debride and tubularize the remaining tendon (Figure 14-9).
    - Remove the tenosynovium. This decompresses the retrofibular space and any low-lying muscle belly and the peroneus quartus.

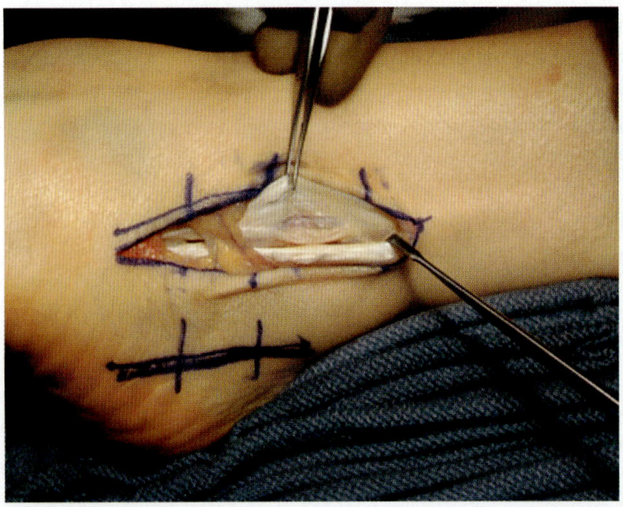

Figure 14-4. Tenosynovitis is removed.

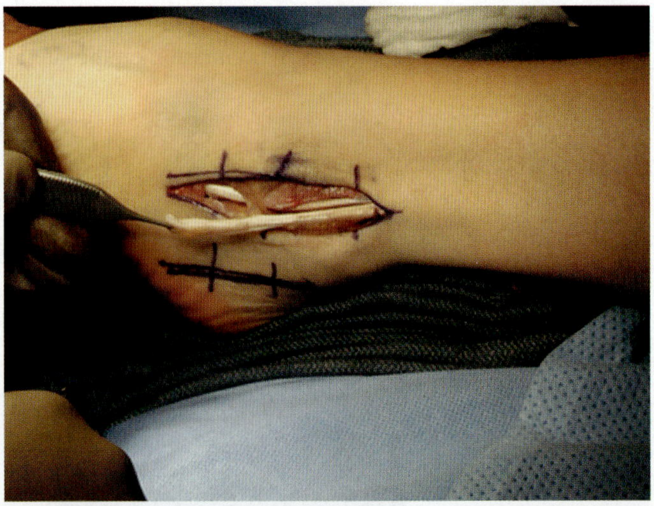

Figure 14-5. Areas of tendinotic tissues are identified and debrided.

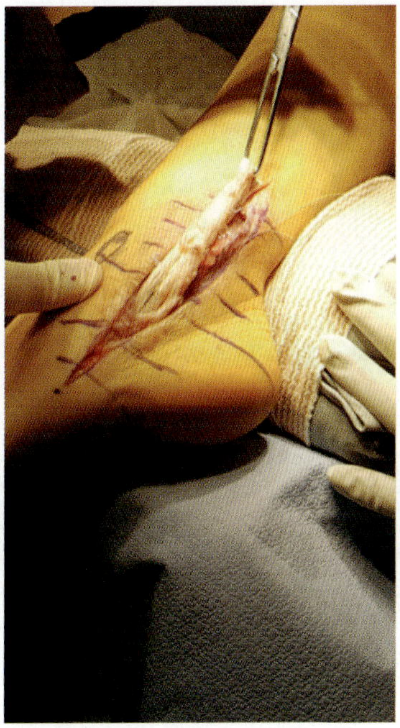

Figure 14-6. Areas of tendinotic tissues are identified and debrided, and the tendon is mobilized.

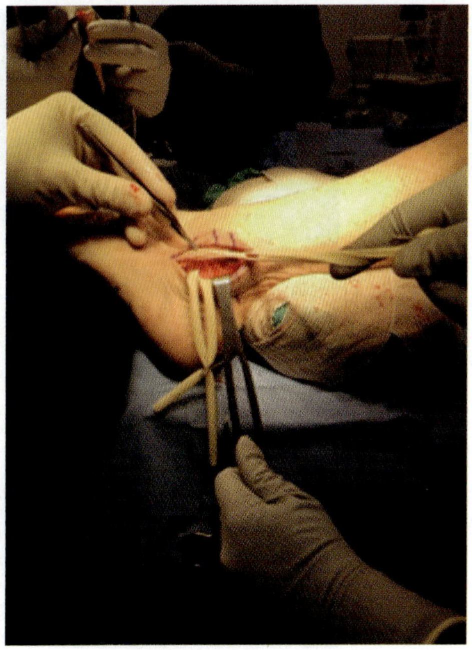

Figure 14-7. A Penrose drain is placed around the tendon to mobilize it.

  - Repair the torn tendon using a #2 orthocord in a buried manner (Figures 14-10 and 14-11).
  - Perform a tenosynovectomy of the peroneus longus.
- If >50% is torn or if the remaining tendon is of very poor quality, replace the tendon using a hamstring (gracilis) tendon autograft (Figures 14-12 to 14-14). See Chapter 11 for hamstring harvest.
- If a tendon transfer is needed:
  - Make a second incision over the base of the fifth metatarsal.
  - Debride the base of the fifth metatarsal with a rongeur.

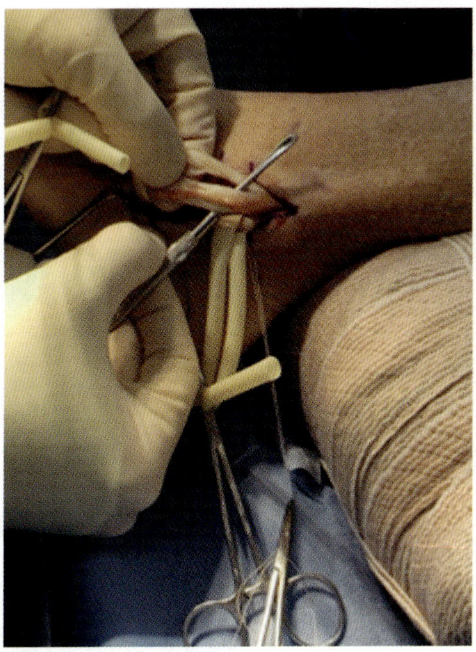

Figure 14-8. Split tears are identified.

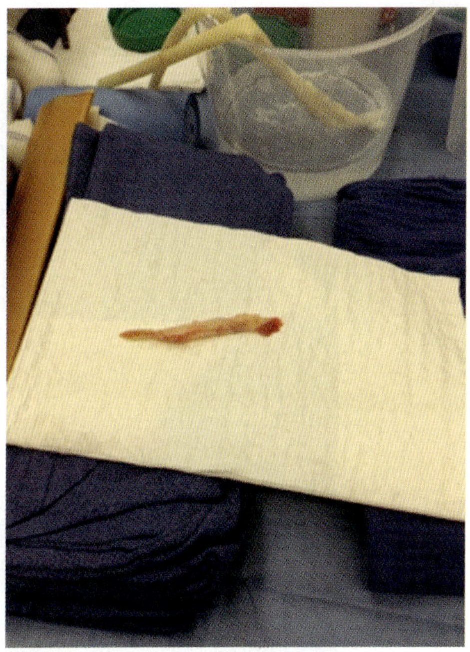

Figure 14-9. Poor-quality tendon is removed.

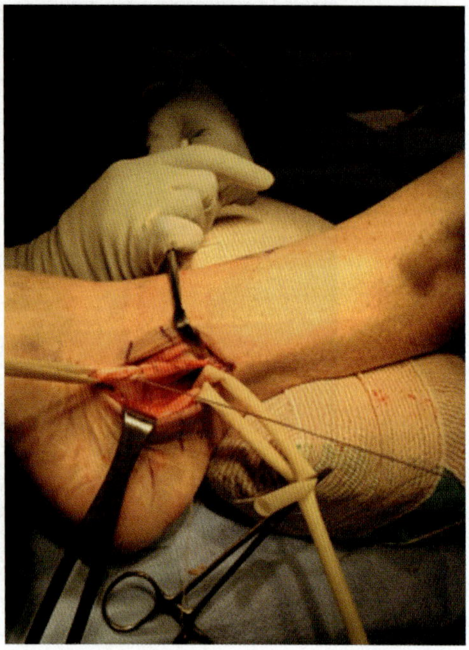

Figure 14-10. The tendon is repaired using a #2 orthocord if <50% is determined to be tendinotic.

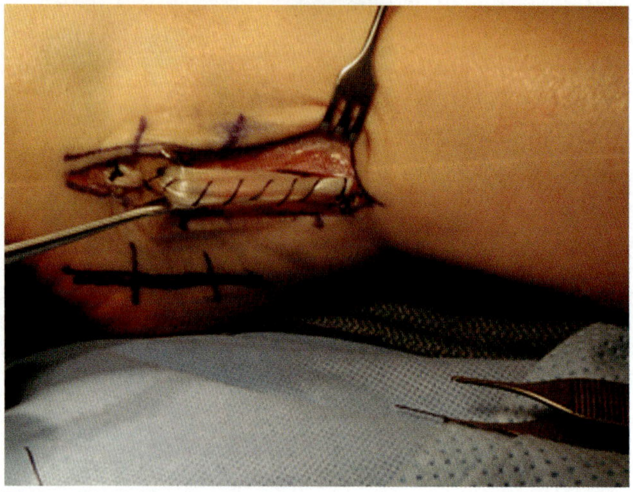

Figure 14-11. The repaired tendon is shown.

- Place a G2 anchor in the base of the fifth metatarsal.
- Bring one end of the gracilis down to the end of the fifth metatarsal.
- Shuttle the gracilis underneath the skin to the distal fibula.
- Use a Pulvertaft-type maneuver to bring the gracilis through the native peroneal tendon.
- Bring the other limb of the gracilis back down to the base of the fifth metatarsal and suture it to the original peroneus brevis stump.
- Tubularize the two limbs of the reconstructed tendon using a 0-Vicryl.

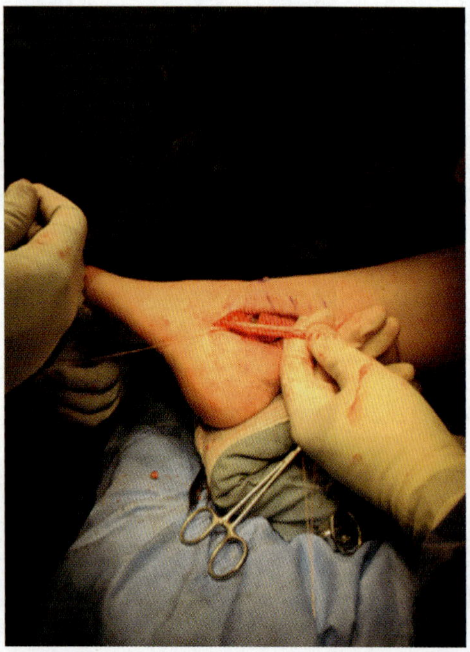

Figure 14-12. If a gracilis is needed, it is first secured to the distal portion of the tendon.

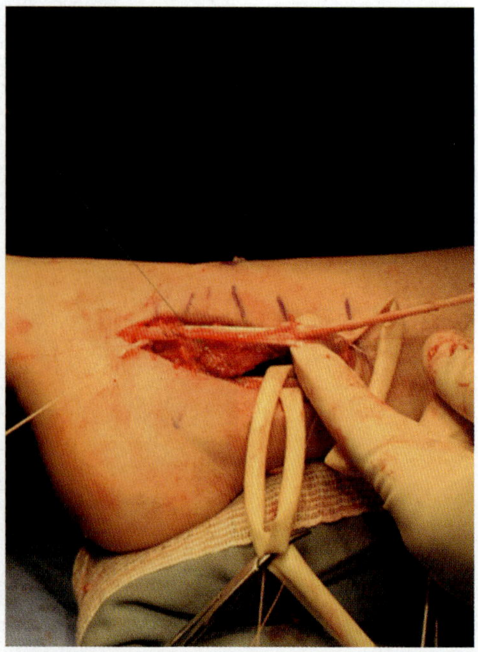

Figure 14-13. The gracilis is brought proximally and secured to the native tendon.

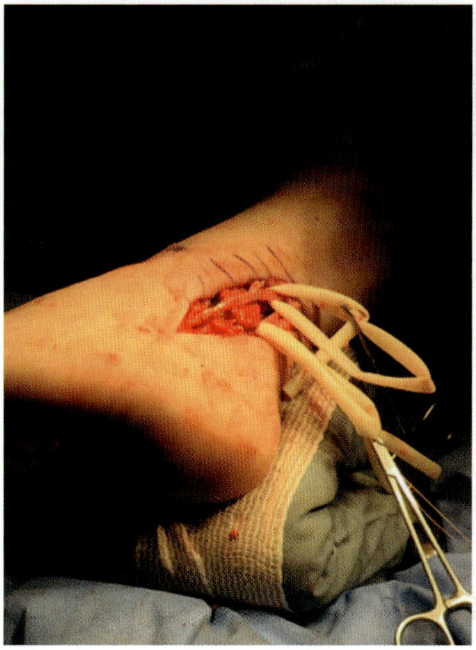

Figure 14-14. The gracilis is secured in place on the proximal end of the native tendon.

- If the patient has an enlarged peroneal tubercle, perform an exostectomy using a rongeur, burr, or an oscillating rasp.
- If there is still subluxation of the tendon, do a fibular groove deepening using a 4.0 burr. Create a concave posterior fibula for distal 2.5 cm. Make four drill holes in the posterolateral aspect of the fibula with a 2.0 drill bit (Figures 14-15 and 14-16).
- Bring the superior peroneal retinaculum through the drill holes.
- Repair this area with a 3-0 Ethibond through the drill holes (Figure 14-17).

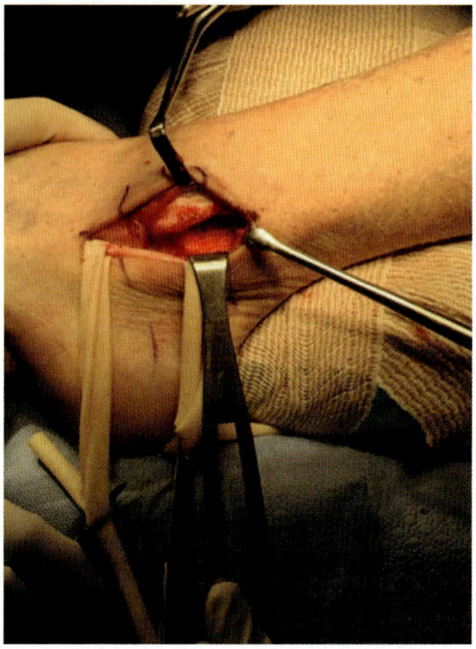

Figure 14-15. The fibular groove is examined to determine whether a groove deepening is needed.

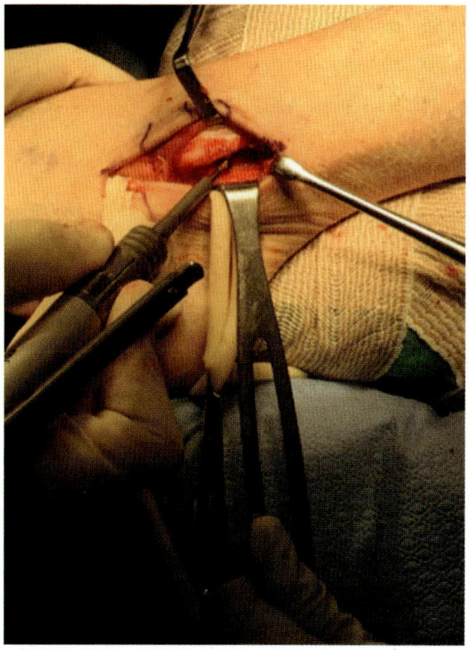

Figure 14-16. A fibular groove deepening is performed using a 4-0 burr, if needed.

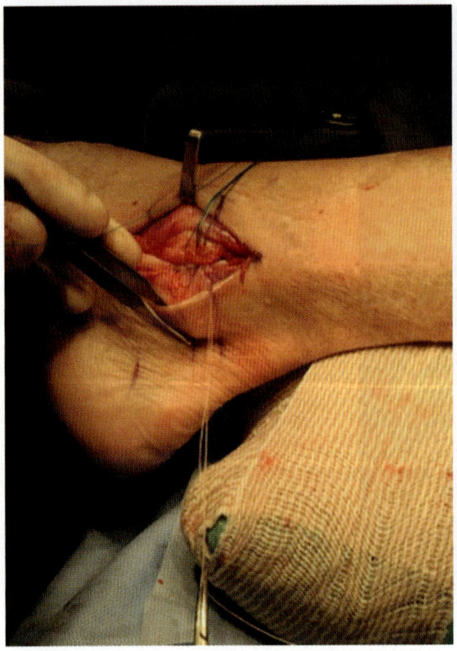

Figure 14-17. The retinaculum is repaired using a 3-0 Ethibond.

Closing

- Thoroughly irrigate the wound with normal sterile saline solution.
- Repair the subcutaneous tissues with a 3-0 Vicryl.
- Close the skin using a 3-0 nylon.
- Apply Steri-strips and sterile dressing to the wound.
- Place the patient in a non-weight-bearing splint.
- Mobilize the patient in a boot after 2 weeks with protective weight-bearing.
- Restrict inversion and eversion for 6 weeks.
- The patient should start physical therapy at 6 weeks.
- Increase weight-bearing as guided by the therapist.
- The patient can progress out of the boot and into sneakers at 3 months.
- The patient can return to sports at 4 to 6 months postoperatively depending on the extent of repair and recovery.

Chapter 15
Dislocating Peroneal Tendons

SYDNEY C. KARNOVSKY
MARK C. DRAKOS

Sterile Instruments/Equipment

- Tourniquet
- 3-0 Vicryl, 3-0 nylon sutures
- Bump
- 2-0 drill
- 3-0 Ethibond
- 4-0 burr
- Penrose drain
- Rongeur available
- Oscillating rasp available

Positioning

- Place the patient in a supine position. Position a large bump under the hip to create a sloppy lateral-type position.
- Place a nonsterile tourniquet on the operative thigh. Prep and drape the lower extremity in a sterile manner.
- Exsanguinate the lower extremity and inflate the tourniquet 250 mm Hg.

Surgical Approach

- Identify the fibula just posterior to bone.
- Make a 6-cm incision on the lateral aspect of the patient's ankle (Figure 15-1).
- Incise the peroneal retinaculum to expose the peroneal tendons and the superior peroneal tendon sheath (Figure 15-2).
- Identify the dislocated tendon(s) and determine whether they will need a fibular groove deepening. If they have a shallow groove or there is an absence of a groove, this will be necessary (Figures 15-3 and 15-4).
- Debride the tendons. Remove the tenosynovium; inspect for tears; and if the tendon is torn, repair the tendon (see Chapter 14).

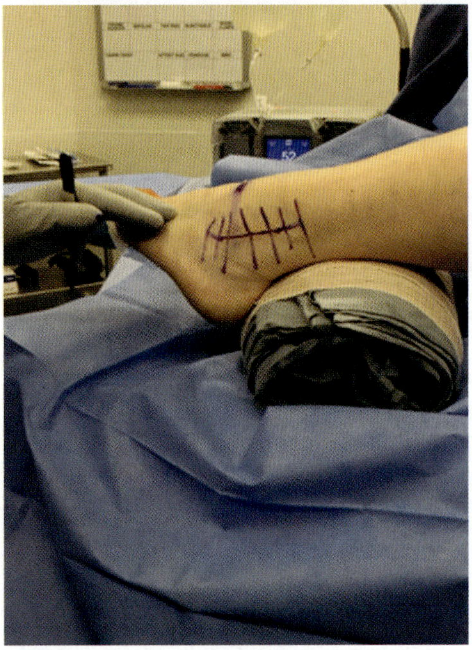

Figure 15-1. The site of the incision is identified and marked on the patient's ankle.

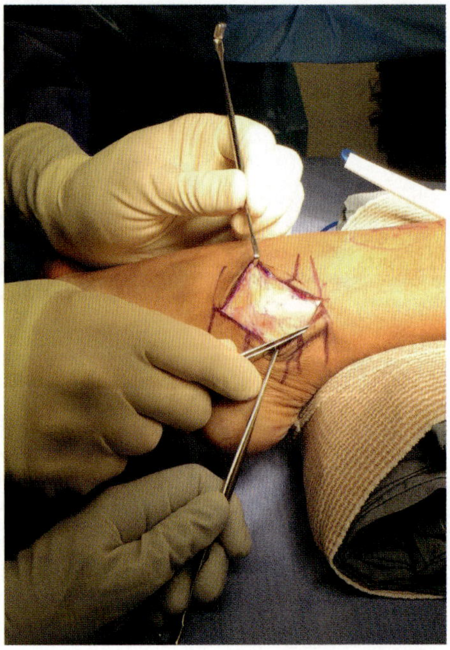

Figure 15-2. The peroneal retinaculum is incised.

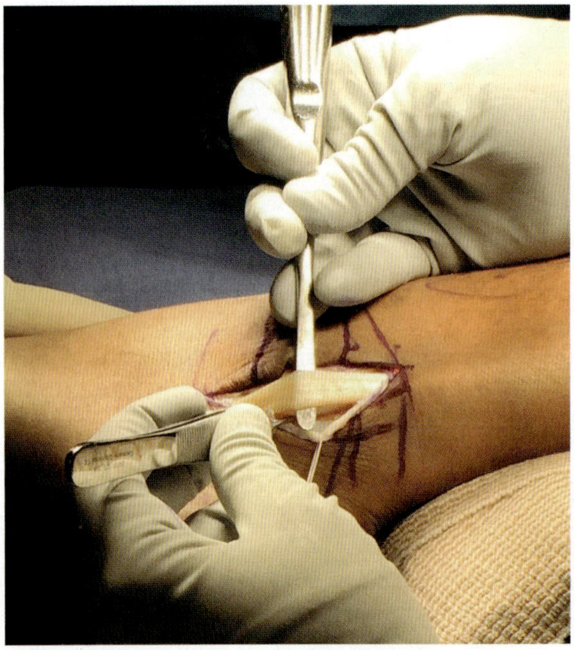

Figure 15-3. The peroneal tendons are exposed. They are debrided, if needed.

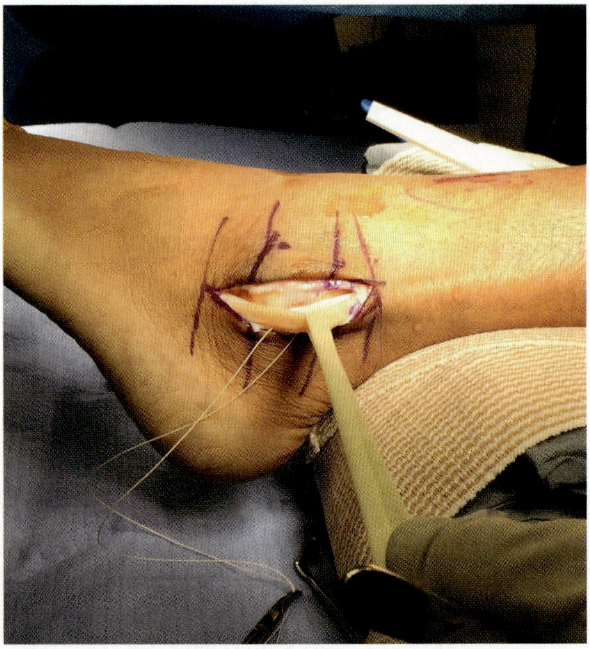

Figure 15-4. A Penrose drain is used to secure the tendons in place.

- If the patient has an enlarged peroneal tubercle, perform an exostectomy using a rongeur, burr, or an oscillating rasp to remove it (Figure 15-5).
- Perform a fibular groove deepening using a 4-0 burr. Create a concave posterior fibula for the distal 2.5 cm that ensures the tendons will sit in the correct place (Figures 15-6 to 15-8).

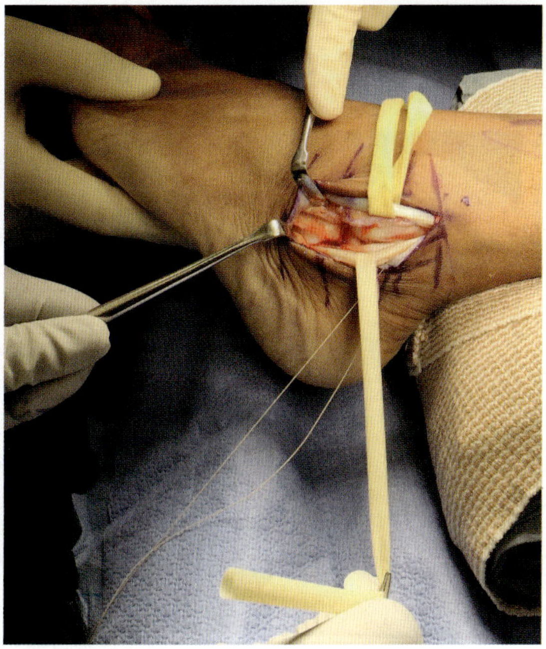

Figure 15-5. The peroneal tubercle is removed.

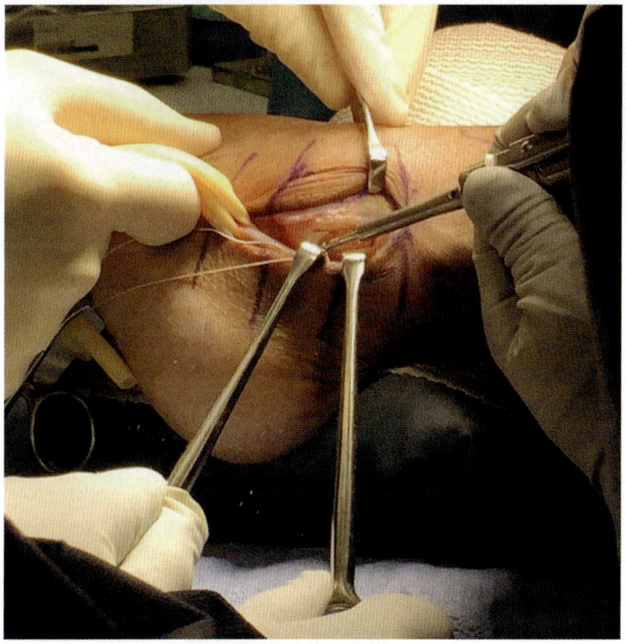

Figure 15-6. A 4-0 burr is used to perform a fibular groove deepening.

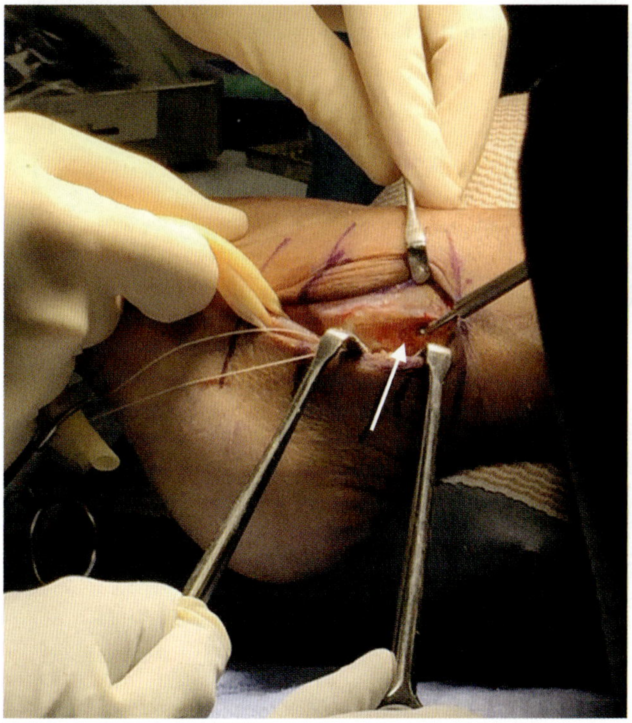

Figure 15-7. The newly created fibular groove is shown.

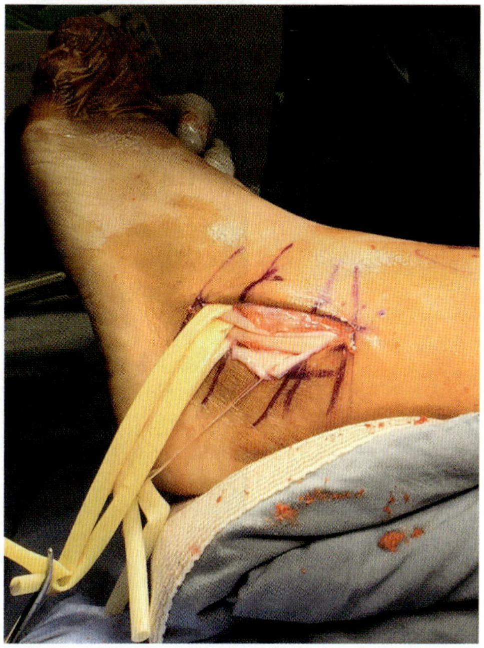

Figure 15-8. The peroneal tendons are shown fitting into the new fibular groove.

- Using a 2-0 drill bit, drill four holes in the posterolateral aspect of the fibula (Figure 15-9).
- Put in three 3-0 Ethibond stitches through the drill holes in the superior peroneal retinaculum and repair the peroneal retinaculum (Figures 15-10 and 15-11).

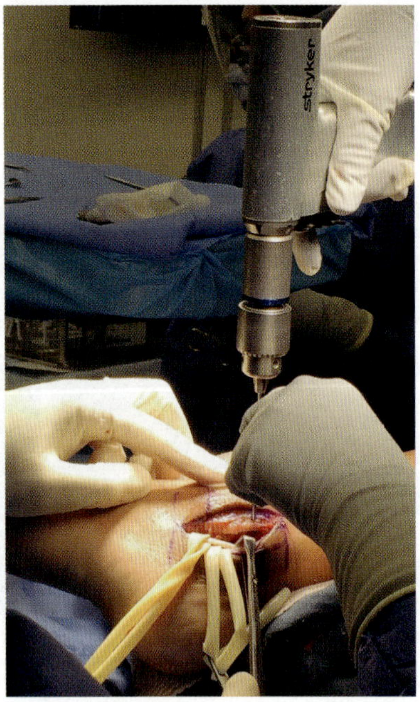

Figure 15-9. A drill is used to make four drill holes into the fibula.

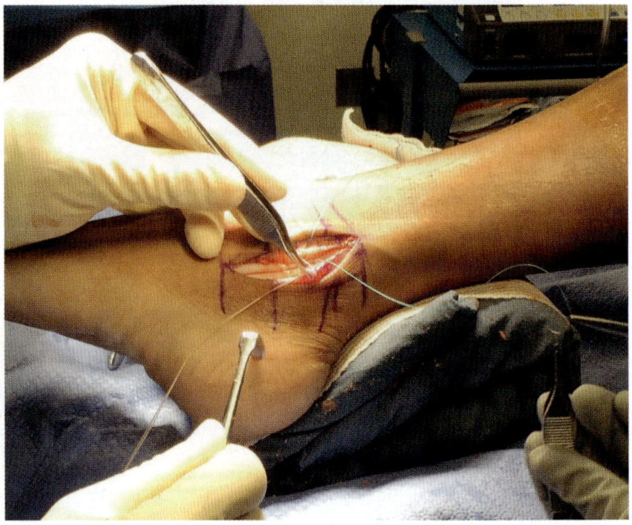

Figure 15-10. Three Ethibond 3-0 stitches are led through the drill holes.

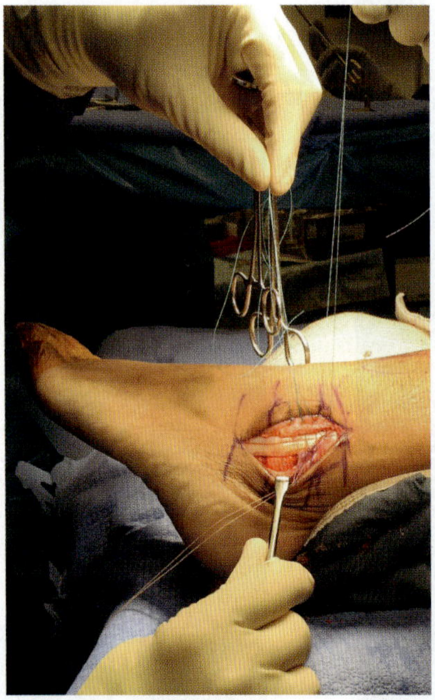

Figure 15-11. The peroneal retinaculum is repaired.

Closing

- Thoroughly irrigate the wound with normal sterile saline solution.
- Repair the subcutaneous tissues with a 3-0 Vicryl (Figure 15-12).
- Close the skin using a 3-0 nylon (Figure 15-13).

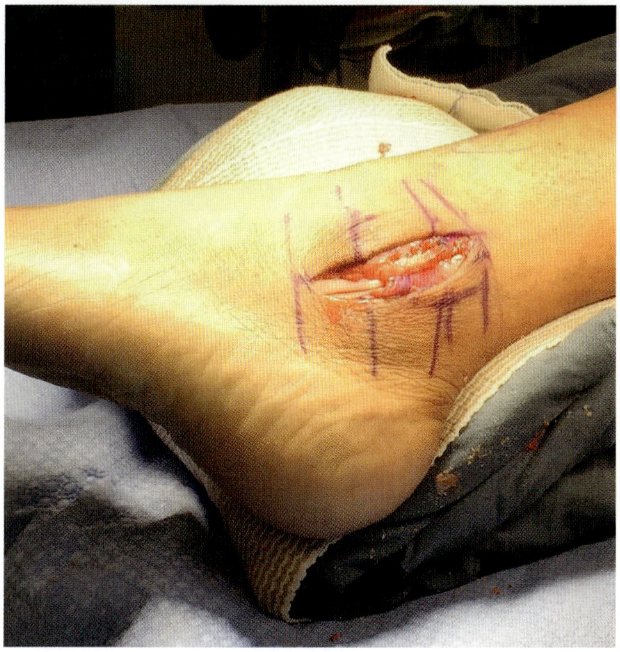

Figure 15-12. The subcutaneous tissues are repaired using a 3-0 Vicryl.

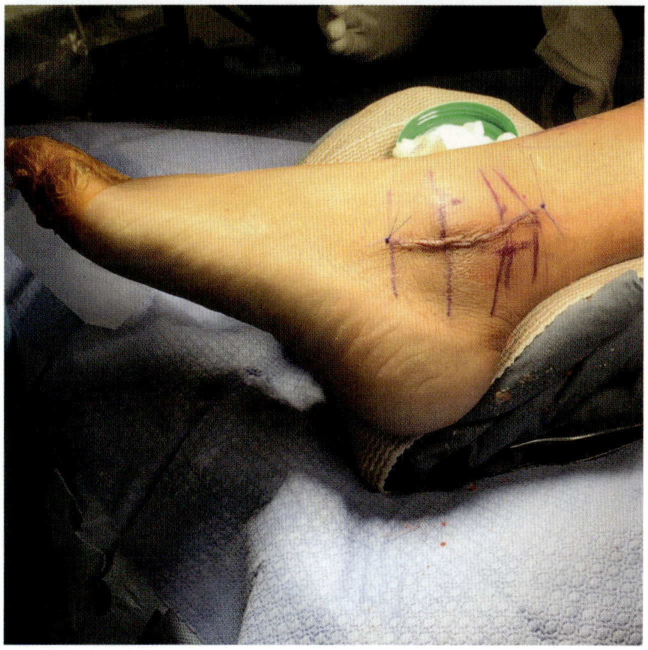

Figure 15-13. The skin is closed using a 3-0 nylon.

- Apply Steri-strips and sterile dressing to the wound.
- Place the patient in a non-weight-bearing splint.
- Mobilize the patient in a CAM walker boot after 2 weeks with protective weight-bearing.
- Restrict inversion and eversion for 6 weeks postoperatively.
- The patient should start physical therapy at 6 weeks postoperatively.
- Increase weight-bearing as guided by the physical therapist.
- The patient can progress out of the boot and into sneakers at 2 months postoperatively.
- The patient can return to sports at 3 to 4 months postoperatively depending on the extent of the repair and recovery, as long as there was no tendon tear.

Chapter 16
Tibialis Anterior Tendinopathy

SYDNEY C. KARNOVSKY
MARK C. DRAKOS

Sterile Instruments/Equipment

- Tourniquet
- #2 orthocord
- 3-0 Vicryl, 0 Vicryl, 3-0 nylon sutures
- Drill
- Bio-Tenodesis screw

Positioning

- Place the patient in a supine position.
- Place a nonsterile tourniquet on the operative thigh. Prep and drape the lower extremity in a sterile manner.
- Exsanguinate the lower extremity and inflate the tourniquet 250 mm Hg.

Surgical Approach

- Identify the tibialis anterior tendon (Figure 16-1).

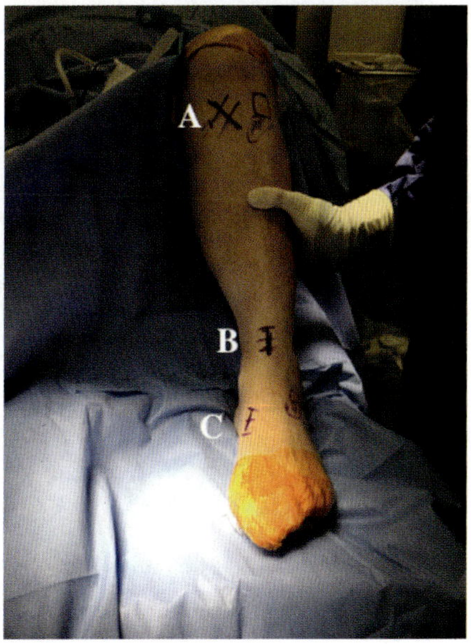

Figure 16-1. The incision sites are labeled. A, The hamstrings. B, The proximal native tibialis anterior stump. C, The tibialis anterior insertion at the medial cuneiform.

- In all chronic cases, use a hamstring autograft to augment and reconstruct the tendon (see Chapter 11 for hamstring harvest techniques).
- Locate the area of the tibialis anterior rupture and make a 2- to 3-cm incision.
- Remove the damaged area of the tendon (Figure 16-2).

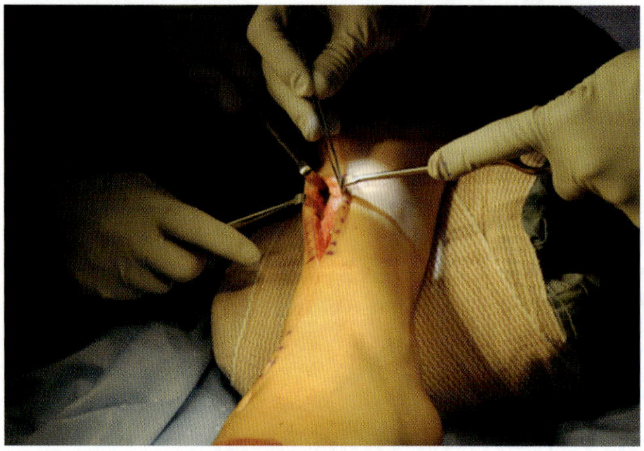

Figure 16-2. An incision is made over the area of the damaged tendon.

- Resect the tibialis anterior stump back to normal-looking tendon (Figures 16-3 to 16-7).
  - Note: Cheat high during this portion of the operation.
- Make a 2-cm incision over the medial cuneiform (Figure 16-8).

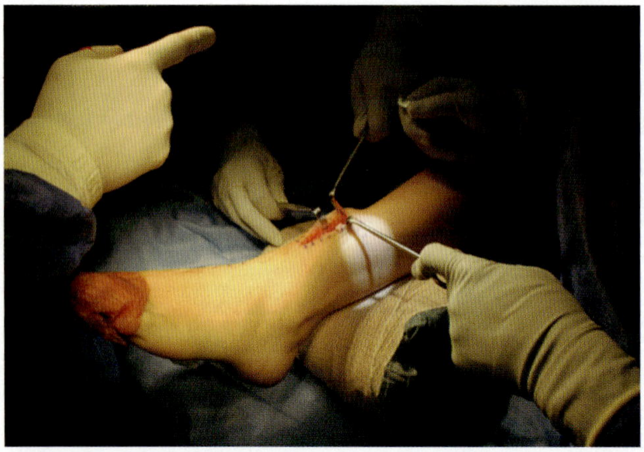

Figure 16-3. The tibialis anterior tendon stump is located.

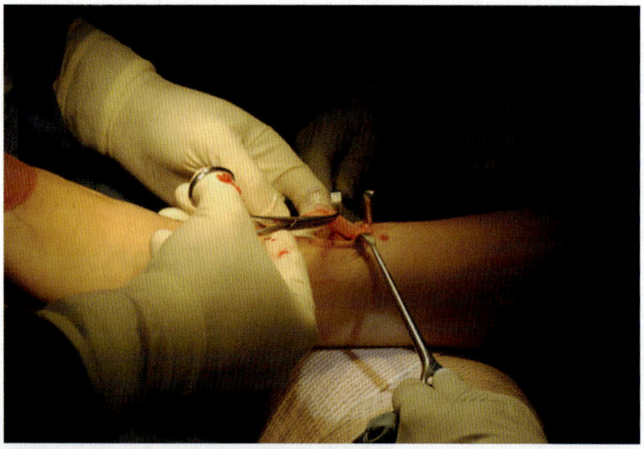

Figure 16-4. The tendon stump is resected back to normal-looking tendon.

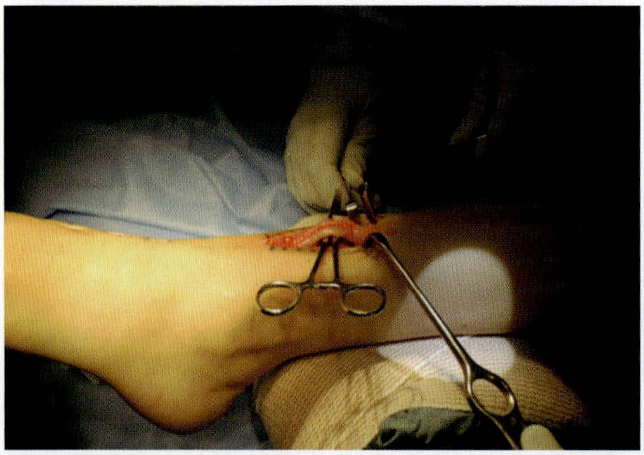

Figure 16-5. The degenerated tendon is removed.

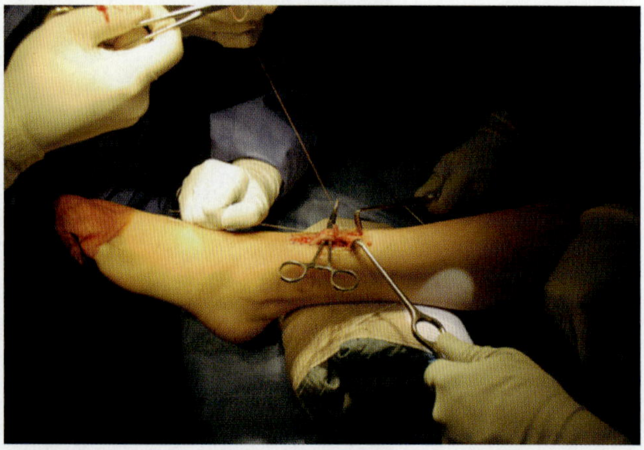

Figure 16-6. The proximal tendon is tagged with a stitch.

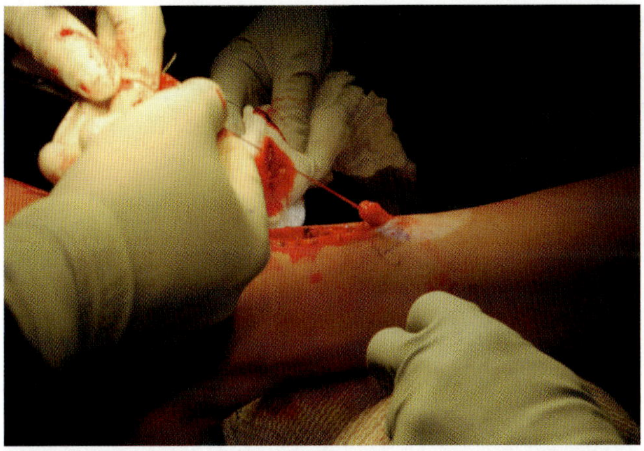

Figure 16-7. The tendon is mobilized.

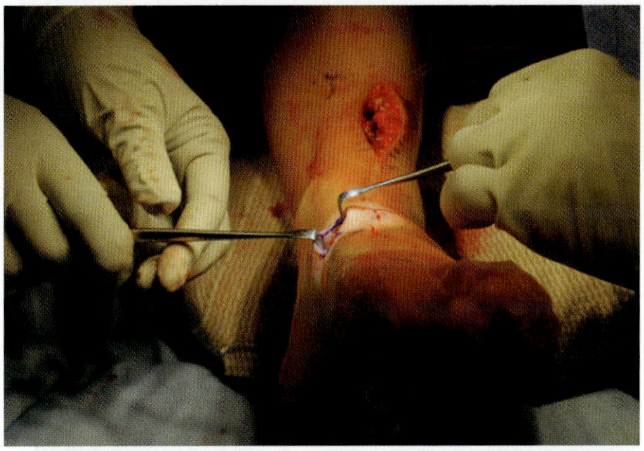

Figure 16-8. The tendon insertion site is exposed over the medial border of the medial cuneiform.

- Locate the tibialis anterior attachment remnant.
  - Note that there is usually some stump on this side as well.
- Drill a bone tunnel obliquely in the medial cuneiform in the same vector as in the native tibialis anterior tendon. The diameter should be within 0.5 mm of the diameter of the hamstring graft. Drill to approximately 20 mm (Figures 16-9 and 16-10).
- Place the hamstring graft in the tunnel (Figure 16-11).

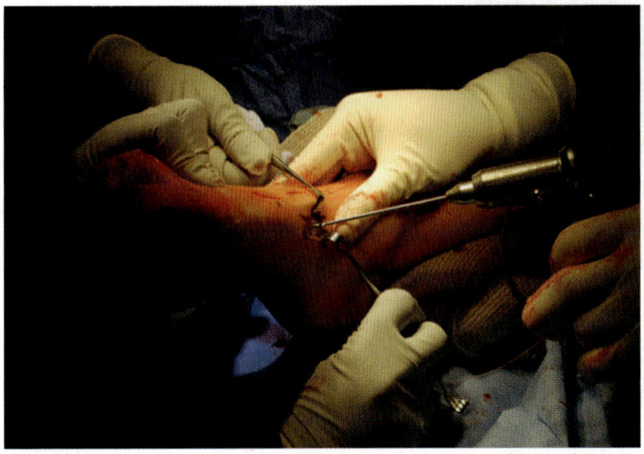

Figure 16-9. A bone tunnel is drilled at the insertion site on the medial cuneiform.

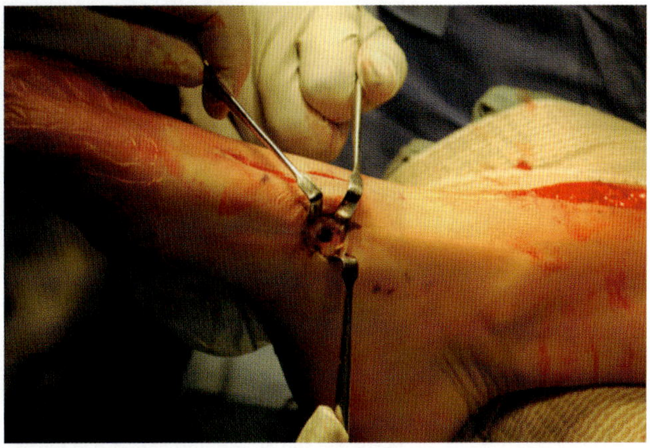

Figure 16-10. The bone tunnel is prepared for the hamstring graft.

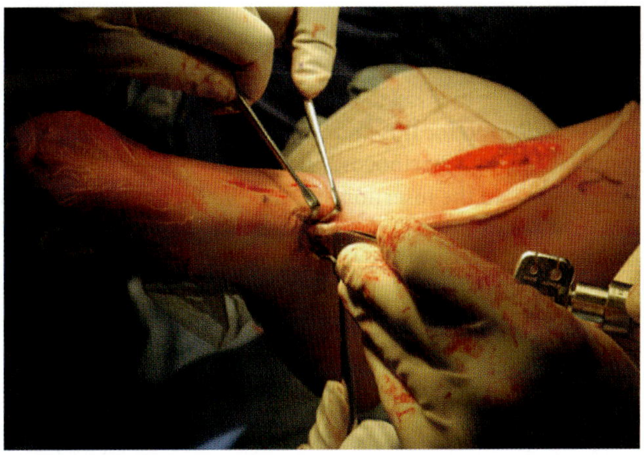

Figure 16-11. The hamstring graft is brought into the bone tunnel.

- Use a Bio-Tenodesis screw to secure the distal end of the hamstring graft to the medial cuneiform within the tunnel (Figures 16-12 and 16-13).
- Pass the graft subcutaneously and proximally to the tendon stump (Figure 16-14).

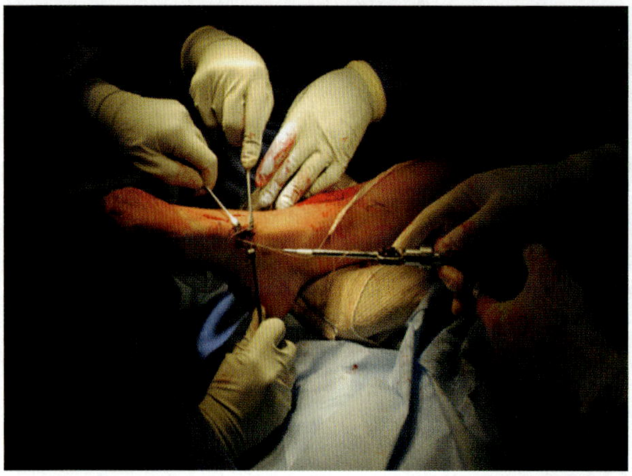

Figure 16-12. The hamstring graft is secured in the bone tunnel with a Bio-Tenodesis screw.

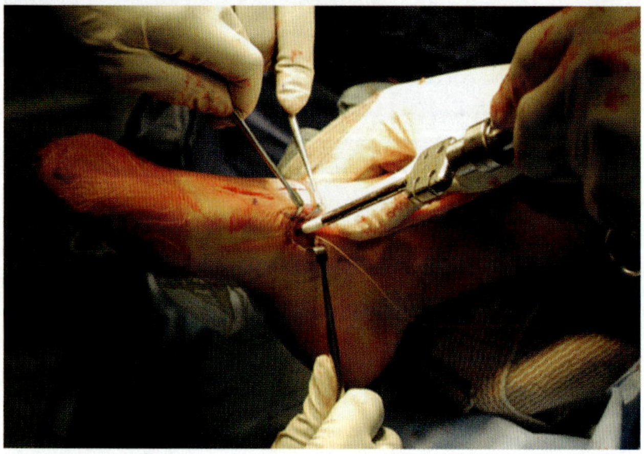

Figure 16-13. The hamstring graft is secured in the bone tunnel with a Bio-Tenodesis screw after insertion.

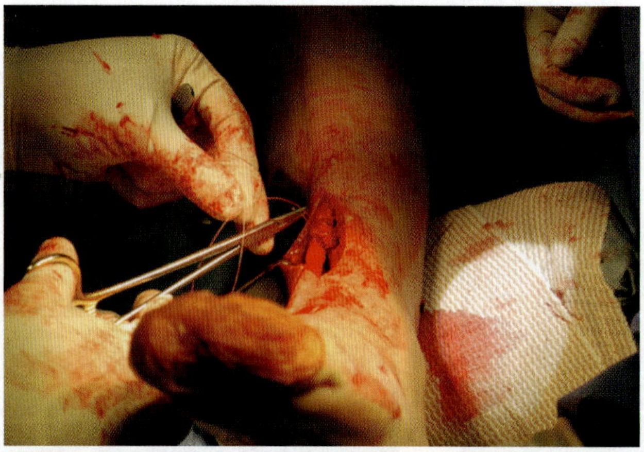

Figure 16-14. The graft is brought subcutaneously and proximally to the tendon stump and secured in place using a Pulvertaft-type maneuver and #2 orthocord sutures.

- Perform an extensor retinaculum release to prevent stenosis of the tendon's path and relieve tension.
- Use a Pulvertaft-type maneuver to bring and secure the graft to the tendon. The foot should be in neutral or up to 5° of dorsiflexion for this and in slight supination.
- Secure the tendon in place using #2 orthocord sutures.
- Tunnel the graft back distally to the insertion site and secure it with stitches to the other limb of the suture from the Bio-Tenodesis screw (Figures 16-15 and 16-16).
- Tubularize the graft using a 3-0 Vicryl suture.

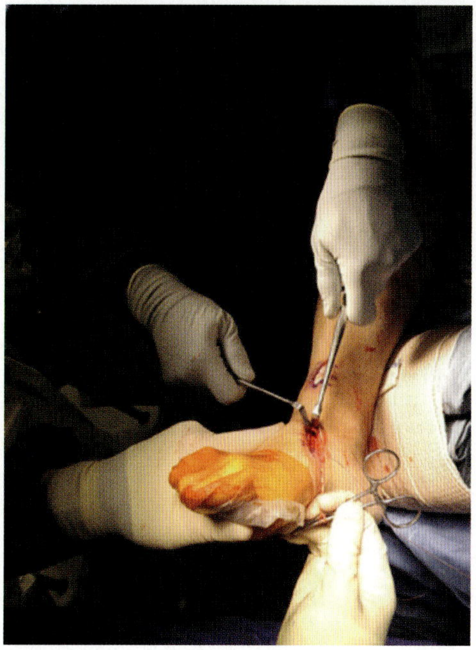

Figure 16-15. The graft is brought back down to create a double-bundle effect.

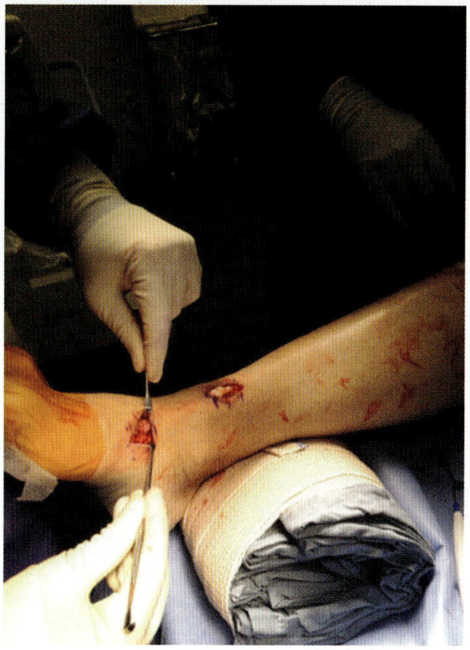

Figure 16-16. The graft is tied to sutures in the Bio-Tenodesis screw and native tendon stump.

Closing

- Thoroughly irrigate the wound with normal sterile saline solution.
- Repair the subcutaneous tissues with a 0-Vicryl.
- Close the skin using a 3-0 nylon.
- Apply Steri-strips and sterile dressing to the wound.
- Place the patient in a non-weight-bearing splint for 2 weeks.
- At 2 weeks postoperatively, transition the patient into either a non-weight-bearing boot or a cast, depending on age. The patient can begin slight range of motion activities, focusing mainly on dorsiflexion.
- Transition the patient into a partial-weight-bearing boot at 6 weeks postoperatively and begin physical therapy at this point, progressing the weight-bearing status as instructed by the physical therapist.
- Transition the patient into a sneaker at 3 months postoperatively.

Chapter 17
Lateral Ankle Instability

ANDREW J. ROSENBAUM

Sterile Instruments/Equipment

- Tourniquet
- Sharp Senn retractors
- Freer elevator
- Wire driver/drill
- Littler dissection scissors
- Small joint arthroscope and ankle distractor (if arthroscopy is to be performed at the time of surgery)
- Implants
  - FiberTak suture anchors (Arthrex, Naples, Florida, USA)
  - InternalBrace (Arthrex, Naples, Florida, USA)

Positioning

- Supine on operating room table
- Bump placed under ipsilateral hip to ensure foot is straight up and down
- Thigh–knee holder and noninvasive ankle distractor applied next if arthroscopy to be performed
  - Use a gel pad to minimize pressure on peroneal nerve and the popliteal space.

Surgical Approach

- Anterior approach begins 1.5 cm proximal to the tip of the fibula and extends 1.5 cm distal distally in line with the fifth metatarsal base (Figure 17-1).
- Avoid superficial peroneal and sural nerve branches.
- Identify the interior extensor retinaculum and tag it with a no. 0 absorbable suture.
- Identify the anterolateral capsule and release in a subperiosteal manner off the distal fibula.
  - Do not stray too far anterior to prevent iatrogenic injury to the superficial peroneal nerve.
  - The posterior landmark is the peroneal sheath, which allows inspection of the tendons.
  - Address any peroneal tendon pathology at the time.
- If additional tissue is needed for repair, elevate the distal fibula periosteum from distal to proximal.

Ligament Stabilization

- Excise any loose ossicle while taking care to preserve the capsule and integrity of the anterior talofibular ligament (ATFL).
- Prepare distal fibula for healing following ligament fixation with a rasp and bone rongeurs.
- Calcaneofibular ligament is not routinely incorporated into the repair, because outcomes are not improved when done in conjunction with ATFL repair.[1]

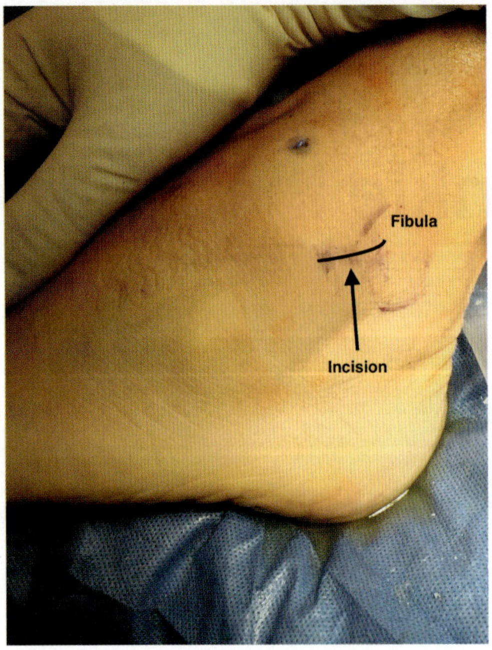

Figure 17-1. Incision used to address lateral ankle instability. A larger incision is used, or this incision is extended, if peroneal tendon pathology necessitating treatment is present. Courtesy of Andrew Rosenbaum, MD.

- The InternalBrace is then placed at the ATFL footprint on the talus.
  - Identify the nonarticulating surface of the lateral border of the talus.
  - Use a 3.5-mm drill in a direction of 45° medial and parallel to the floor, with the foot in neutral to avoid entering the sinus tarsi or ankle joint.
    - Sinus probe is used to ensure the tunnel is blind-ending (Figure 17-2).
  - Tap and then place a 4.75-mm BioComposite SwiveLock preloaded with FiberTape.
  - Weave FiberTape through the ATFL with a free needle.
  - Before docking InternalBrace, perform the Brostrom procedure.
    - Two FiberTak anchors proloaded with SutureTape are used.
    - These are placed proximal and distal to the fibular InternalBrace tunnel (Figure 17-3).

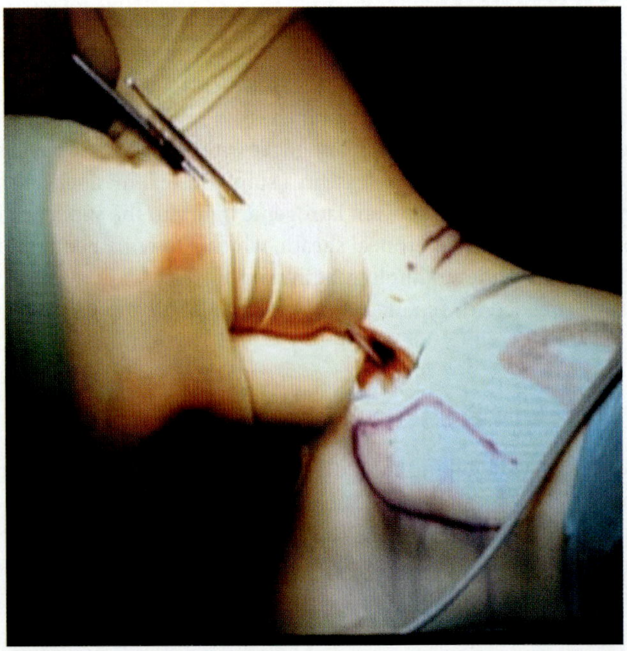

Figure 17-2. Sinus probe used in talar tunnel to ensure that tunnel does not violate subtalar or ankle joint. Reproduced with permission from Mackay GM, Ribbans WJ. The addition of an "Internal Brace" to augment the Brostrom technique for lateral ankle ligament instability. *Tech Foot Ankle Surg*. 2016;15(1):47-56. Figure 8. doi:10.1097/BTF.0000000000000111.

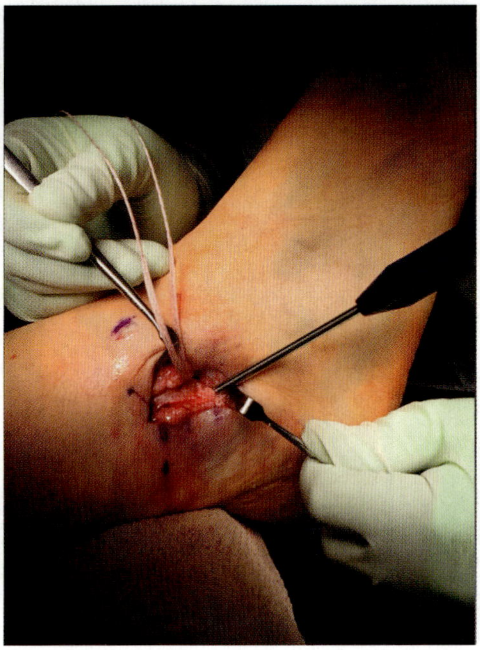

Figure 17-3. Placement of distal FiberTak anchor in fibula. Courtesy of Andrew Rosenbaum, MD.

- Fibula InternalBrace tunnel is then prepared with a 3.5-mm drill at the origin of the ATFL.
  - 14-mm from the tip of the fibula (Figure 17-4)
- SutureTape is delivered through lateral capsuloligamentous tissue (Figure 17-5).
- With the ankle held in neutral dorsiflexion and slight eversion, the SutureTape is secured with surgical knots.
- The FiberTape on the InternalBrace is then tensioned with the foot in the same position and the 3.5-mm BioComposite SwiveLock is inserted into the fibular tunnel.
  - Proper tensioning of the InternalBrace is critical.
  - A hemostat is routinely placed between the FiberTape and underlying tissue before anchor tightening to minimize construct laxity (Figure 17-6).
- FiberTape cut flush with fibular fixation (Figure 17-7)

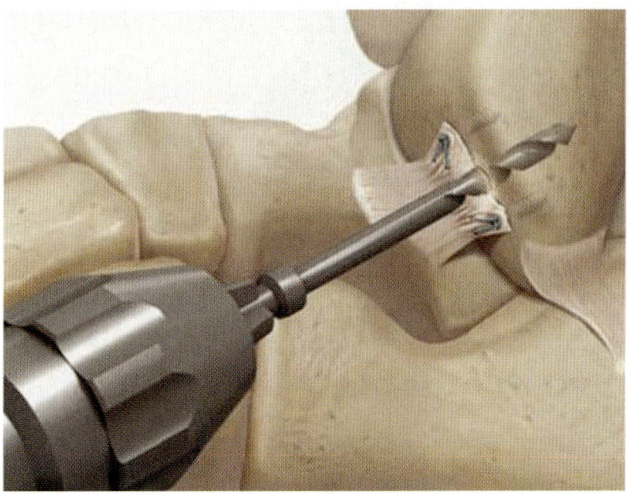

Figure 17-4. Location of fibular tunnel for InternalBrace. Reproduced with permission from Mackay GM, Ribbans WJ. The addition of an "Internal Brace" to augment the Brostrom technique for lateral ankle ligament instability. *Tech Foot Ankle Surg*. 2016;15(1):47-56. Figure 4. doi:10.1097/BTF.0000000000000111.

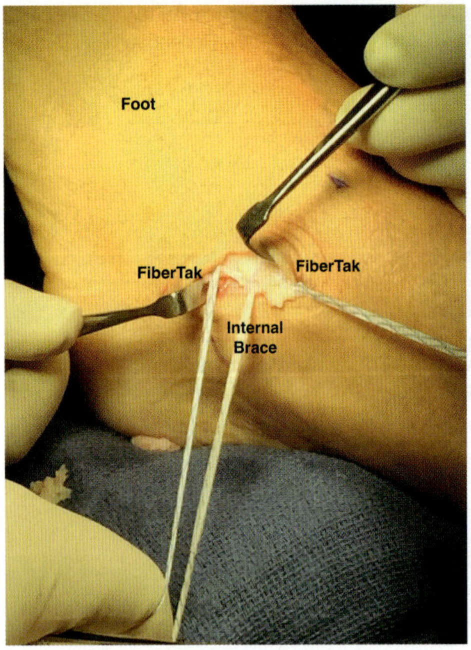

Figure 17-5. Lateral capsuloligamentous tissue being pulled over the fibula with traction on the SutureTape. The FiberTape from the InternalBrace is located between the SutureTape. Surgical knots are used to secure the SutureTape, with the ankle in neutral dorsiflexion and slight eversion. Courtesy of Andrew Rosenbaum, MD.

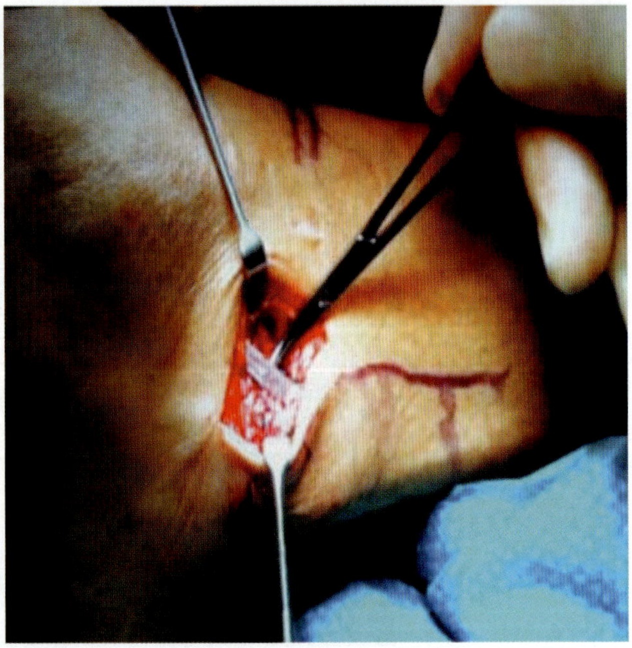

Figure 17-6. Hemostat placed under the FiberTape to prevent excessive tension during attachment. Reproduced with permission from Mackay GM, Ribbans WJ. The addition of an "Internal Brace" to augment the Brostrom technique for lateral ankle ligament instability. *Tech Foot Ankle Surg*. 2016;15(1):47-56. Figure 11. doi:10.1097/BTF.0000000000000111.

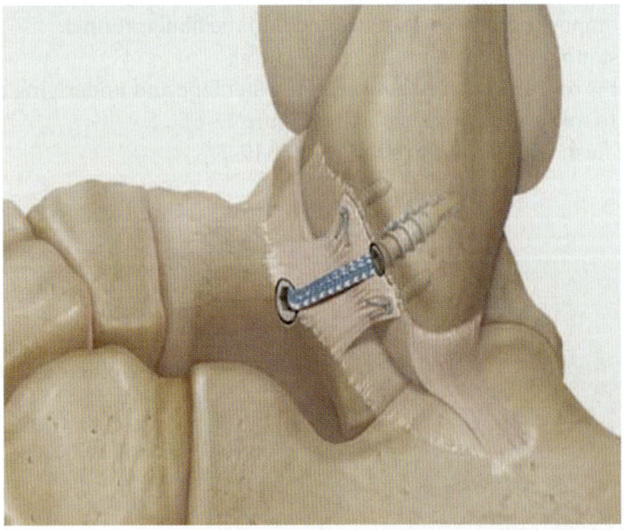

Figure 17-7. Final construct including two anchors and the InternalBrace. Reproduced with permission from Mackay GM, Ribbans WJ. The addition of an "Internal Brace" to augment the Brostrom technique for lateral ankle ligament instability. *Tech Foot Ankle Surg*. 2016;15(1):47-56. Figure 12C. doi:10.1097/BTF.0000000000000111.

Postoperative Protocol

Weeks 1 to 2

- Weight-bearing as tolerated in CAM boot
- Sutures removed in 14 to 16 days
- Start active range of motion (ROM) (ankle dorsiflexion/plantarflexion).
- Okay to ride stationary bike, elliptical in CAM boot

Weeks 3 to 6

- Outpatient physical therapy begins.
- Start using ankle brace.
- Bike, walk, elliptical without the boot

Weeks 6 to 8

- Continue active ROM and begin active inversion and eversion.
- Proprioceptive training: single-leg stance, balance beam, standing on uneven surfaces

Weeks 8 to 10

- Activity-specific training
- Return to sport

Reference

1. Maffulli N, Del Buono A, Maffulli GD, et al. Isolated anterior talofibular ligament Brostrom repair for chronic lateral ankle instability. *Am J Sports Med.* 2013;41(4):858-864.

Chapter 18
Medial Ankle Instability

ANDREW POSNER
KYLE ANGELICOLA-RICHARDSON
ANDREW J. ROSENBAUM

Sterile Instruments/Equipment

- Beanbag or bump
- Knee holder
- Thigh tourniquet
- Ankle arthroscopy equipment (if needed)
- Suture anchors
- Semitendinosus allograft (if needed)

Positioning

- Supine
- Bump the hip on the operative limb, allowing the foot to remain in neutral.
- Place thigh tourniquet.
- Use knee holder to support the distal femur, allowing the foot to move freely for arthroscopy before open reconstruction.
- Prep and drape in the normal sterile manner, extended proximal to the knee.
- After completion of arthroscopy, the knee holder is removed and the foot can rest freely.

Surgical Approach

- Ankle arthroscopy
  - Knee holder used to support the distal femur and get the foot into a hanging position (Figure 18-1)

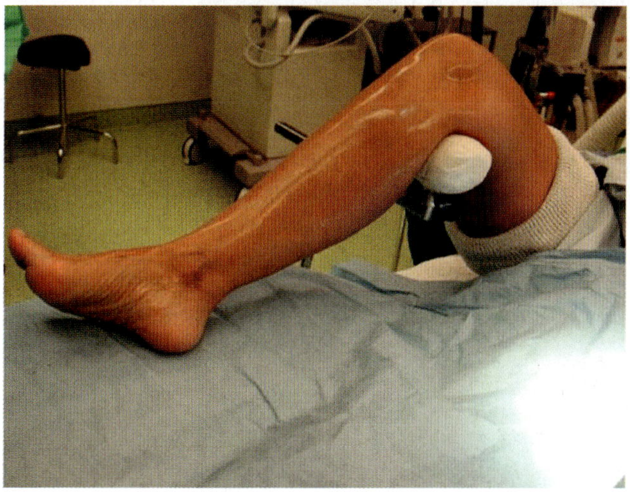

Figure 18-1. Use knee holder to support the distal femur, allowing the foot to move freely for arthroscopy before open reconstruction. Reprinted with permission from Wiesel SW. *Operative Techniques in Orthopaedic Surgery*. 1st ed. Philadelphia, PA: Wolters Kluwer, Lippincott Williams & Wilkins; 2010. Figure 104-4b.

- Incision
  - Anteromedial, longitudinal, curved incision (Figure 18-2)
  - Begin 1 cm proximal to medial malleolus. Continue incision across anterior third of medial malleolus, finish 2 to 4 cm distal to the tip of the medial malleolus, heading toward medial aspect of the navicular.
- Superficial dissection
  - Mobilize skin flaps.
  - Identify and protect great saphenous vein and nerve just anterior to medial malleolus.
  - Expose periosteum and capsule.

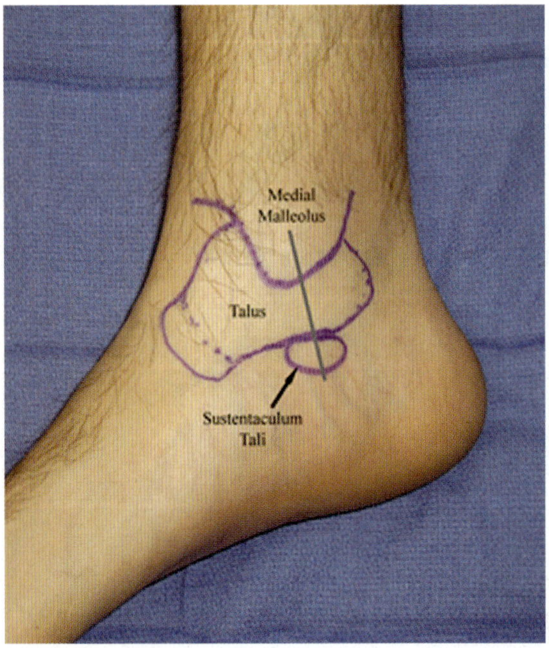

Figure 18-2. Approach for deltoid ligament reconstruction. Reprinted with permission from Wiesel SW. *Operative Techniques in Orthopaedic Surgery*. 1st ed. Philadelphia, PA: Wolters Kluwer, Lippincott Williams & Wilkins; 2010. Figure 103-2.

- Deep dissection (Figure 18-3)
  - Posterior tibial tendon should be displaced from the sheath and preserved.
  - Incise anterior joint capsule to visualize joint.
  - Identify remaining fibers of deltoid ligament.
    - Superficial portion: fan-shaped, commonly torn mid-substance or avulsed from medial malleolus
    - Deep portion: short, heavy, clinically more significant; may be avulsed from the talus (most common), torn from the tip of malleolus, torn mid-substance

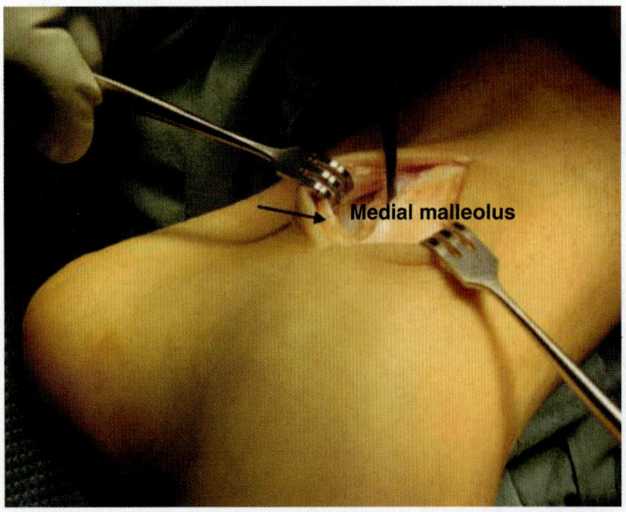

Figure 18-3. Medial approach. Posterior tibial tendon (arrow) is retracted posteriorly. Reprinted with permission from Giza E, Wuellner J. Acute deltoid rupture: history, diagnosis, and a repair technique. *Tech Foot Ankle Surg*. 2014;13(2):73-80. doi:10.1097/BTF.0000000000000045.

Reduction and Fixation Techniques

- Perform ankle arthroscopy to evaluate for and treat concurrent intra-articular pathology (Figures 18-4 and 18-5).
- Reconstruction of the superficial deltoid ligament: proximal tear or avulsion (Figure 18-6)
  - Expose anterior border of medial malleolus with short incision between the tibiospring and tibionavicular ligaments. A fibrous septum is usually present between these two ligaments.
  - Roughen the medial surface of the medial malleolus and place suture anchor 6 mm proximal to the tip (FiberTak, Arthrex, Naples, FL, USA).
  - Refix the tibiospring and tibionavicular ligaments to the medial malleolus and secure with an overlying no. 0 absorbable suture.

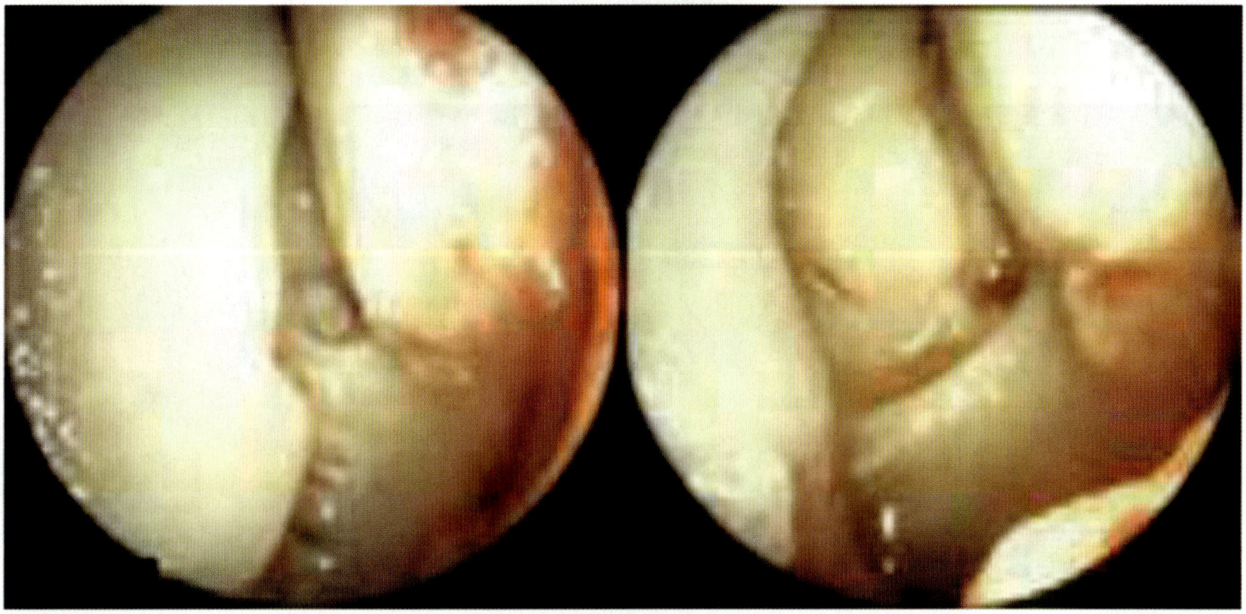

Figure 18-4. Arthroscopic visualization, separation of the talus from the medial malleolus, where foot eversion and pronation signifies deltoid ligament incompetence. Reprinted with permission from Wiesel SW. *Operative Techniques in Orthopaedic Surgery*. 1st ed. Philadelphia, PA: Wolters Kluwer, Lippincott Williams & Wilkins; 2010. Figure 104.TechFig2ab.

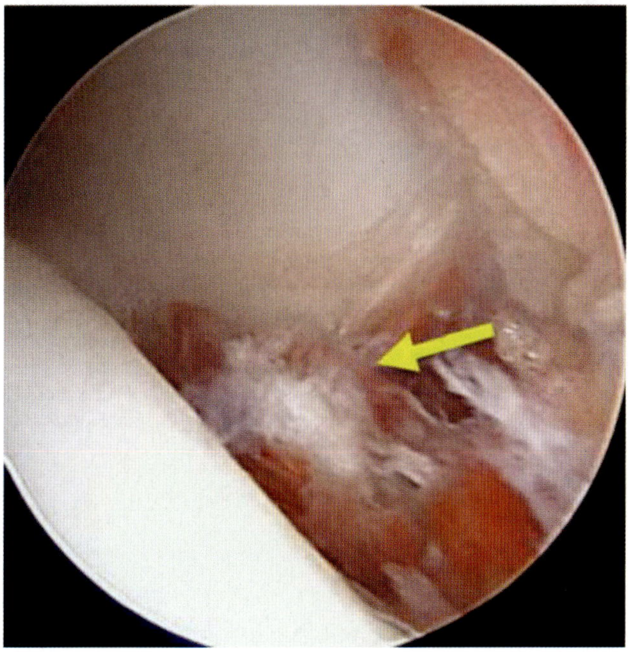

Figure 18-5. Arthroscopic visualization demonstrating medial ankle instability and deltoid complex avulsion off of the medial malleolus (yellow arrow). Reprinted with permission from Hsu AR. Treatment of deltoid injuries associated with ankle fractures. *Tech Foot Ankle Surg*. 2018;17(3):115-120. doi:10.1097/BTF.0000000000000180.

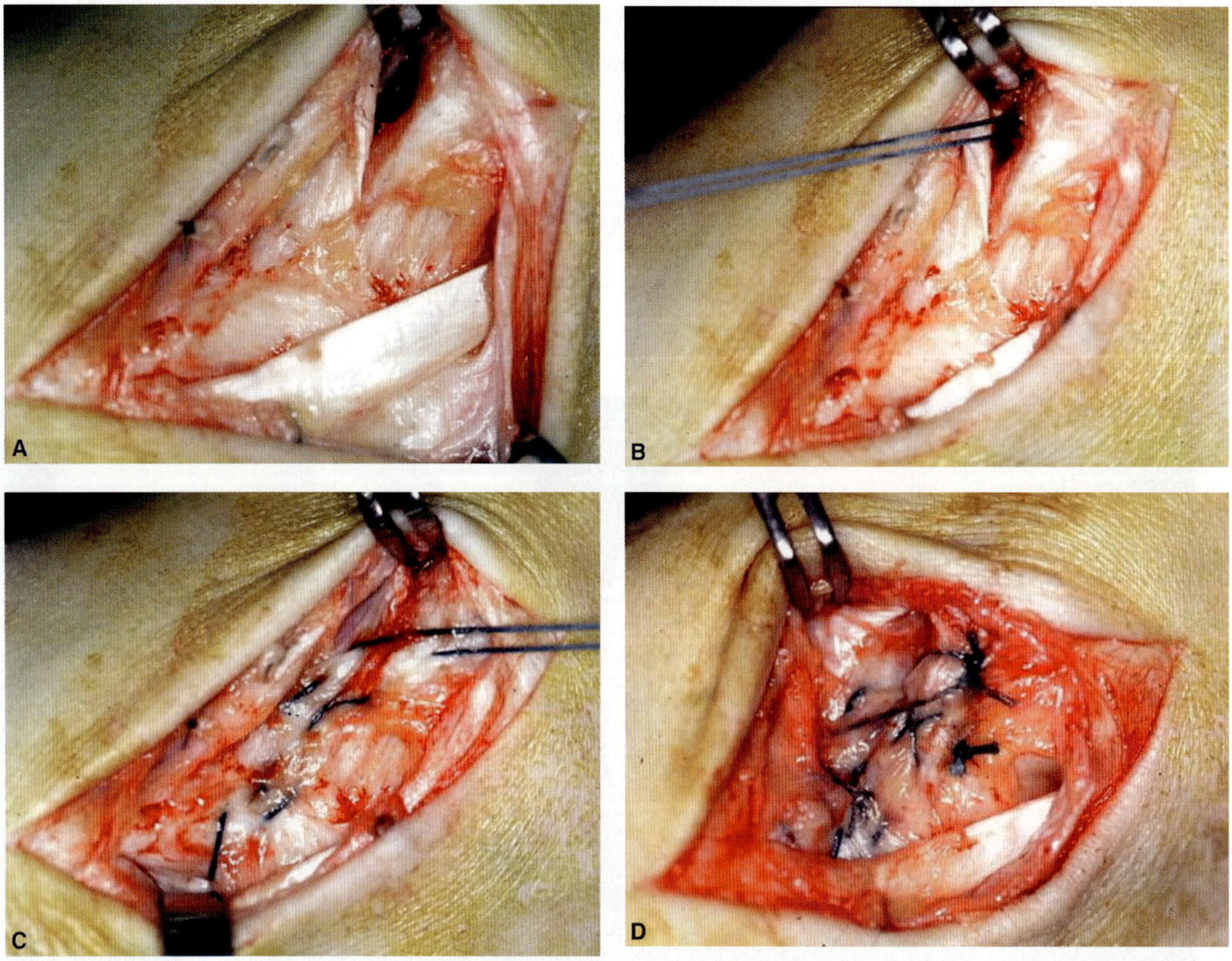

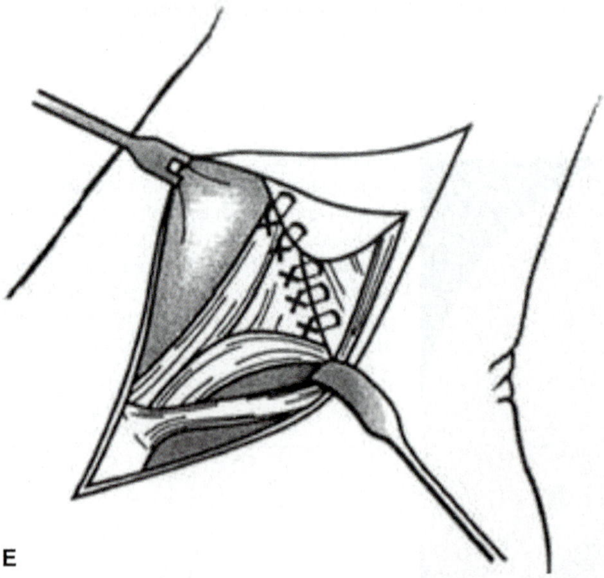

E

Figure 18-6. A, The rupture between the tibionavicular and tibiospring ligaments. B, Anchor placed 6 mm above the tip of the medial malleolus. C, Refixation of the tibionavicular and tibiospring ligaments to the medial malleolus. D, Final reconstruction with overlying no. 0 resorbable sutures. E, Principle of reconstruction. Reprinted with permission from Wiesel SW. *Operative Techniques in Orthopaedic Surgery*. 1st ed. Philadelphia, PA: Wolters Kluwer, Lippincott Williams & Wilkins; 2010. Figure 104.TechFig4d.1-6.

- Reconstruction of the superficial deltoid ligament: intermediate tear (Figure 18-7)
    - Divide the proximal and distal flaps.
    - Place two suture anchors proximal to the medial malleolus, and refix them to the distal flap and the tibionavicular ligament, respectively. Place one suture anchor on the navicular tuberosity and refix it to the proximal flap. Secure reconstructed tibionavicular and tibiospring ligaments with an overlying no. 0 absorbable suture.

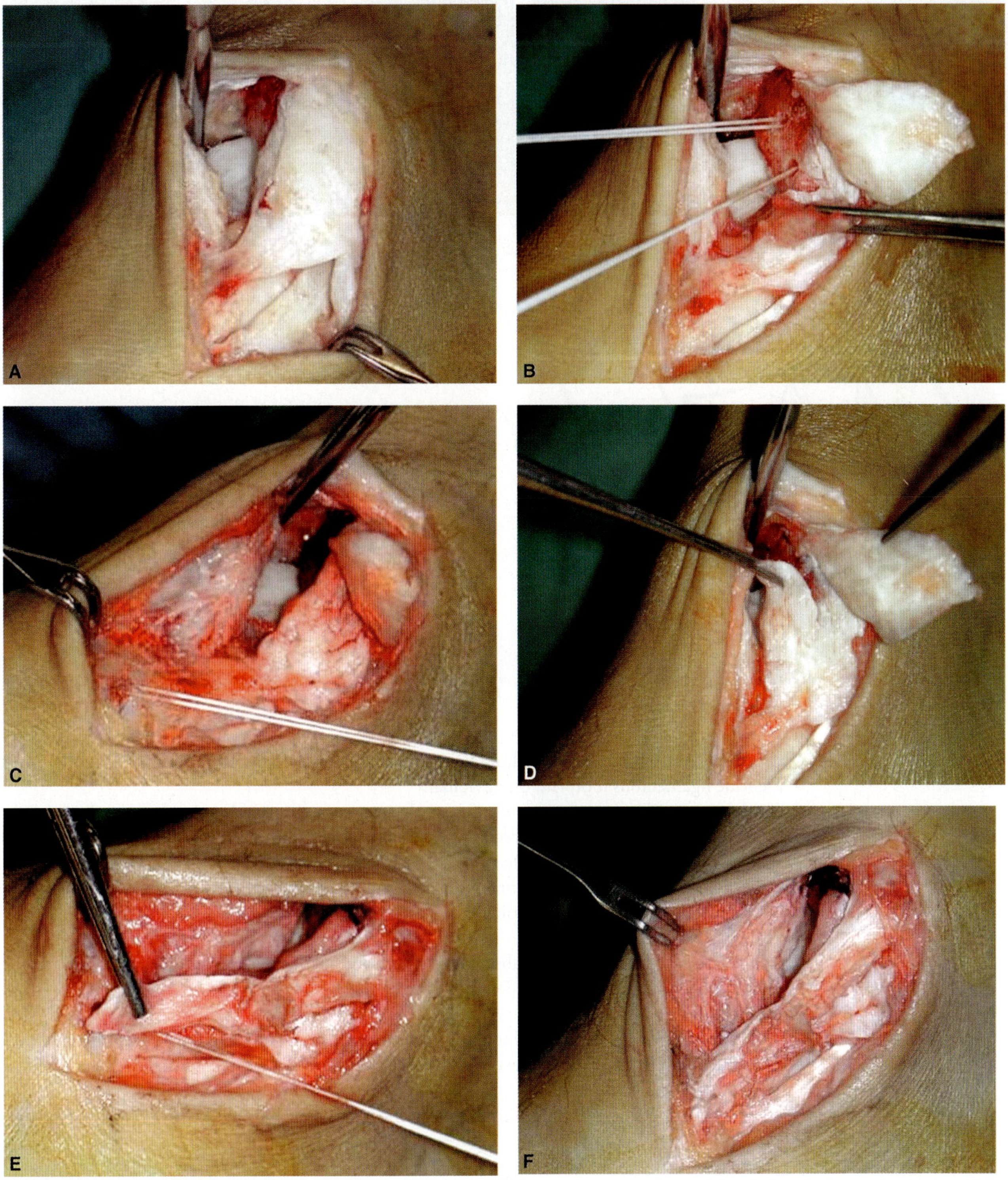

Figure 18-7. A, The superficial deltoid ligament with intermediate tear. B, Two anchors are in the medial malleolus. C, One anchor is placed into the tuberosity of the navicular. D, The deep flap is reattached to the medial malleolus using the distal anchor suture. E, The superficial flap is reattached to the tuberosity of the navicular. F, Sutures are tightened and ligament reconstruction is reconstructed. G, The superior medial malleolus anchor is used to reconstruct the tibionavicular ligament. H, Final reconstruction with overlying no. 0 resorbable sutures. I, Principle of reconstruction. Reprinted with permission from Wiesel SW. *Operative Techniques in Orthopaedic Surgery*. 1st ed. Philadelphia, PA: Wolters Kluwer, Lippincott Williams & Wilkins; 2010. Figure 104.TechFig5a-i.

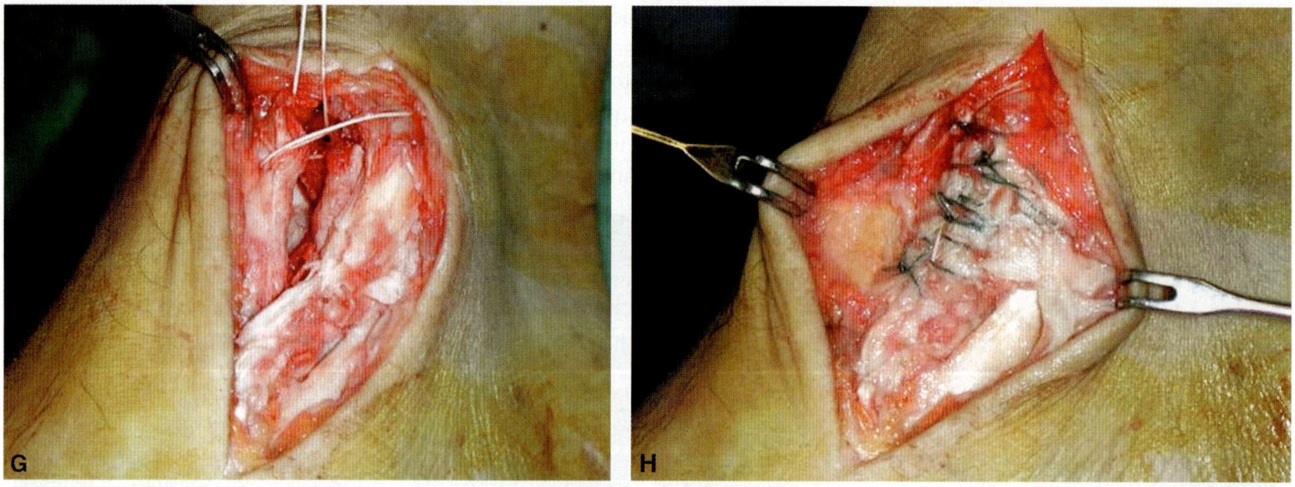

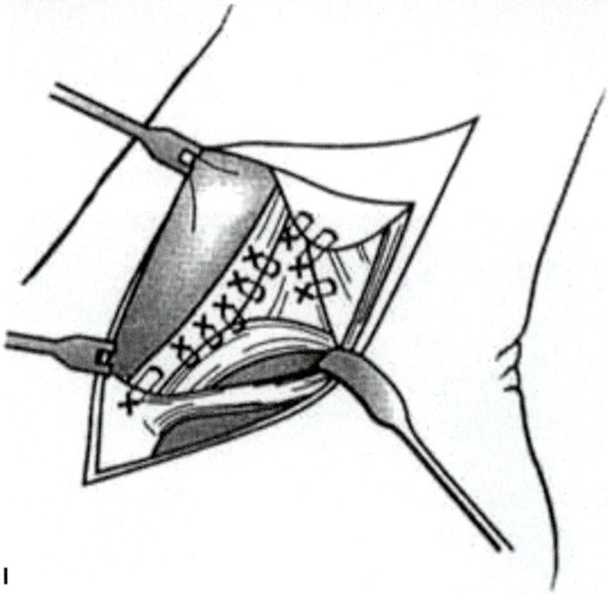

Figure 18-7. *(continued)*

- Reconstruction of the superficial deltoid ligament: distal tear or avulsion (Figure 18-8)
  - Debride ligamentous footprint on navicular.
  - Place suture anchor in navicular tuberosity, place two nonabsorbable sutures in the tibiospring ligament. Tighten the sutures to reconstruct tibionavicular and tibiospring ligaments, and secure with an overlying no. 0 absorbable suture.
- Reconstruction of deep deltoid ligament: allograft reconstruction with tibial, talar (deep deltoid), and calcaneal limbs (superficial deltoid) (Figures 18-9 to 18-12)
  - Use semitendinosus allograft.
  - Tubularize each limb with a nonabsorbable suture and measure diameter of each limb for tunnel preparation.
  - Tibial limb:
    - Place guidewire at the intercollicular groove and aim at about 5 to 6 cm above the joint line lateral to the anterior tibial crest. A 6-mm reamer is used to create a tunnel over the wire to a depth of 30 to 40 mm.
    - Secure unsplit end with interference screw and TightRope button (Arthrex, Naples, Florida, USA).
  - Talar limb:
    - Insert guidewire into the medial nonarticulating portion of the talus.
      - 12 mm posterior from the anteromedial corner of the trochlea
    - Drill a 5-mm tunnel over wire to a depth of 17 to 20 mm.
    - Pass graft medial to lateral, secure with a 5-mm interference screw at medial end of the tunnel, and countersink 1 to 2 mm.

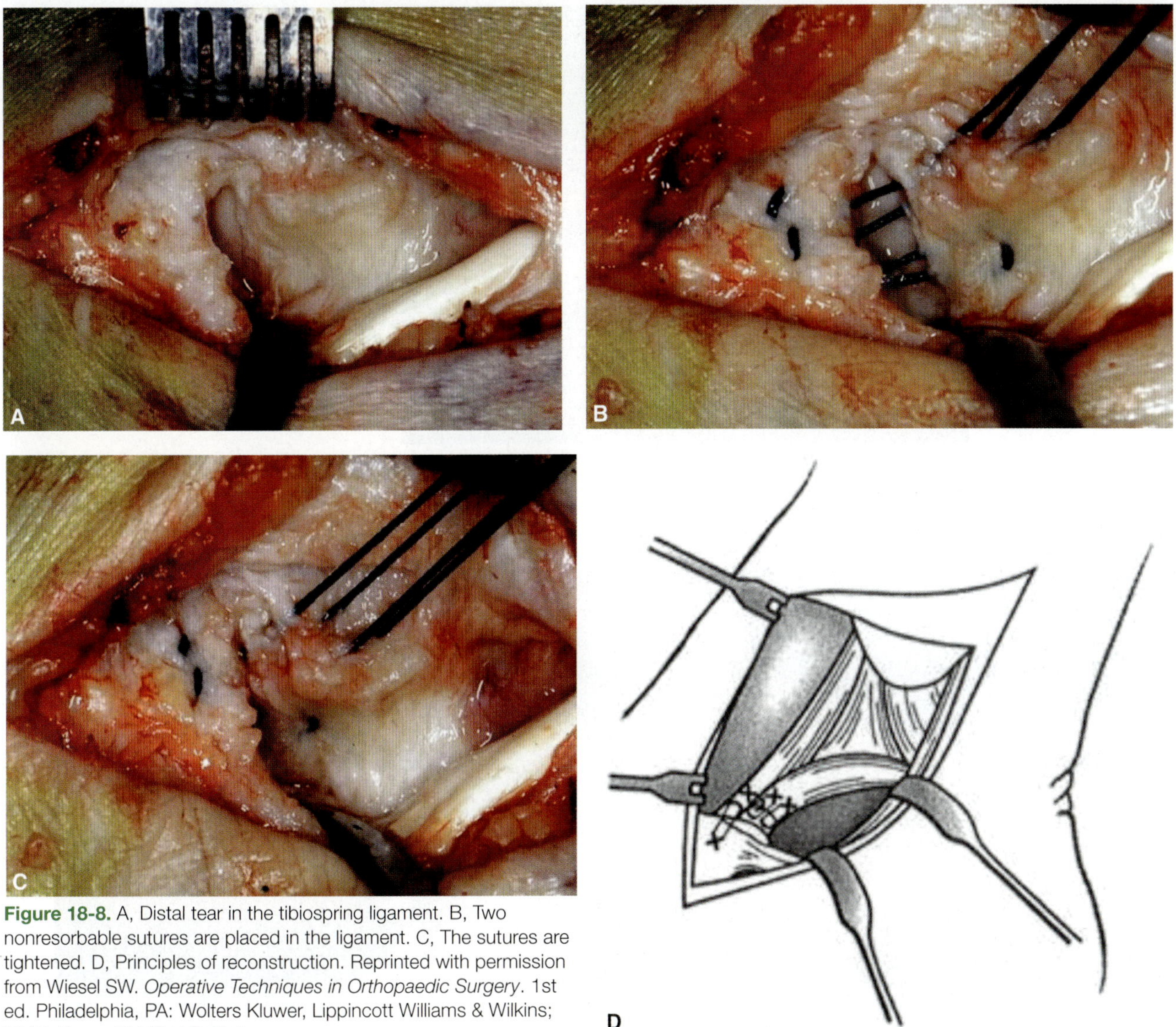

Figure 18-8. A, Distal tear in the tibiospring ligament. B, Two nonresorbable sutures are placed in the ligament. C, The sutures are tightened. D, Principles of reconstruction. Reprinted with permission from Wiesel SW. *Operative Techniques in Orthopaedic Surgery*. 1st ed. Philadelphia, PA: Wolters Kluwer, Lippincott Williams & Wilkins; 2010. Figure 104.TechFig6-d.

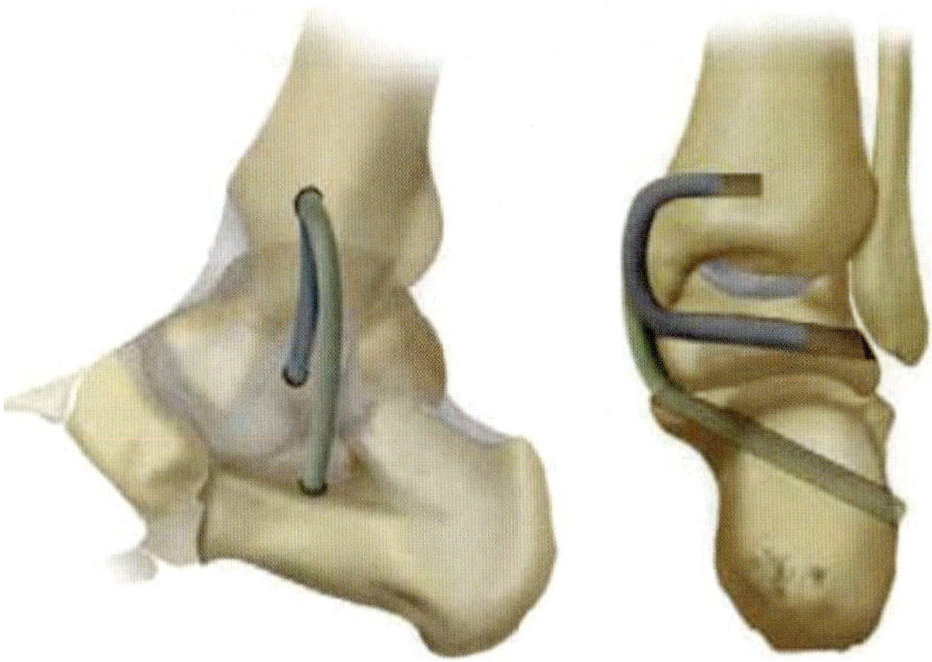

Figure 18-9. Principles of reconstruction.

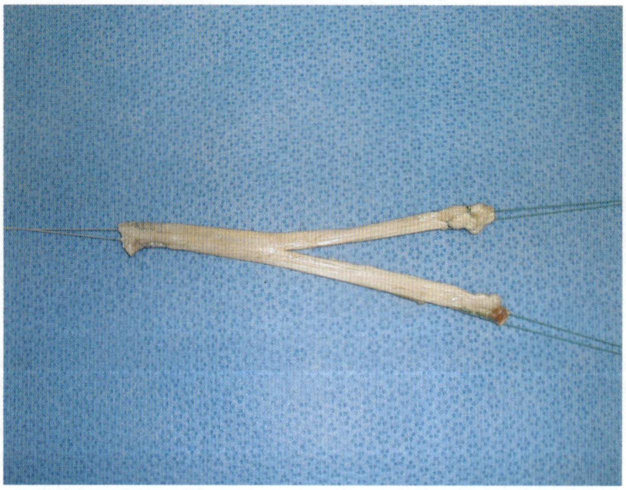

Figure 18-10. Forked allograft tendon with Krackow stitch in all limbs. Reprinted with permission from Wiesel SW. *Operative Techniques in Orthopaedic Surgery*. 1st ed. Philadelphia, PA: Wolters Kluwer, Lippincott Williams & Wilkins; 2010. Figure 103.TechFig1b.

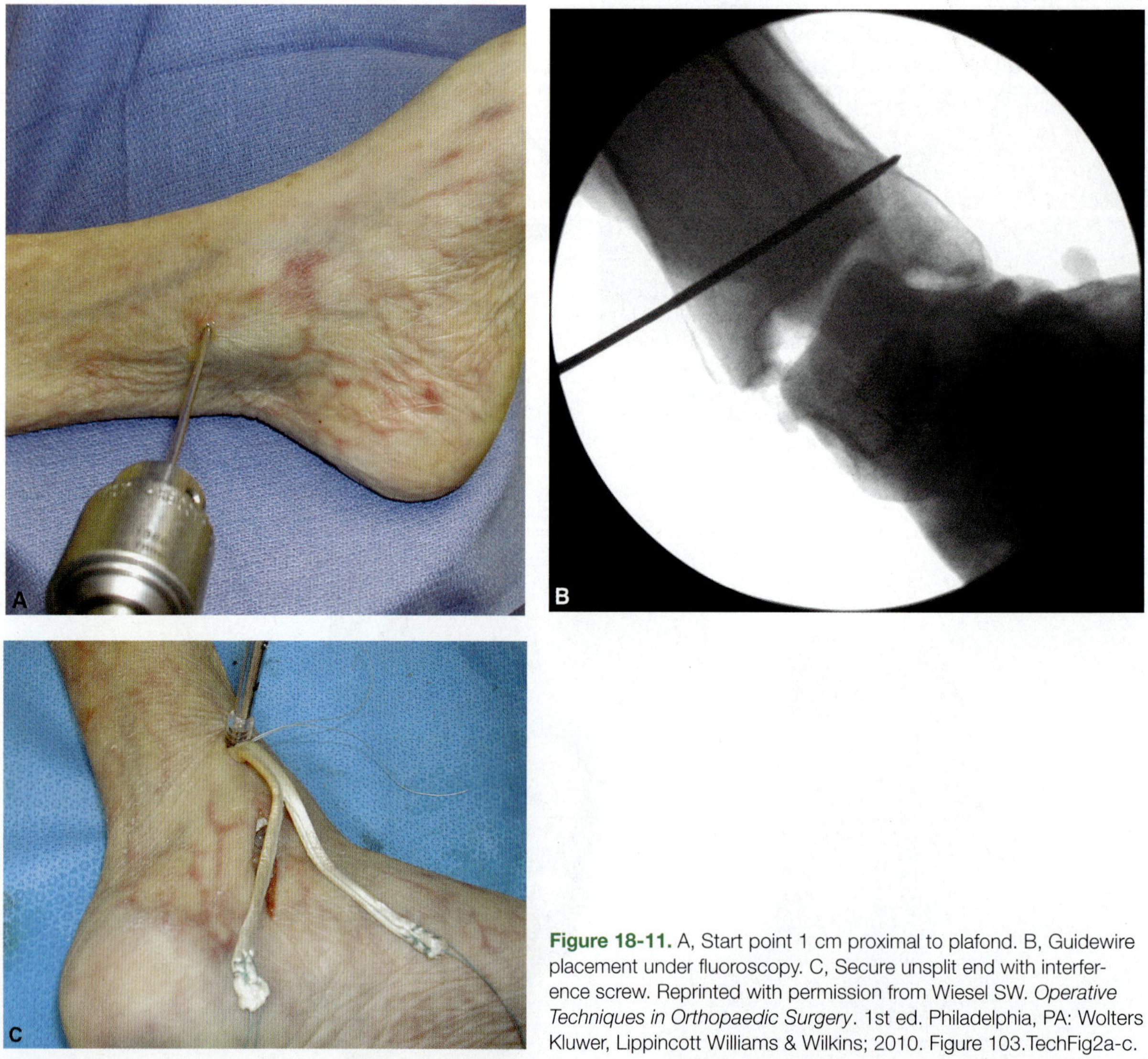

Figure 18-11. A, Start point 1 cm proximal to plafond. B, Guidewire placement under fluoroscopy. C, Secure unsplit end with interference screw. Reprinted with permission from Wiesel SW. *Operative Techniques in Orthopaedic Surgery*. 1st ed. Philadelphia, PA: Wolters Kluwer, Lippincott Williams & Wilkins; 2010. Figure 103.TechFig2a-c.

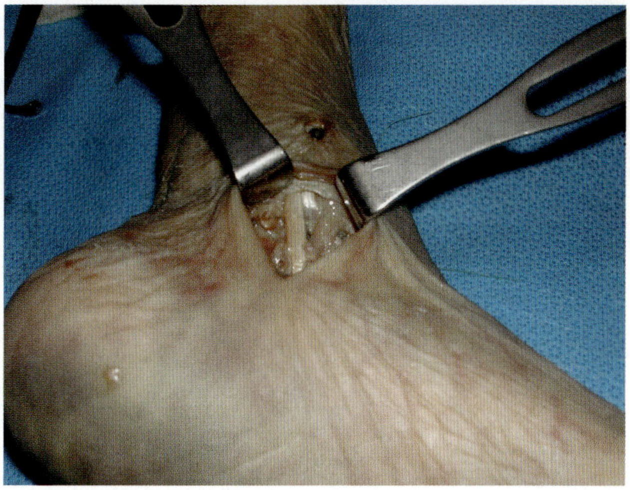

Figure 18-12. Completed deltoid ligament reconstruction. Reprinted with permission from Wiesel SW. *Operative Techniques in Orthopaedic Surgery*. 1st ed. Philadelphia, PA: Wolters Kluwer, Lippincott Williams & Wilkins; 2010. Figure 103.TechFig4b.

- Calcaneal limb:
  - Tunnel from midportion of sustentaculum to 1 cm superior to peroneal tubercle laterally. Use fluoroscopy to ensure that the subtalar joint has not been breached.
  - Pass last end of graft lateral to medial and secure with a 5-mm interference screw medially.

Postoperative Protocol

- 0 to 2 weeks: non-weight-bearing in a well-padded Jones splint
- 0 to 6 weeks: weight-bearing as tolerated in short leg fiberglass cast in neutral
- 6 to 10 weeks: weight-bearing as tolerated in CAM boot. Boot is removed for physical therapy. Active and passive range of motion initiated.
- 10 to 12 weeks: transition to regular shoe wear with ASO brace. Begin proprioceptive training.
- 12 weeks: advance activities as tolerated. ASO brace is used for first year following surgery during exercise and sports.

Suggested Readings

Giza E, Wuellner J. Acute deltoid rupture: history, diagnosis, and a repair technique. *Tech Foot Ankle Surg*. 2014;13(2):73-80.

Hsu AR. Treatment of deltoid injuries associated with ankle fractures. *Tech Foot Ankle Surg*. 2018;17(3):115-120.

Wiesel S. *Operative Techniques in Orthopaedic Surgery*. 1st ed. Philadelphia, PA: Wolters Kluwer, Lippincott Williams & Wilkins; 2010.

Chapter 19
Arthroscopic Management of Osteochondral Lesions of the Talus

YOSHIHARU SHIMOZONO
JOHN G. KENNEDY

Indications

- Symptomatic osteochondral lesions of the talus (OLT)
  - Failed conservative treatment for more than 3 months
  - Lesion size: <150 mm^2 in area or 15 mm in diameter.[1,2] Recently, lesions <100 mm^2 are regarded as the optimal size.[3]
  - Without significant bone loss (Berndt and Harty stages 2-4)

Sterile Instruments/Equipment

- Thigh tourniquet
- Ankle distractor
- Standard arthroscopic equipment
- Irrigation system (pressure: 50-60 mm Hg, fluid flow: 0.5 L/min)
- A 2.4/2.7-mm arthroscope with 30°/70° viewing angle
- A 3.5/4.5-mm shaver for soft-tissue debridement
- A small-size curette
- Microfracture pics or a 2.0-mm Kirschner wire for bone marrow stimulation (BMS)

Positioning

- The patient is positioned in the supine position with the ipsilateral hip flexed and supported by a well-padded leg holder (Figure 19-1).
- A sterile ankle distraction strap is placed around the hindfoot and midfoot (Figure 19-2).

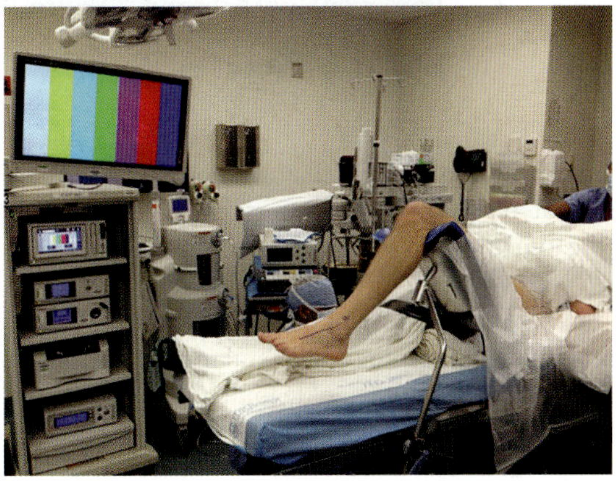

Figure 19-1. A small bump can be additionally placed under the ipsilateral pelvis to facilitate the neutral alignment of the foot and ankle.

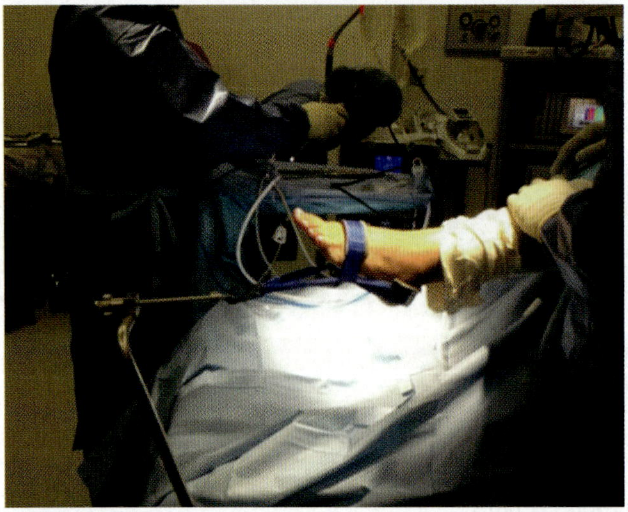

Figure 19-2. Ankle with sterile distraction strap. It is connected to a sterile bar using a band and allows the surgeon to achieve the desired degree of distraction of the ankle joint.

Knowledge About Portals

- Anteromedial, anterolateral, and, occasionally, posterolateral portals
- Before any incision, mark anatomic landmarks including lateral malleolus, medial malleolus, peroneus tertius, anterior tibial tendon, and superficial peroneal nerve (Figure 19-3). The superficial peroneal nerve is identified with plantar flexion and inversion of the foot (Figure 19-4).

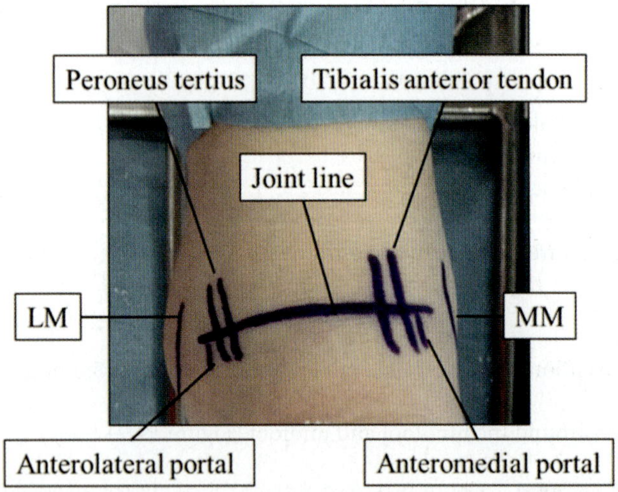

Figure 19-3. Anterior portals and landmarks. LM, lateral malleolus; MM, medial malleolus.

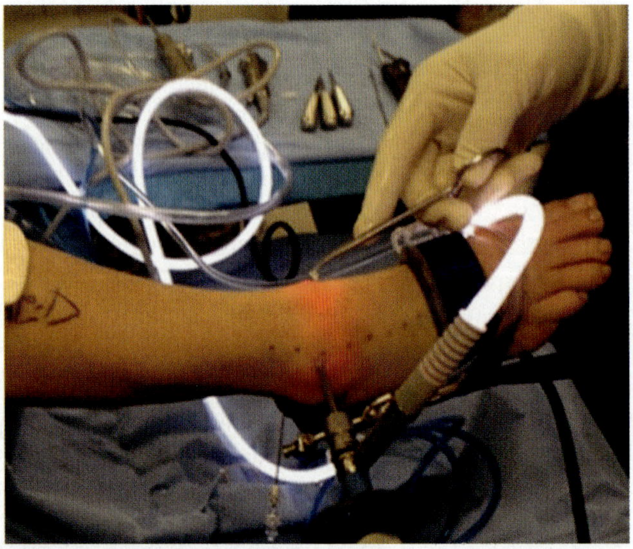

Figure 19-4. Marking the course of the superficial peroneal nerve is important before starting.

- Anteromedial portal is 1 mm medial to the medial border of anterior tibial tendon.
- Anterolateral portal is 1 mm lateral to the peroneus tertius. The location of the superficial peroneal nerve is found by flexing the fourth toe down. This can accentuate the subcutaneous course of the nerve.
- Posterolateral portal is 1 mm anterior to the lateral border of the Achilles tendon at the level between the horizontal lines of medial malleolus and lateral malleolus tips. This portal is sometimes needed to approach the posterior aspect of the ankle joint. Care should be taken about the location of the sural nerve (Figure 19-5).

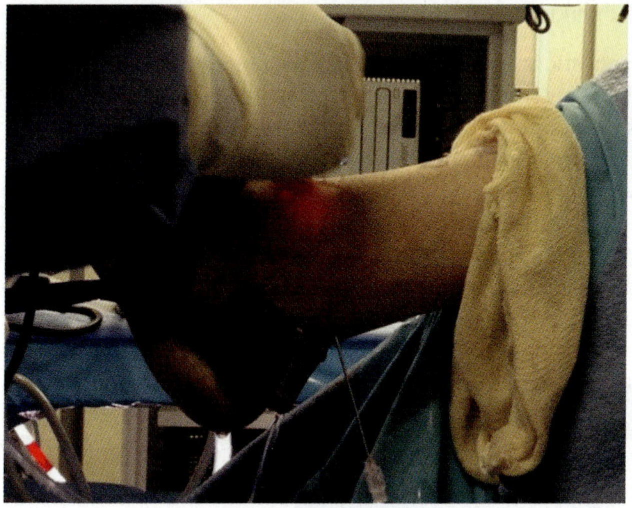

Figure 19-5. Posterolateral portal is useful both for inflow and for posterior visualization.

Operative Technique

Making the Portals

- The portals are usually made in the following order: anteromedial portal, anterolateral portal, posterolateral portal.
- A 22-gauge needle is inserted from the site of the previously marked anteromedial portal to the ankle joint and 10 mL saline is injected into the ankle joint (Figure 19-6). This allows to judge the joint orientation and to verify the correct portal position if saline is injected smoothly with overall ankle joint inflation.

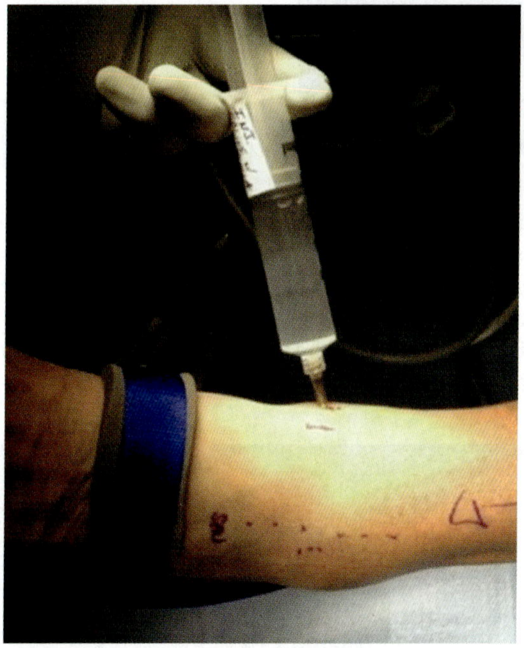

Figure 19-6. The needle is used to locate the optimal position for the portal.

- Skin cut using a #11 blade and subcutaneous blunt dissection using a mosquito clamp
- A 2.7-mm arthroscope sleeve with trocar is carefully advanced into the ankle joint, and then switched out for a 2.7-mm arthroscope.
- A 22-gauge needle is inserted from the site of the previously marked anterolateral portal to the ankle joint. Once needle is confirmed, skin cut and subcutaneous blunt dissection are performed. This can be done under direct arthroscopic visualization using the transillumination technique to avoid neurovascular injury.

Diagnostic Arthroscopy

- An organized diagnostic arthroscopy is performed initially from the anteromedial portal. A probe is placed through the anterolateral portal to palpate the talar surface.
- Cartilage lesions are examined by probing. Any loose, unstable, or degenerative cartilage needs to be removed and requires the microfracture technique.
- In some lesions where the overlying cartilage appears normal, the retrograde drilling technique is applied to preserve the intact hyaline cartilage, while stimulating the subchondral bone revascularization.
- The location of pathology guides surgical treatment strategies. A nine-zone grid of the articular cartilage based on magnetic resonance imaging allows for accurate descriptions of the location of osteochondral lesion (OCLs) (Figure 19-7).[4]

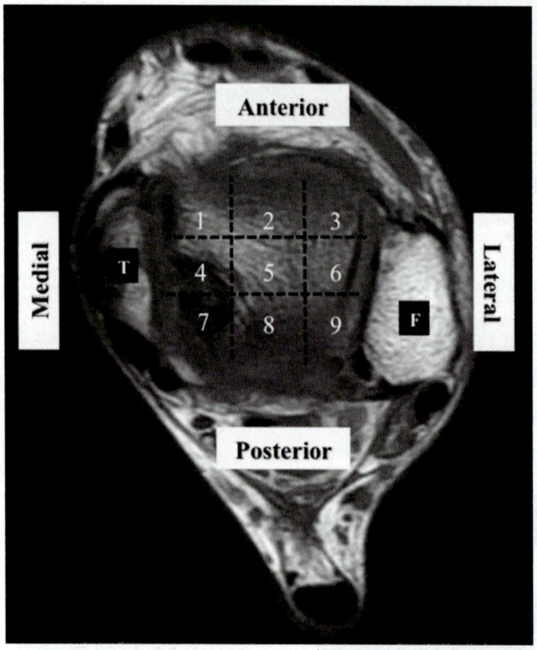

Figure 19-7. Anatomic nine-zone grid of the axial talar dome, with zones 1, 4, and 7 positioned on the medial talus and zones 1, 2, and 3 positioned anteriorly.

- In general, during the surgical procedure, the arthroscope is placed on the side opposite to the lesions and the instruments are inserted through the portal on the same side as the lesions.
- Concomitant disorders are common. They should be treated at the same time.
  - Soft- and bony-tissue impingement, ligament injuries (Figure 19-8)
  - The procedures for cartilage lesions should be performed last, when performed with other intra-articular procedures.

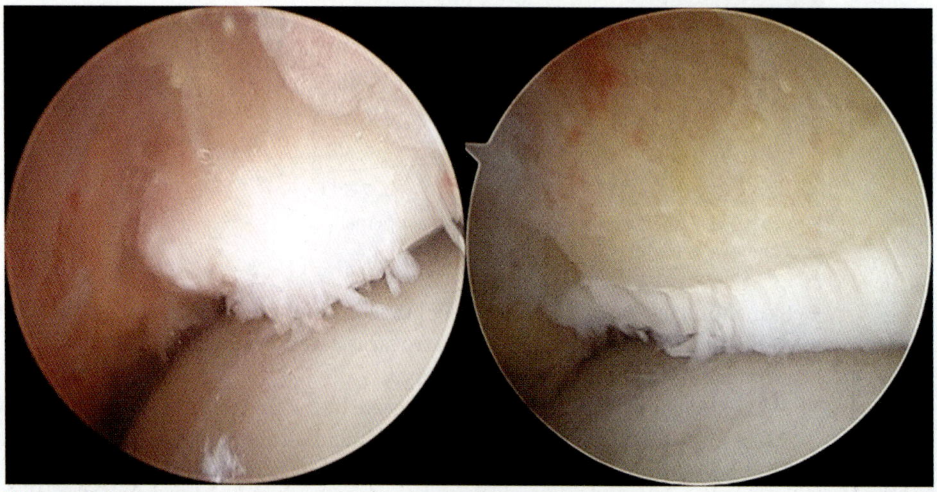

Figure 19-8. Tibial bony impingement (left), after resection of the osteophyte using a shaver and burr (right).

Retrograde Drilling

- For medial lesions, a 0.45 K-wire is introduced via the lateral process of the talus. Under the guidance of the fluoroscopy, the K-wire is directed into the center of the lesion.
- Care should be taken not to penetrate the articular cartilage surface with direct visualization of the arthroscope.
- A 3.5-mm cannulated drill is introduced over the K-wire into the lesion fluoroscopically. The angled curette is then inserted into the drill hole and the cystic lesion is debrided entirely (Figure 19-9).
- The remaining cavity is filled with calcium sulfate, to support the overlying cartilage (Figure 19-10).[5]
- For lateral lesions, the insertion site of a K-wire is the anteromedial talus at the junction of the deltoid and the tibiospring ligament. The remaining procedure is similar to that for medial lesions.

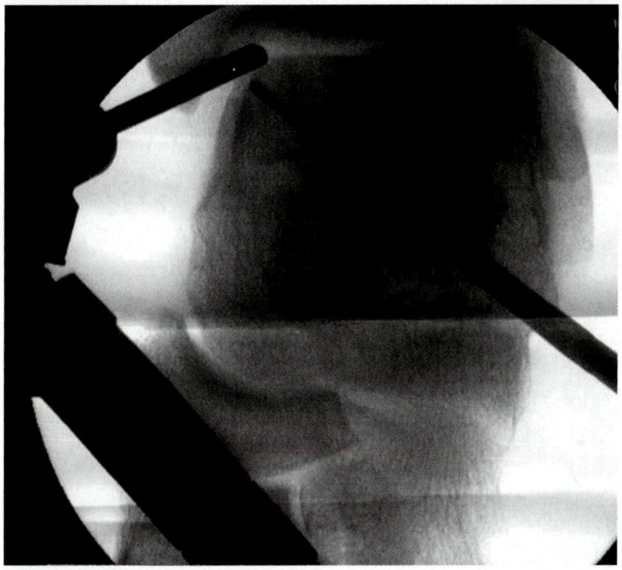

Figure 19-9. Fluoroscopic view of debridement of the cystic lesion with a curette via a drill hole.

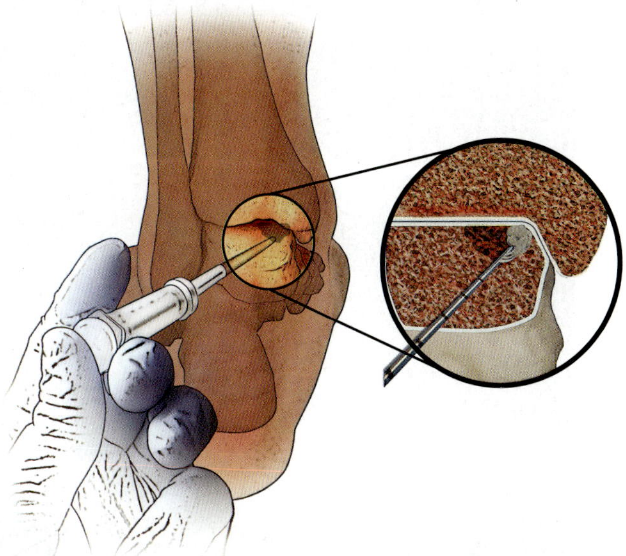

Figure 19-10. The cystic cavity is filled with calcium sulfate.

Microfracture

Debridement of Unstable Cartilage, Necrotic Bone, and Calcified Layer

- Almost all appropriately sized OLTs in any location can be treated arthroscopically through standard portals. Rarely, accessory portals may be required to get optimal access.
- The articular cartilage is evaluated with a probe. All degenerated or unstable cartilage is removed with a sharp curette (Figure 19-11).
- Necrotic bone and the calcified layer are removed with the curette and the motorized suction shaver.
- Care is taken to avoid iatrogenic cartilage injury using multiple instruments and changing portals for better visualization.
- Debridement should be performed carefully. Failure to excise loose fragment and dead cartilage will lead to failure.
- Finally, the stable rim of the remaining cartilage is confirmed (Figure 19-12).

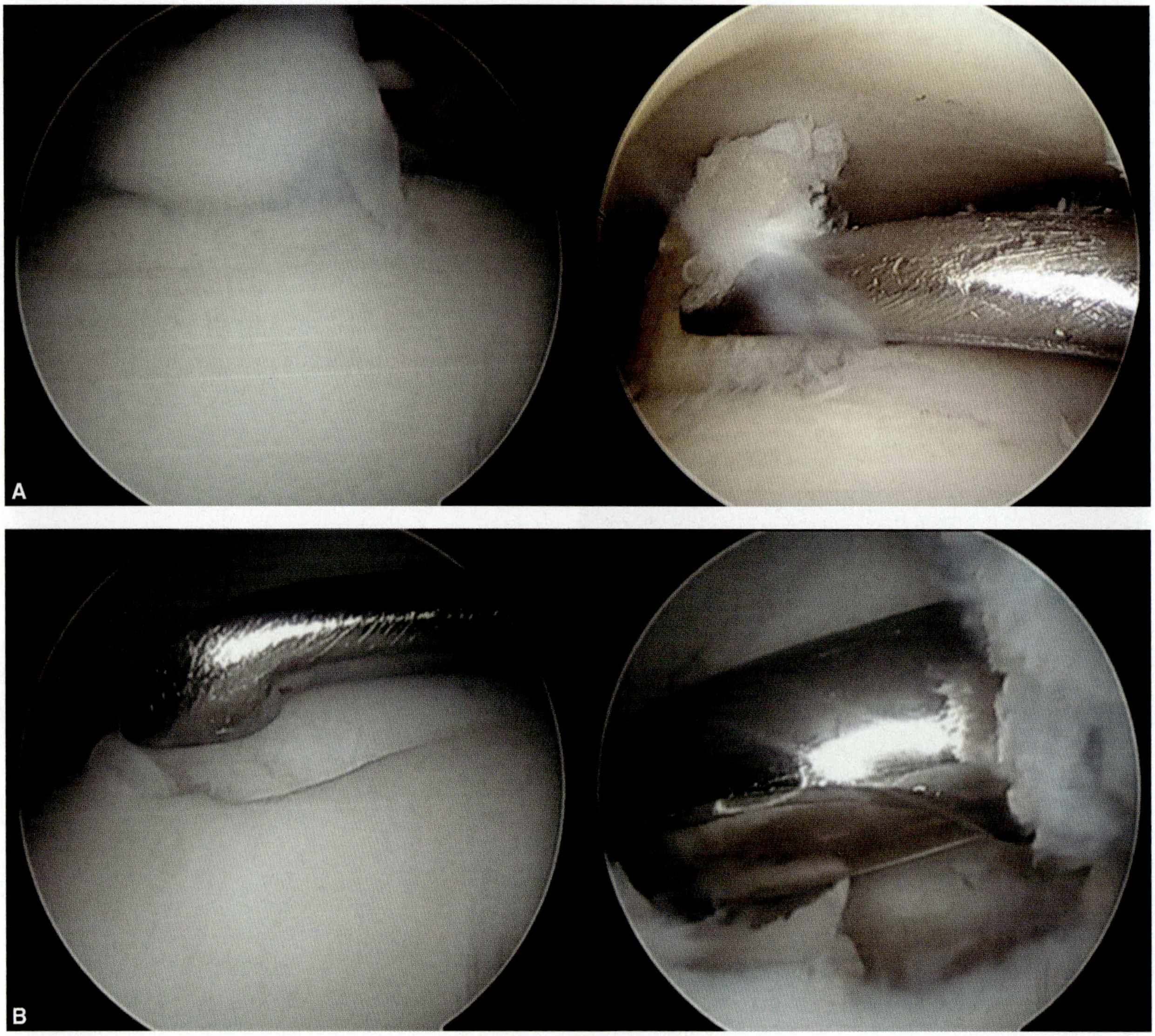

Figure 19-11. A, Unstable articular cartilage fragment on the talar dome (left). A probe is used to elevate an unstable cartilage (right). B, Curettage of the lesion (left). A motorized shaver can assist in removing large flaps, necrotic bone, and calcified layers (right).

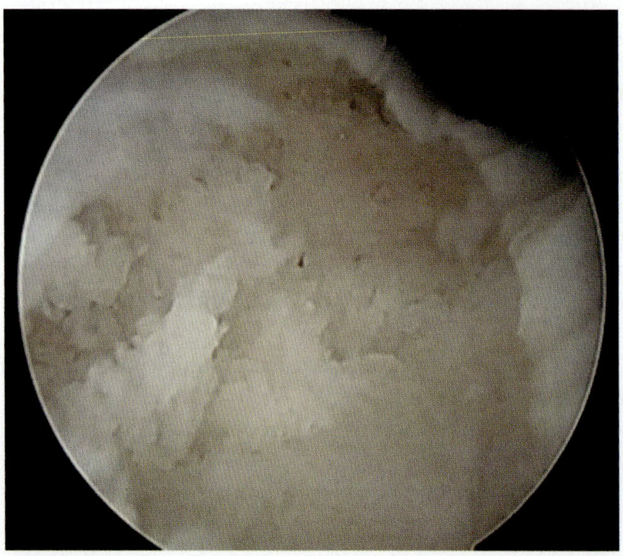

Figure 19-12. The cartilage defect after debridement of degenerated tissue and calcified layer with creation of stable shoulders.

Penetration of Subchondral Bone Plate

- Microfracture is performed to penetrate the subchondral bone plate using microfracture awls (Figure 19-13). The aim of the procedure is to stimulate mesenchymal stem cells to promote fibrous cartilage repair tissue. The holes are traditionally placed 3 to 4 mm apart and at a depth of 3 mm.

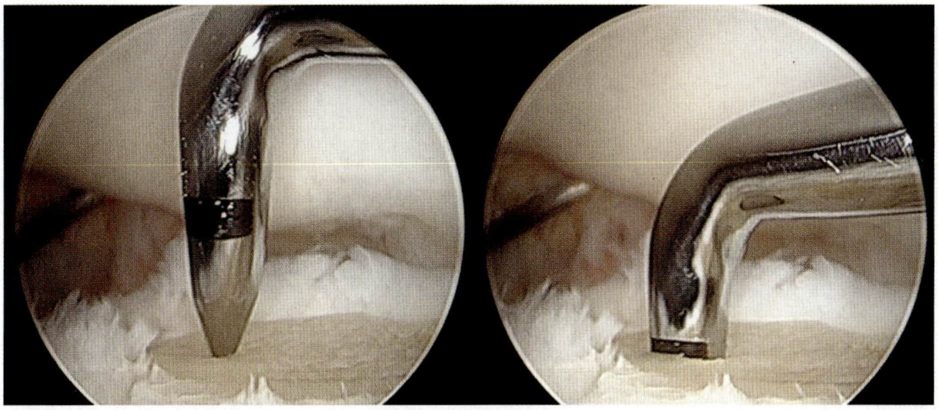

Figure 19-13. Microfracture awl with right-angled tip is used to perform multiple penetrations of the base of the lesion.

- Microfracture awls are commercially available with different angled tips. The surgeon can choose the appropriate angled tip to provide perpendicular tip alignment to the defect surface.
- The subchondral bone plate is damaged by the procedure and it is not likely to adequately remodel. Therefore, microfracture should be performed with small-diameter microfracture awls to reduce the damage to the subchondral bone, resulting in improvement in the quality and longevity of the cartilage repair tissue.
- After creating the holes, it is important to observe blood inflow from the holes by decreasing the inflow pressure (Figure 19-14).

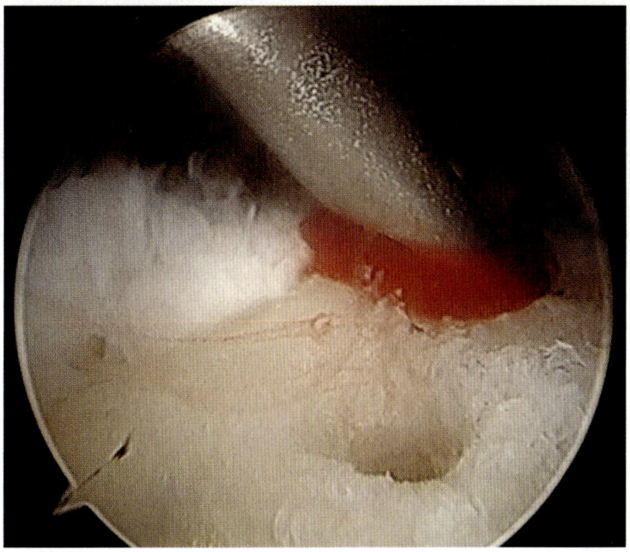

Figure 19-14. Lowered inflow pressure confirms the adequate depth of the holes by observing the marrow elements arising from the holes into the joint.

For Cystic OLT

- Cystic lesions should be completely excised and/or microfractured. A probe is used to open the cyst and remove the gelatinous material within the cysts. After curettage and debridement, microfracture is performed in areas where the subchondral bone is intact. This should be followed by bone grafting from the calcaneus if the loss of subchondral bone is large (Figure 19-15).

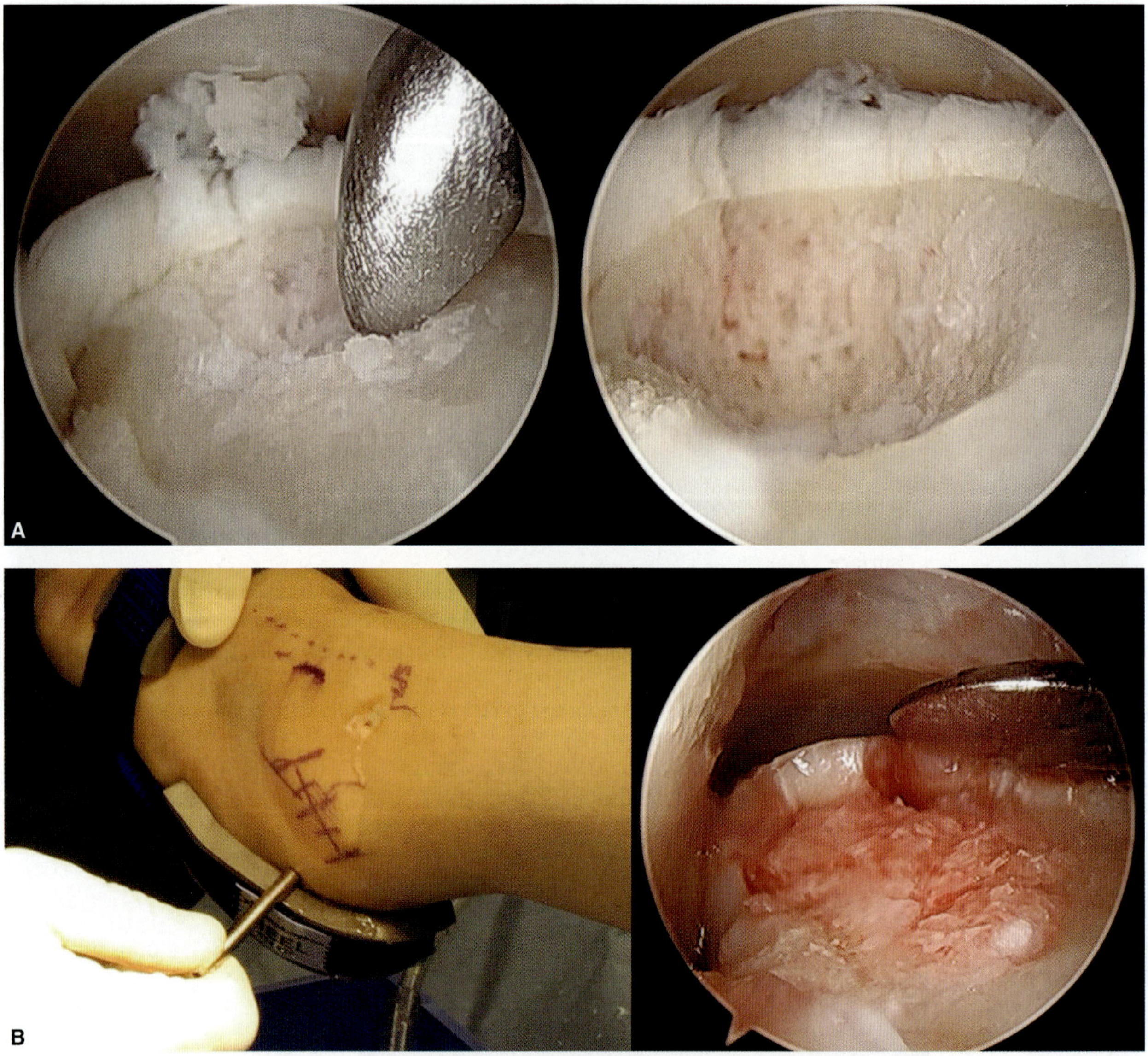

Figure 19-15. A, The cyst is identified by probing, and the curettage is performed. The cystic lesions should be completely excised. B, Calcaneal autograft can be easily obtained using a trephine with a small skin incision (left). Care should be taken to avoid the sural nerve. Bone grafting of smooth surface with adjacent bones by molding (right).

Biologic Adjuvants

- Biologics including platelet-rich plasma (PRP) and concentrated bone marrow aspirate (CBMA) is injected into the bed of the lesion in an attempt to improve the cartilage repair (Figure 19-16).[6]

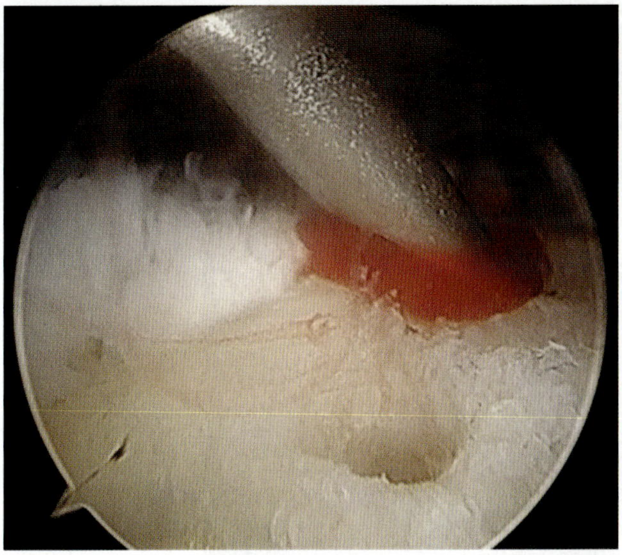

Figure 19-16. Concentrated bone marrow aspirate or platelet-rich plasma is applied over the microfracture defect.

BioCartilage

- BioCartilage (Arthrex, Inc., Naples, FL, USA) is an extracellular matrix cartilage allograft, which contains type II collagen, proteoglycans, and cartilaginous growth factors. It is used as a biologic adjuvant to BMS. The principle of BioCartilage is to serve as a scaffold over cartilage defects by providing a tissue network, and improve the quality of tissue healing.[7]
- After the microfracture procedure, BioCartilage is applied over the defects. The following procedures are performed in a dry arthroscopy technique.
- The BioCartilage is mixed with CBMA or PRP and then the mixture is applied into the defect (Figure 19-17). They are smoothed out within the defect and should be flush or slightly recessed compared to the surrounding articular cartilage surface.
- Finally, fibrin or platelet-poor plasma should be applied over the top of the BioCartilage to cover the defect (Figure 19-18).

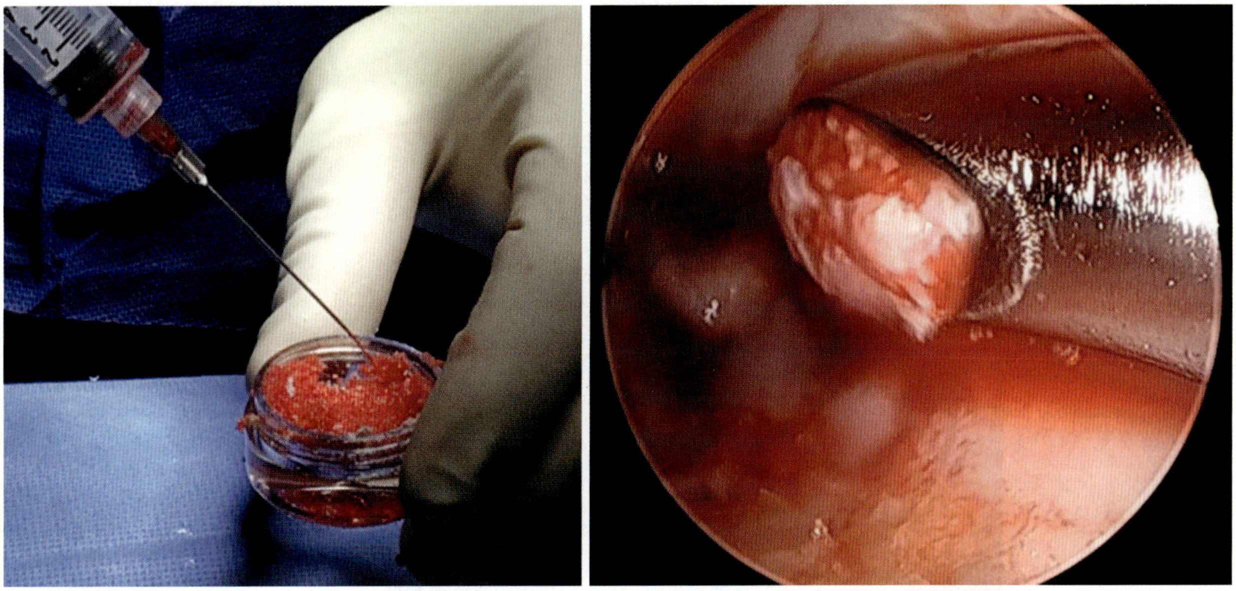

Figure 19-17. Concentrated bone marrow aspirate or platelet-rich plasma is added to BioCartilage (left). BioCartilage is introduced over the defect under dry condition (right).

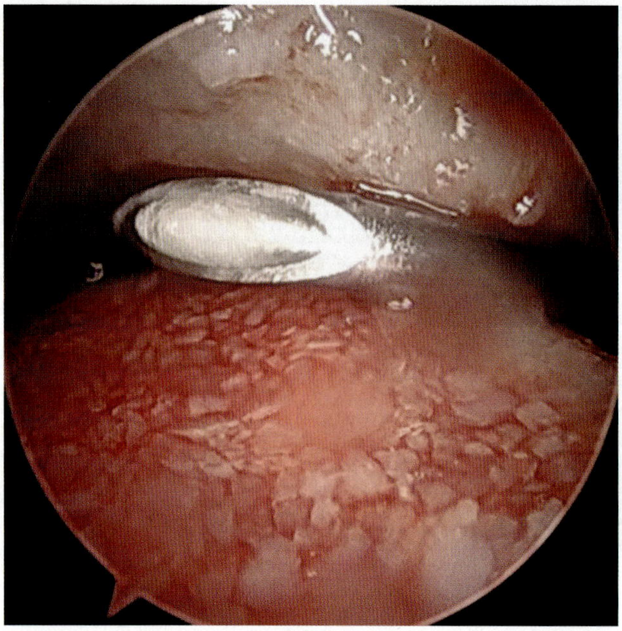

Figure 19-18. Fibrin glue is applied over the top of the BioCartilage.

Trap Door Procedure

- In the juvenile population, the lesions have greater healing potential than the equivalent lesions in adults. In these cases, internal fixation of OCLs, called the trap door procedure, is a good alternative technique.[8]
- This technique is carried out arthroscopically as follows: (1) lifting the osteochondral flap, (2) debridement of the subchondral bone and BMS, (3) grafting using cancellous bone or demineralized bone allograft, and (4) fixation of the flap with Bio-Compression screw(s) (Arthrex) or chondral dart(s) (Arthrex).
- The location of the defect is identified by palpating the cartilage with a probe. An osteochondral flap is created by making a sharp rim with a beaver knife. The posterior side of the flap is left intact.
- With a probe, the osteochondral flap is lifted up (Figure 19-19). An attached bone of the osteochondral flap is drilled to promote the revascularization and the sclerotic bone of the bed is debrided with a curette and microfractured using awls.

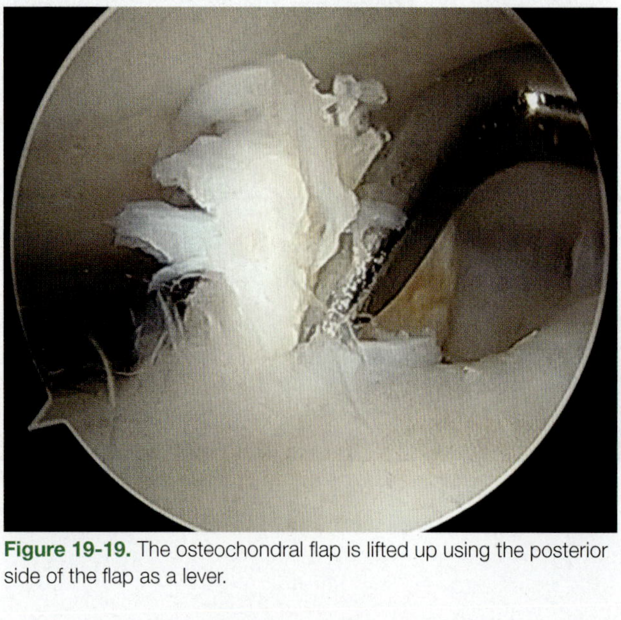

Figure 19-19. The osteochondral flap is lifted up using the posterior side of the flap as a lever.

- The defect is filled with cancellous bone autograft or demineralized bone matrix allograft (Figure 19-20). Cancellous bone is harvested from the calcaneus, as mentioned.
- Finally, the osteochondral flap is reduced and fixed with Bio-Compression screw(s) or chondral dart(s) (Figure 19-21). By bringing the ankle in plantar flexion, the fixation procedure can be performed throughout arthroscopically. If it is difficult to perform arthroscopically when the lesion is located in a posterior position, a transmalleolar approach can be applied.

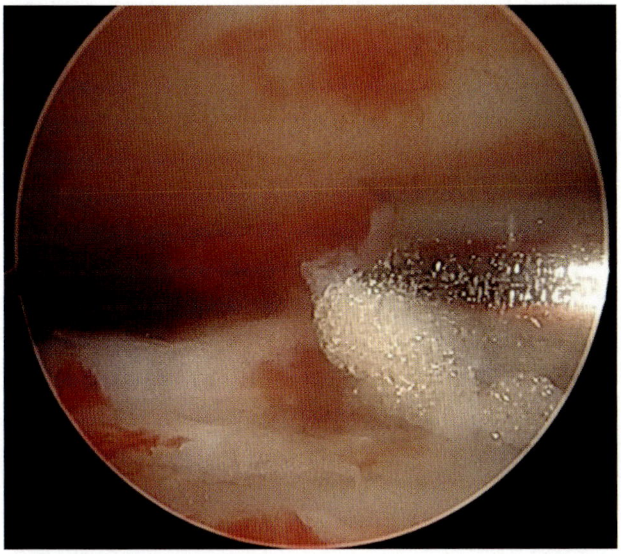

Figure 19-20. Demineralized bone matrix allograft is transported to the defect.

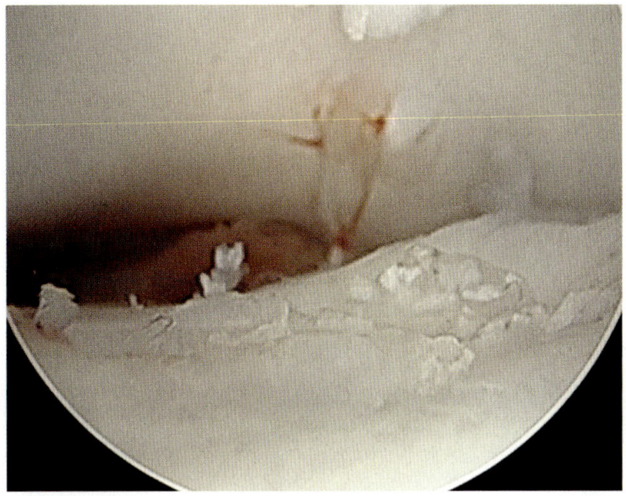

Figure 19-21. The flap is fixed with a chondral dart.

References

1. Chuckpaiwong B, Berkson EM, Theodore GH. Microfracture for osteochondral lesions of the ankle: outcome analysis and outcome predictors of 105 cases. *Arthroscopy*. 2008;24:106-112.
2. Choi WJ, Park KK, Kim BS, Lee JW. Osteochondral lesion of the talus: is there a critical defect size for poor outcome? *Am J Sports Med*. 2009;37(10):1974-1980.
3. Ramponi L, Yasui Y, Murawski CD, et al. Lesion size is a predictor of clinical outcomes after bone marrow stimulation for osteochondral lesions of the talus: a systematic review. *Am J Sports Med*. 2017;45(7):1698-1705.
4. Elias I, Zoga AC, Morrison WB, Besser MP, Schweitzer ME, Raikin SM. Osteochondral lesions of the talus: localization and morphologic data from 424 patients using a novel anatomical grid scheme. *Foot Ankle Int*. 2007;28(2):154-161.
5. Kennedy JG, Suero EM, O'Loughlin PF, Brief A, Bohne WH. Clinical tips: retrograde drilling of talar osteochondral defects. *Foot Ankle Int*. 2008;29(6):616-619.
6. Smyth NA, Murawski CD, Haleem AM, Hannon CP, Savage-Elliott I, Kennedy JG. Establishing proof of concept: platelet-rich plasma and bone marrow aspirate concentrate may improve cartilage repair following surgical treatment for osteochondral lesions of the talus. *World J Orthop*. 2012;3(7):101-108.
7. Fortier LA, Chapman HS, Pownder SL, et al. BioCartilage improves cartilage repair compared with microfracture alone in an equine model of full-thickness cartilage loss. *Am J Sports Med*. 2016;44(9):2366-2374.
8. Kerkhoffs GM, Reilingh ML, Gerards RM, de Leeuw PA. Lift, drill, fill and fix (LDFF): a new arthroscopic treatment for talar osteochondral defects. *Knee Surg Sports Traumatol Arthrosc*. 2016;24(4):1265-1271.

Chapter 20
Autologous Osteochondral Transplantation

YOSHIHARU SHIMOZONO
JOHN G. KENNEDY

Indications

- Large osteochondral lesions of the talus (OLTs), generally considered as lesion size >150 mm^2 in area or 15 mm in diameter.[1,2] Recently, smaller lesions >100 mm are regarded as the optimal size.[3]
- Secondary procedure for failed arthroscopic bone marrow stimulation technique[4]
- OLTs with large cystic subchondral defects (Berndt and Harty stage 5)[5]

Sterile Instruments/Equipment

- Thigh tourniquet
- Standard surgical instruments for osteotomy and exposure of the ankle joint
- Specially designed instruments for autologous osteochondral transplant (AOT) procedure
  - Recipient sizer, recipient harvester, donor harvester, and tamp
- K-wires, cannulated drill set, and screws (3.5/4.0 mm)
- Fluoroscopy

Positioning

- The patient is positioned in the supine position. The level of the heel is set around the edge of the table.

Operative Technique

- The surgical approach is determined by the location of the OLT. If the lesions are located in the anterior aspect of the talar dome, a mini-open arthrotomy can be applied. However, if the lesions are located in the central or posterior position, the osteotomy is required to expose the lesions because a perpendicular approach to the lesions is important for implantation.

Tibial Osteotomy

Medial Malleolar Osteotomy

- As most of the medial OLT are located in the center of the posterior position, a medial malleolar osteotomy is usually required for medial lesions.
- A skin incision is made over the medial malleolus after palpation of the medial corner of the joint line (Figure 20-1).
- Expose medial corner of anterior aspect of tibia to prepare a chevron-type osteotomy. A provisional K-wire is inserted to visualize the osteotomy site under the guidance of fluoroscopy (Figure 20-2).

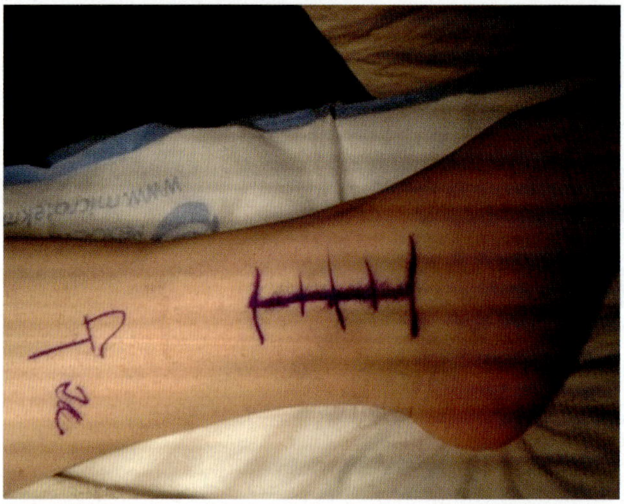

Figure 20-1. A longitudinal incision centered over the medial malleolus.

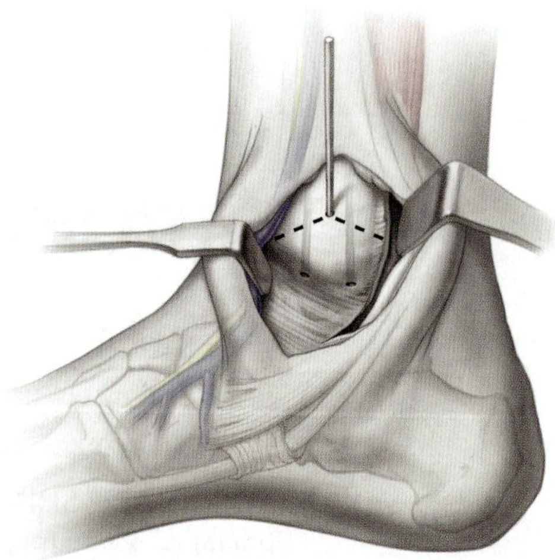

Figure 20-2. A provisional K-wire is drilled to visualize the osteotomy site fluoroscopically. A chevron-type osteotomy is then made in the medial malleolus. Illustrations copyright of and reproduced with permission from J. G. Kennedy, MD. Reproduction without express written consent is prohibited.

- Before performing the osteotomy, two parallel fixation holes are predrilled in the medial malleolus for a later anatomic screw fixation (Figure 20-3).
- A chevron-type osteotomy is performed using a bone saw and an osteotome. This type of osteotomy provides appropriate alignment, stability after fixation, and large surface area for healing. Cold saline should be used to prevent thermal necrosis at the osteotomy site. The bone saw is stopped at the subchondral bone, and the osteotomy is completed by an osteotome to protect the posterior tibial tendon and minimize the articular cartilage damage (Figure 20-4).
- The malleolar fragment is retracted in the plantar direction to allow adequate visualization and access to the medial talar dome (Figure 20-5).

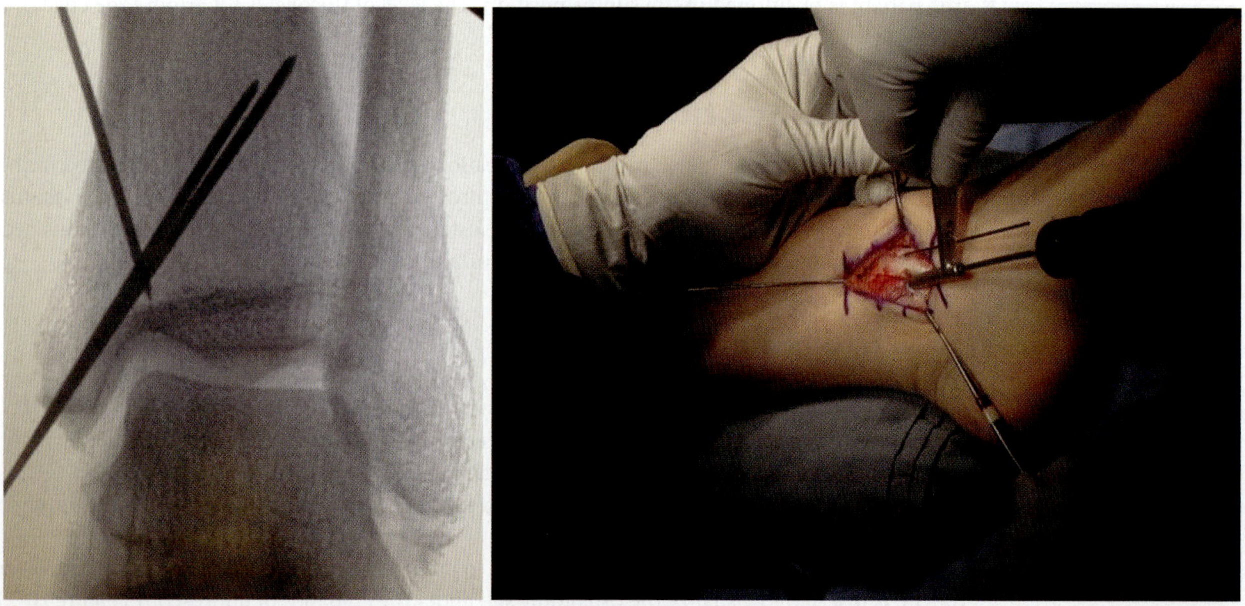

Figure 20-3. The osteotomy site is determined under the guidance of fluoroscopy (left). Predrilling the medial malleolus with two parallel fixation holes crossing the proposed osteotomy (right).

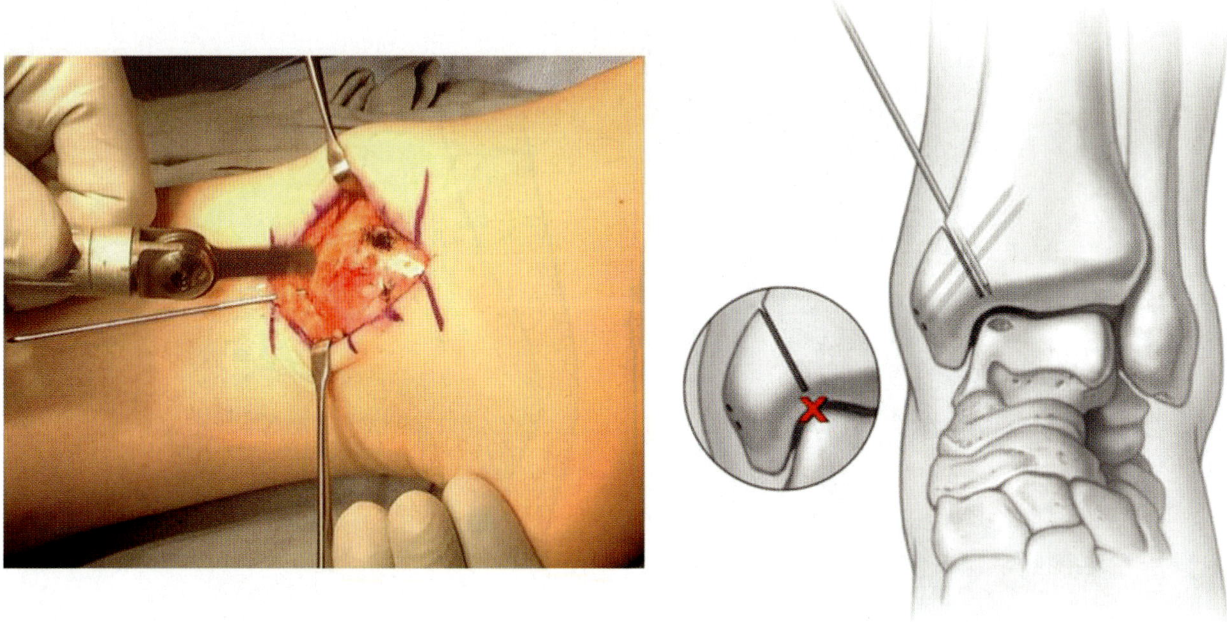

Figure 20-4. Medial malleolar osteotomy started with bone saw parallel to the K-wire (left). The remainder of osteotomy is completed with a sharp osteotome (right). Illustrations copyright of and reproduced with permission from J. G. Kennedy, MD. Reproduction without express written consent is prohibited.

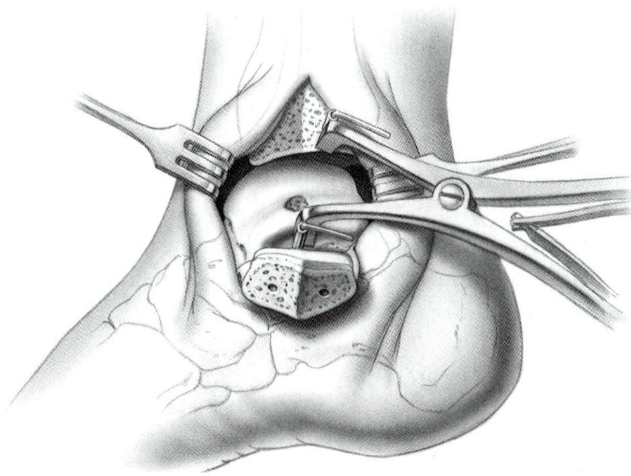

Figure 20-5. Plantar displacement of the osteotomized medial malleolus allows exposure of the medial aspect of the talar dome. Illustrations copyright of and reproduced with permission from J. G. Kennedy, MD. Reproduction without express written consent is prohibited.

Anterolateral Tibial Osteotomy

- Anterolateral lesions can be approached by arthrotomy with plantar flexing the ankle joint. However, central or posterior lesions require an osteotomy of the tibia or fibula. Access to centrolateral lesions and most posterolateral lesions can be obtained by an anterolateral tibial osteotomy (Figure 20-6).[6]
- A trapezoidal osteotomy minimizes articular damage.
- The site of the proposed osteotomy is predrilled for subsequent fixation with a 4-mm titanium screw.

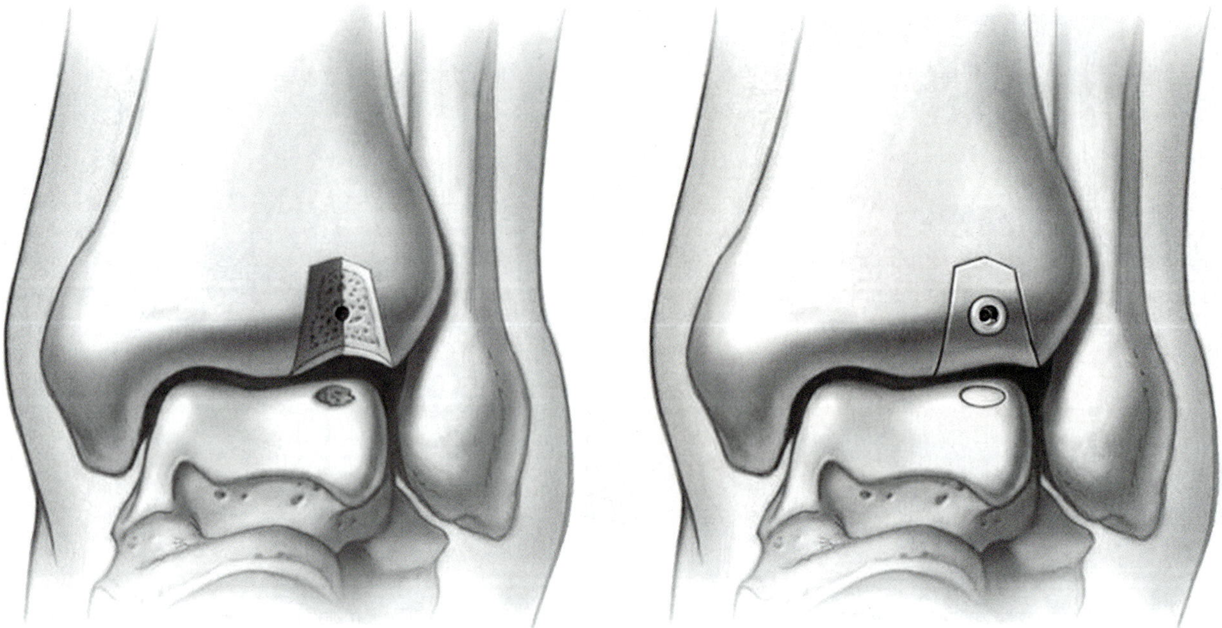

Figure 20-6. Anterolateral tibial osteotomy (left). Fixation of the osteotomy following the osteochondral graft implantation (right). Illustrations copyright of and reproduced with permission from J. G. Kennedy, MD. Reproduction without express written consent is prohibited.

Determining the Graft Size

- Debride the damaged cartilage and bone from the talus using a curette and rongeur. Debridement should be performed thoroughly to achieve a viable and stable cartilage rim.
- The lesion size is measured, and the required graft size and number are determined. The options of recipient size are generally 6, 8, and 10 mm in the AOT instruments set. The appropriate-sized recipient trephine is placed into the defect site. The orientation of the recipient harvester trephine should be maintained perpendicular to the lesion. The lesion is then removed using the trephine to 10 mm depth (Figure 20-7).
- Bone marrow stimulation is added to the surrounding healthy bone using a 0.45 K-wire. The base of the graft site is overdrilled by a further 2 mm using an acorn-shaped drill tip, resulting in a total graft depth of 12 mm (Figure 20-8).

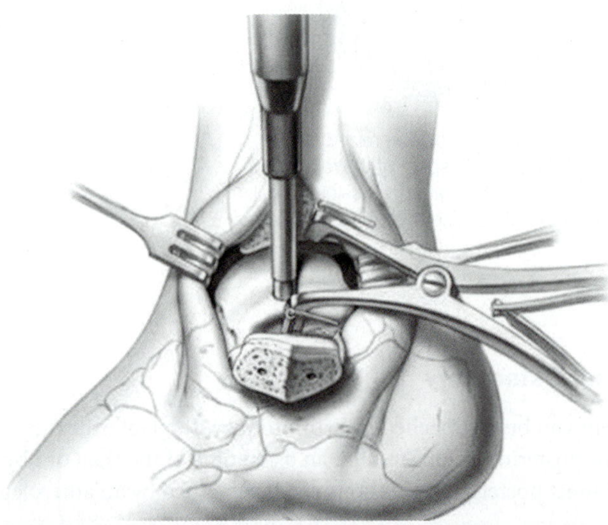

Figure 20-7. The recipient harvester trephine is placed in the talar defect. Illustrations copyright of and reproduced with permission from J. G. Kennedy, MD. Reproduction without express written consent is prohibited.

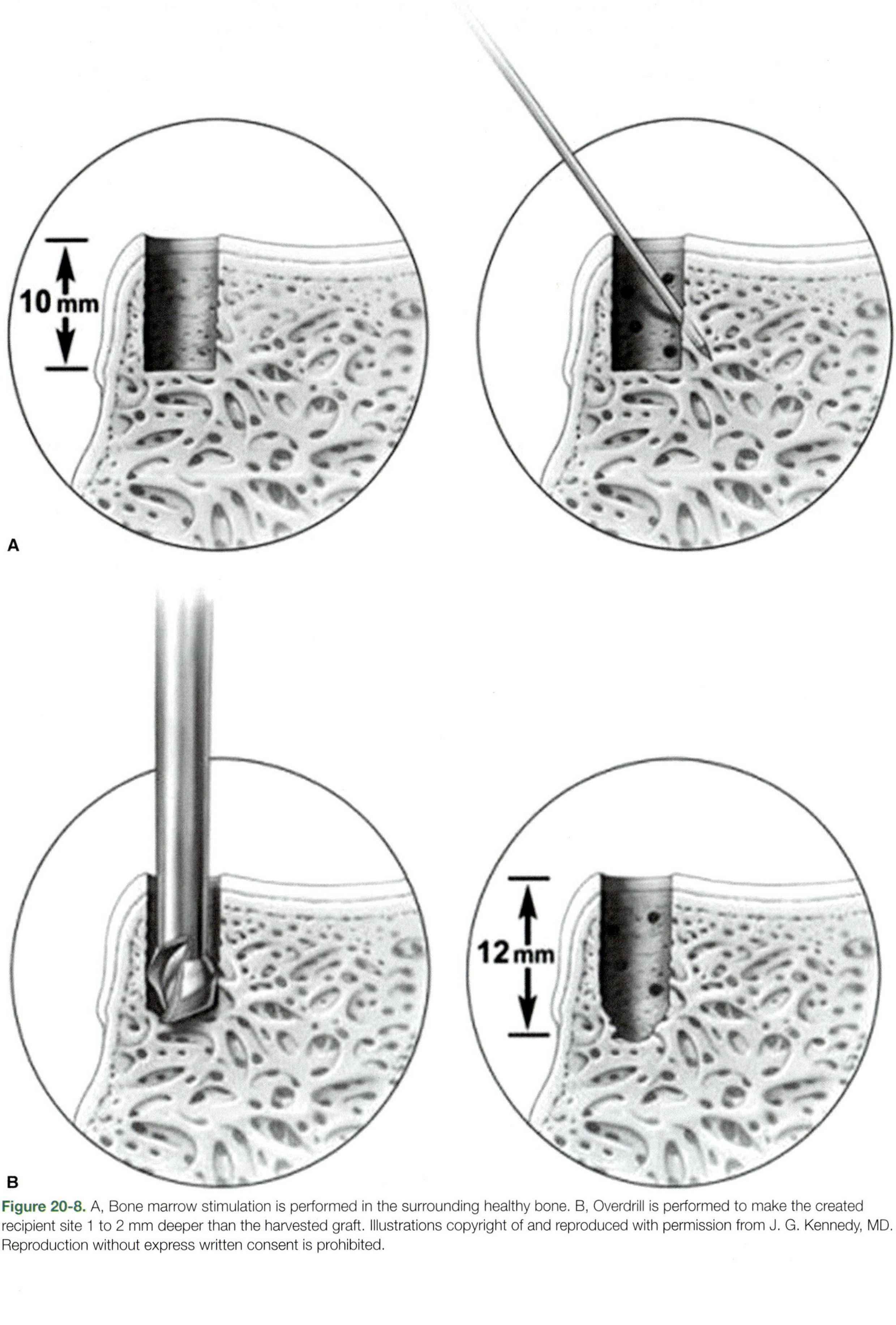

Figure 20-8. A, Bone marrow stimulation is performed in the surrounding healthy bone. B, Overdrill is performed to make the created recipient site 1 to 2 mm deeper than the harvested graft. Illustrations copyright of and reproduced with permission from J. G. Kennedy, MD. Reproduction without express written consent is prohibited.

- The graft should be in a bullet shape, which provides the graft stability and maintains the graft surface congruity throughout the incorporation process (Figure 20-9).[7]

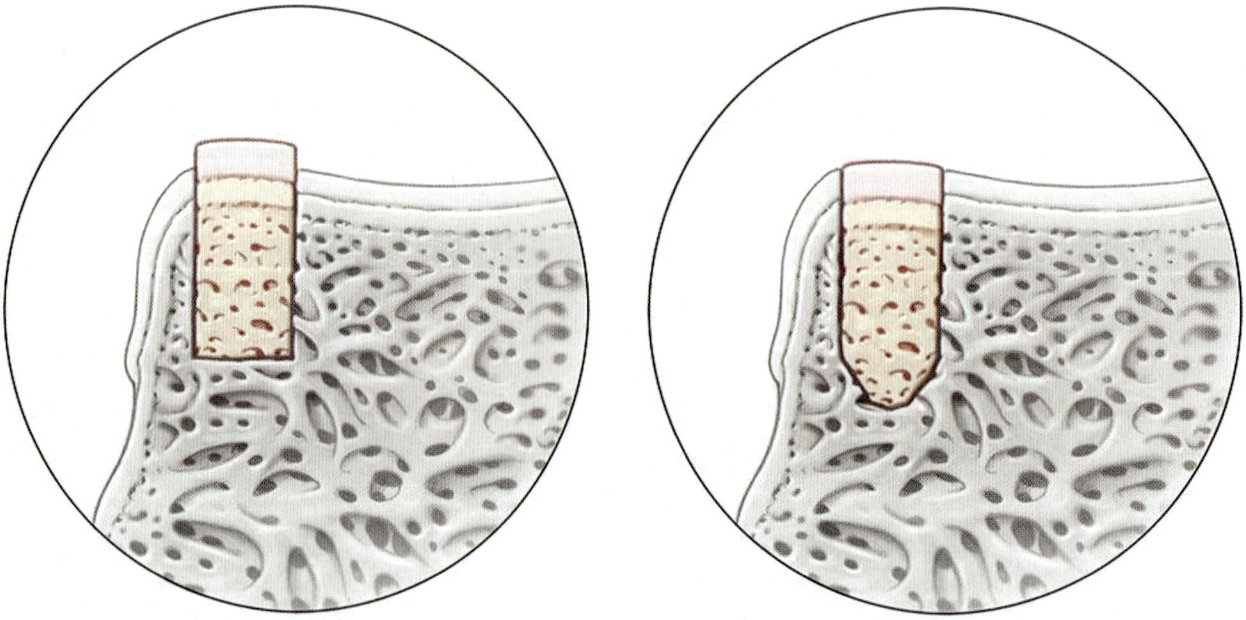

Figure 20-9. This technique may prevent incongruency between the native and graft surface throughout the incorporation process. Illustrations copyright of and reproduced with permission from J. G. Kennedy, MD. Reproduction without express written consent is prohibited.

Graft Harvest

- The ipsilateral knee is most commonly used as the graft harvest site. The authors prefer the non–weight-bearing portion of the superior lateral femoral condyle (Figure 20-10).
- A mini-open arthrotomy with a lateral parapatellar approach and lateral retinacular release is performed. After exposure of the lateral femoral condyle, the appropriate site and orientation of the graft should be established so that the graft matches the talar defect as closely as possible.

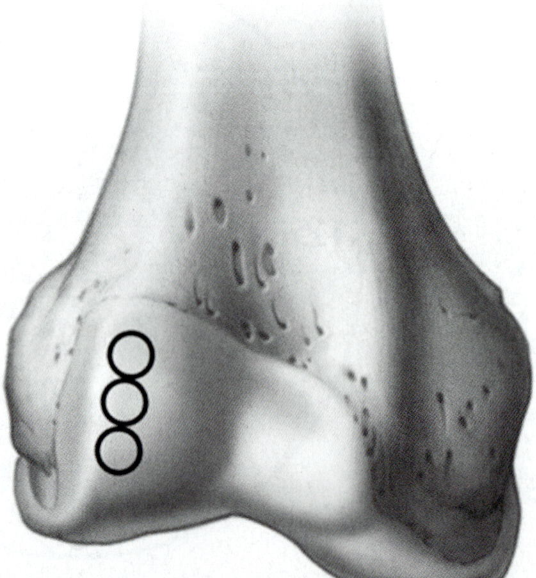

Figure 20-10. The non–weight-bearing portion of the lateral femoral condyle. Illustrations copyright of and reproduced with permission from J. G. Kennedy, MD. Reproduction without express written consent is prohibited.

- The donor trephine is 1 mm larger than the recipient trephine for a precise press-fit.
- The graft is measured and trimmed to match the depth of the recipient site using a rongeur (Figure 20-11).
- The authors then prefer to bathe the graft in concentrated bone marrow aspirate (CBMA) or platelet-rich plasma (PRP) (Figure 20-12).

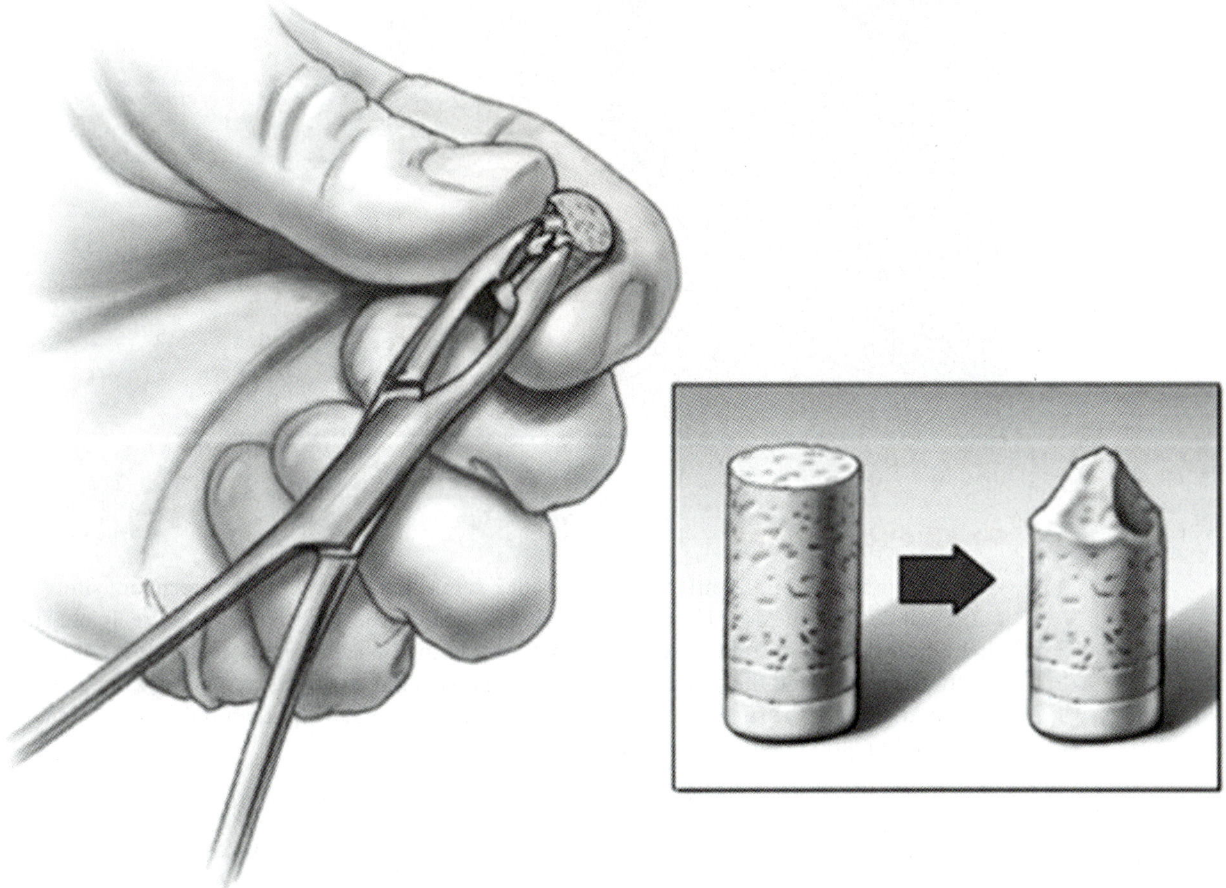

Figure 20-11. The graft is trimmed in a bullet shape. Illustrations copyright of and reproduced with permission from J. G. Kennedy, MD. Reproduction without express written consent is prohibited.

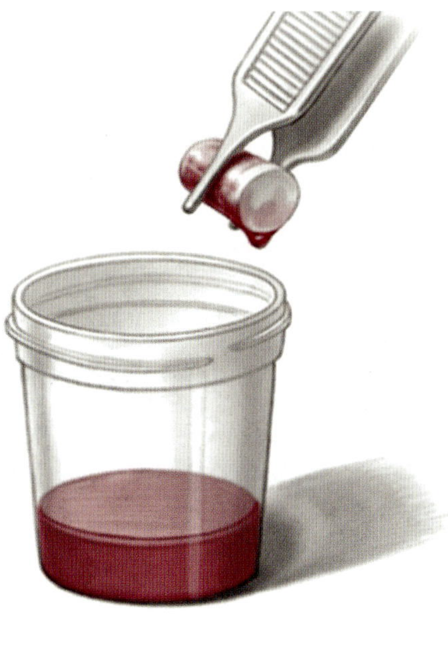

Figure 20-12. The graft is bathed in concentrated bone marrow aspirate or platelet-rich plasma. Illustrations copyright of and reproduced with permission from J. G. Kennedy, MD. Reproduction without express written consent is prohibited.

- The donor site can be backfilled with a synthetic bone plug or an allograft. This procedure provides the articular surface on the defect and prevents hemarthrosis by reducing bleeding (Figure 20-13).

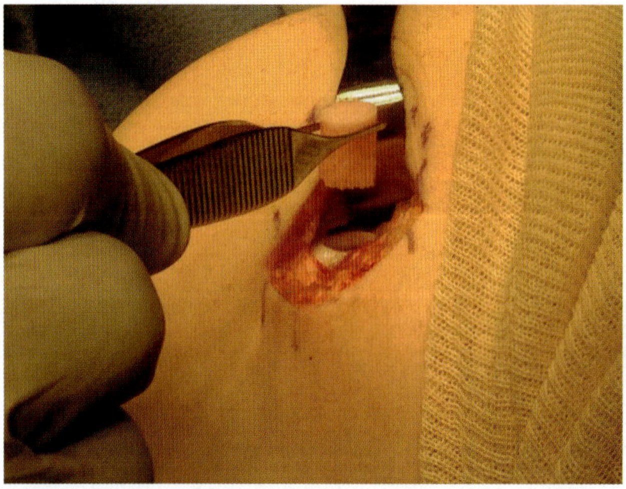

Figure 20-13. The allograft plug is seated into the donor site defect.

Graft Placement

- Before implantation, 1.0 mL of CBMA or PRP is injected into the created recipient site (Figure 20-14). The osteochondral graft plug is then transferred to the created recipient site. At this point, the graft congruency is critically important. To achieve this, the graft is held with a mosquito snap, and the highest point of the graft is marked with a surgical marking pen. The highest point of the surrounding talar cartilage is also marked and then the graft is implanted so that both marks are in line (Figure 20-15).

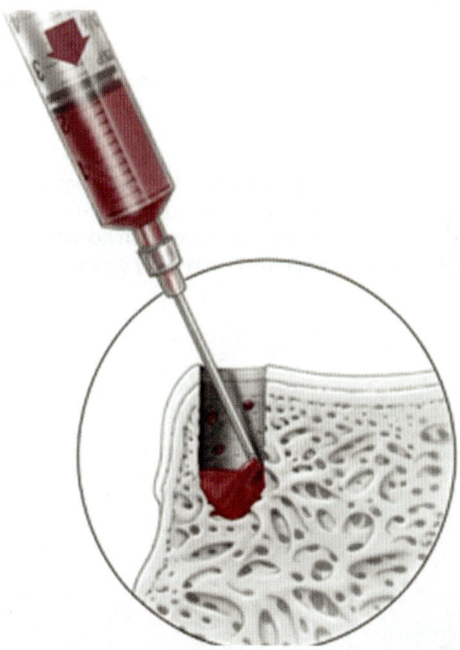

Figure 20-14. Concentrated bone marrow aspirate or platelet-rich plasma is injected into the created recipient site. Illustrations copyright of and reproduced with permission from J. G. Kennedy, MD. Reproduction without express written consent is prohibited.

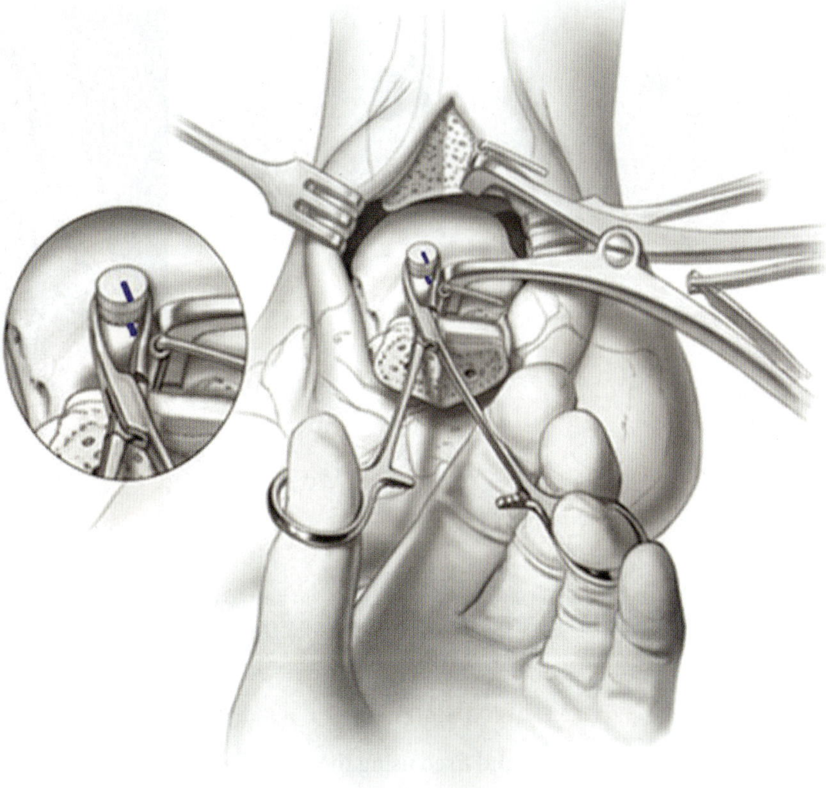

Figure 20-15. A mosquito snap is utilized to rotate the graft gently until the marks are in line. Illustrations copyright of and reproduced with permission from J. G. Kennedy, MD. Reproduction without express written consent is prohibited.

- Final graft placement should be checked to confirm that the graft surface is flush (Figure 20-16).
- If two grafts are required because a lesion is large, a figure-eight "nested" technique should be used to minimize the empty space that will be filled with fibrocartilage (Figure 20-17).[6]

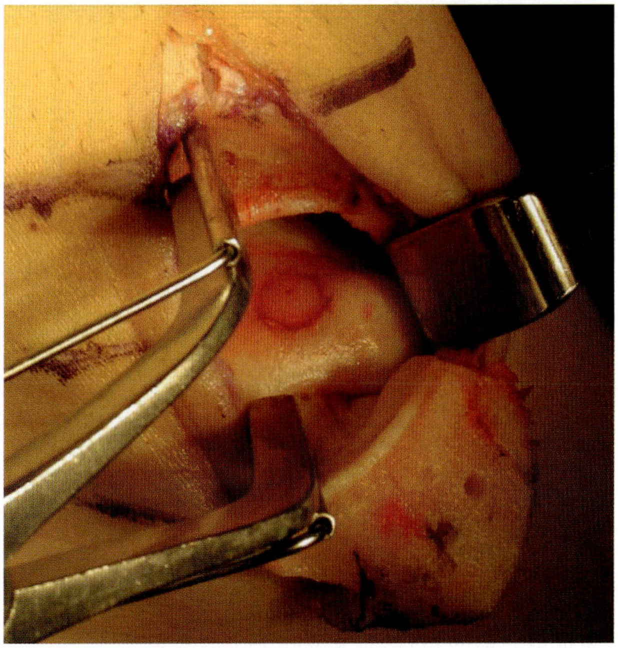

Figure 20-16. The final graft position.

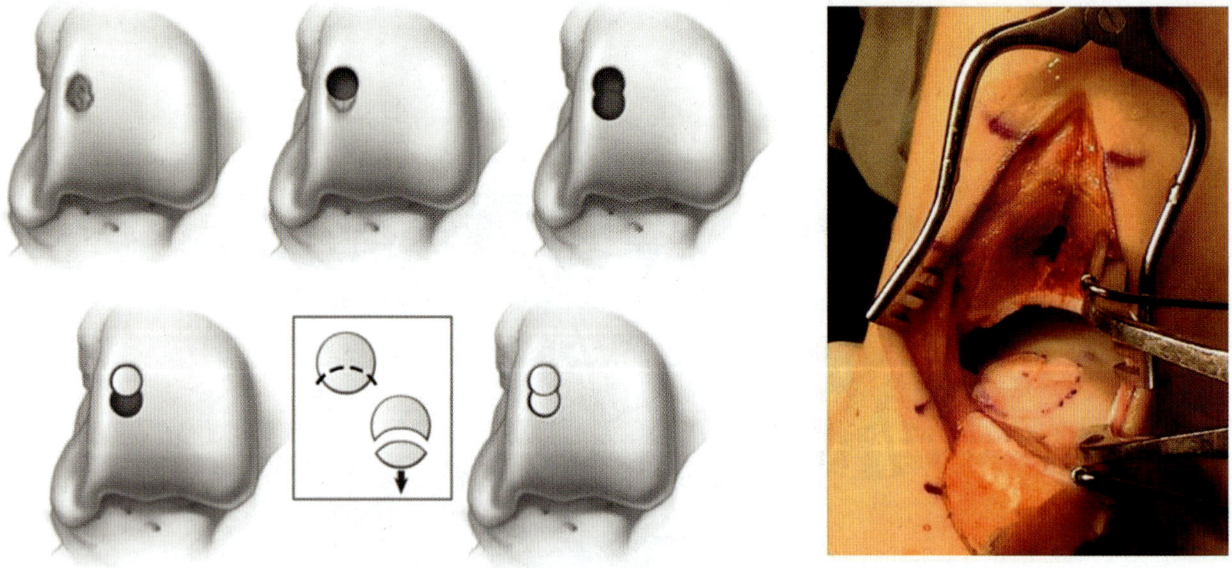

Figure 20-17. Figure-eight "nested" technique. The two plugs are contoured to each other. Illustrations copyright of and reproduced with permission from J. G. Kennedy, MD. Reproduction without express written consent is prohibited.

Fixation of Medial Malleolus

- The osteotomy is replaced and fixed using the predrilled holes with partially threaded cancellous screws. Because the use of only two screws has the potential to allow the malleolus to shift postoperatively, a third transverse screw with a washer should be added (Figure 20-18).

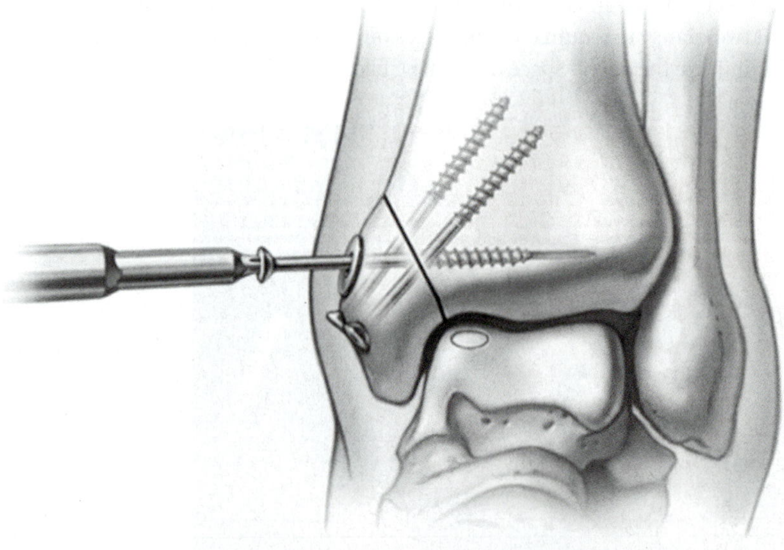

Figure 20-18. Medial malleolar fixation with three screws. Illustrations copyright of and reproduced with permission from J. G. Kennedy, MD. Reproduction without express written consent is prohibited.

Postoperative Protocol

- 0 to 4 weeks: non–weight-bearing in CAM walker boot
    - At 2 weeks, start the range of motion exercise for the ankle joint dorsiflexion active motion.
- 4 to 6 weeks: weight-bearing is increased by 10% per day in CAM walker boot.
    - At approximately 6 weeks, full weight-bearing is achieved.

- 6 weeks: physical therapy is started.
- 10 weeks: sports-specific physical therapies can be considered.
- 4 to 6 months: competitive sports—return to play

References

1. Chuckpaiwong B, Berkson EM, Theodore GH. Microfracture for osteochondral lesions of the ankle: outcome analysis and outcome predictors of 105 cases. *Arthroscopy*. 2008;24:106-112.
2. Choi WJ, Park KK, Kim BS, Lee JW. Osteochondral lesion of the talus: is there a critical defect size for poor outcome? *Am J Sports Med*. 2009;37(10):1974-1980.
3. Ramponi L, Yasui Y, Murawski CD, et al. Lesion size is a predictor of clinical outcomes after bone marrow stimulation for osteochondral lesions of the talus: a systematic review. *Am J Sports Med*. 2017;45(7):1698-1705.
4. Yoon HS, Park YJ, Lee M, Choi WJ, Lee JW. Osteochondral autologous transplantation is superior to repeat arthroscopy for the treatment of osteochondral lesions of the talus after failed primary arthroscopic treatment. *Am J Sports Med*. 2014;42:1896-1903.
5. Scranton PE Jr, Frey CC, Feder KS. Outcome of osteochondral autograft transplantation for type-V cystic osteochondral lesions of the talus. *J Bone Joint Surg Br*. 2006;88(5):614-619.
6. Kennedy JG, Murawski CD. The treatment of osteochondral lesions of the talus with autologous osteochondral transplantation and bone marrow aspirate concentrate: surgical technique. *Cartilage*. 2011;2(4):327-336.
7. Kock NB, Van Susante JL, Buma P, Van Kampen A, Verdonschot N. Press-fit stability of an osteochondral autograft: influence of different plug length and perfect depth alignment. *Acta Orthop*. 2006;77(3):422-428.

Chapter 21
Fifth Metatarsal Stress Fractures

AKASH GUPTA
MARTIN O'MALLEY

Introduction

- In the elite athlete, recognition of fifth metatarsal stress fractures is key to early treatment.
- Fracture occurs because of overuse and lateral overload. Furthermore, there is increased motion of the fifth metatarsal with a base that is anchored by the tendon and ligaments.
- Operative intervention for these patients allows for more aggressive rehabilitation and earlier return to sport.
- Risk factors for this injury include a cavus foot and metatarsus adductus (Figure 21-1). The alignment does not need to be corrected initially; however, the metatarsus adductus may limit the screw size able to be placed.
- In larger athletes, metatarsus adductus is seen along with a prominent base of the fifth metatarsal (Figure 21-2)

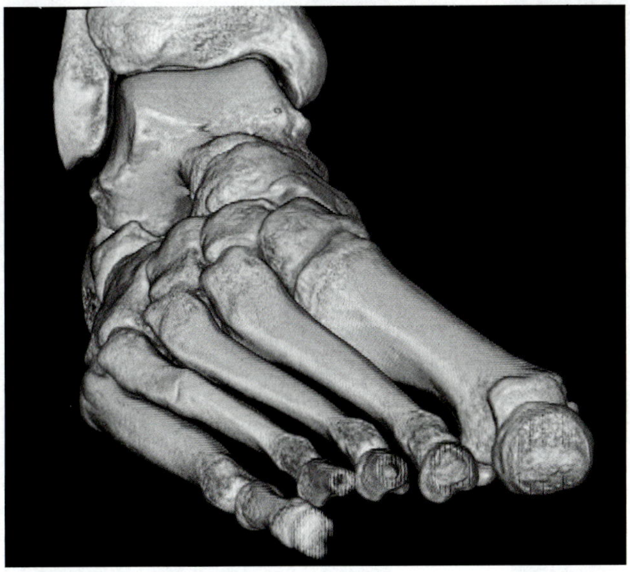

Figure 21-1. Three-dimensional computed tomography reconstruction demonstrating metatarsus adductus.

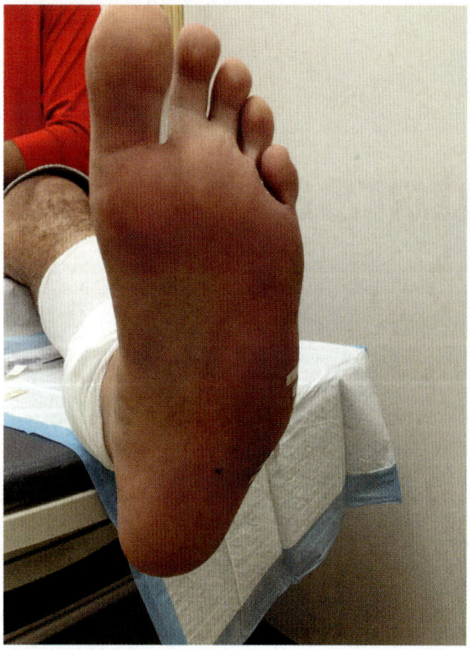

Figure 21-2. Professional basketball player's foot demonstrating a prominent fifth metatarsal base.

Imaging

- X-rays: Routine weight-bearing radiographs (anteroposterior, lateral, and oblique) are typically the initial imaging modality of choice (Figure 21-3). X-rays can allow for assessment of medullary sclerosis and the morphology of the fracture. In addition, measurements can be made such as the fourth-to-fifth intermetatarsal angle, the fifth metatarsal lateral deviation angle, and the calcaneal pitch as described by Lee et al, as well as the metatarsus adductus angle as described by Sgarlato et al.
- Magnetic resonance imaging (MRI): MRI is best at detecting bone edema and stress reaction, which may occur before stress fracture (Figure 21-4). Fifth metatarsal stress reactions present

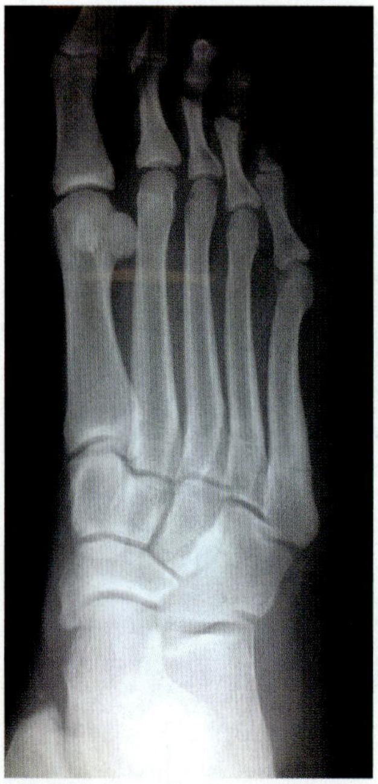

Figure 21-3. Oblique radiograph of the foot demonstrating a proximal fifth metatarsal fracture.

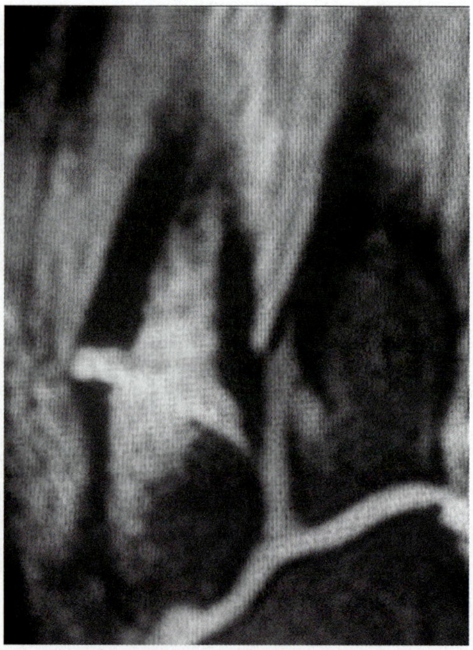

Figure 21-4. T2 magnetic resonance imaging demonstrating bone marrow edema and a stress reaction in the base of the fifth metatarsal.

with symptoms similar to those of stress fractures, but lack an obvious fracture line on computed tomography (CT). By detecting such stress reactions early, steps may be taken to prevent the stress reaction from progressing into a full-blown stress fracture. MRI has the additional advantage of avoiding radiation exposure.
- CT: CT plays an important role in preoperative planning, because it provides the best visualization of the fracture line. It allows the surgeon to determine whether the fracture line is complete, and whether there is a plantar gap. Furthermore, CT can also be used to monitor healing. Of note, repeat CT and MRI scans are often recommended to ensure positive signs of healing before return to sports.

Treatment Algorithm

- The standard method of treatment is percutaneous internal fixation with solid partially threaded screws and with bone marrow aspirate concentrate added to the fracture site.
- In fractures that have a higher risk of nonunion, open bone grafting of the fracture site can also be added to the treatment plan.
- CT scan is performed at 10 weeks, with a goal of 100% union.

Equipment

- Tourniquet
- Headlight
- 22-Gauge needle
- Dental pick and Freer elevator
- K-wires with wire driver
- Bone marrow aspirate set with trocar
- Implants
  - Charlotte Carolina screw system (Wright Medical, Memphis, TN) or a similar alternative with solid partially threaded screws
- Mini C-arm

Positioning

- Supine, with large bump under ipsilateral hip so that foot is internally rotated
- Take care to pad all bony prominences.
- See Chapter 1 for full description.

Technique

Bone Marrow Aspirate

- Bone marrow is aspirated from the ipsilateral iliac crest under local anesthesia and sedation if the patient had an ankle block or was under spinal anesthesia.
- To extract the marrow, a hollow trocar needle is advanced into the cancellous bone of the anterior ilium, just posterior to the anterosuperior spine (Figure 21-5).
- Approximately 60 mL of bone marrow is removed with a standard syringe, prepared, and centrifuged using the Magellan system (Arteriocyte, Cleveland, OH) to produce the bone marrow aspirate concentrate (BMAC).
- 3 to 4 mL of the concentrate is optimal.

Bone Grafting

- For patients who receive open bone grafting, the same entry point created by the aspirate stylet is used.
- The Magellan trocar needle is used to obtain five sleeves of tricortical bone graft from the iliac crest.

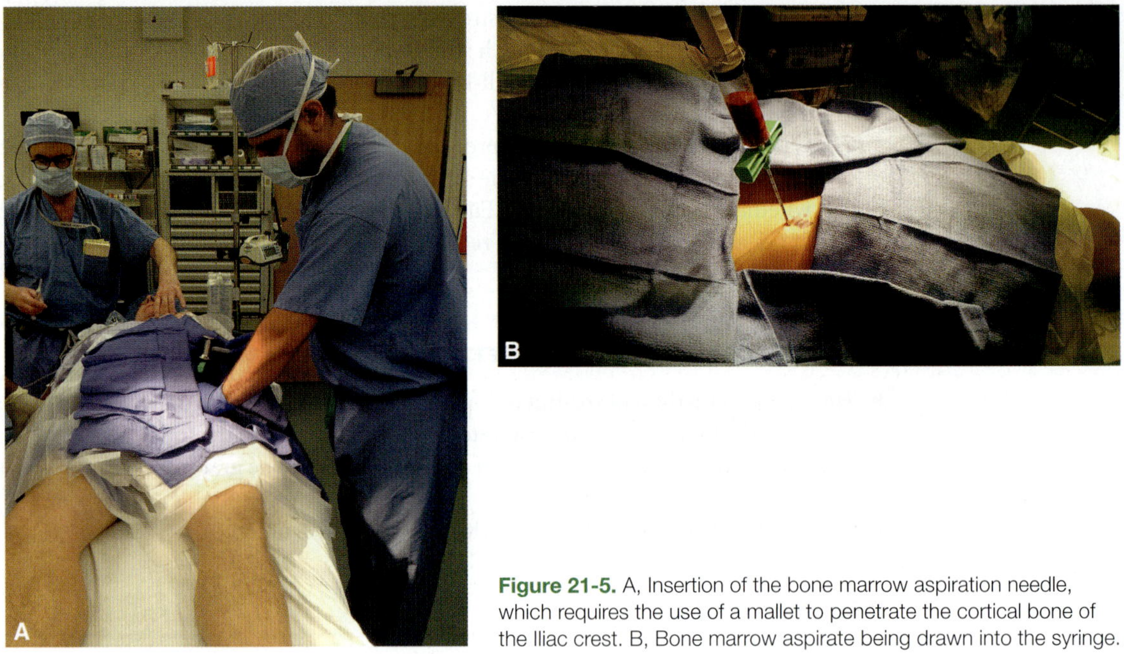

Figure 21-5. A, Insertion of the bone marrow aspiration needle, which requires the use of a mallet to penetrate the cortical bone of the Iliac crest. B, Bone marrow aspirate being drawn into the syringe.

- Using C-arm to determine the side of the fracture, a small 3-cm incision is made directly lateral over the fracture to open the site itself (Figure 21-6).
- The fracture is then cleaned using a dental pick.
- A K-wire can be used to create several holes on either side of the fracture to stimulate a bleeding surface.
- A combination of BMAC and iliac crest bone graft is then impacted into the fracture site just before screw advancement, as described later.
- Once the screw is advanced across the fracture site and good compression is achieved, additional on-lay grafting is done laterally and plantarly before the wound is closed (Figure 21-7).

Fracture Fixation

- Mark out the base of the fifth metatarsal.
- The peroneus brevis runs in a line from just posterior to the tip of the fibula to the dorsolateral cortex of the base of the fifth metatarsal.
- A small incision is made approximately 2.5 cm proximal to the base of the fifth metatarsal, parallel to the plantar surface of the foot.
- Dissection is carried down through the subcutaneous tissue until the peroneus brevis can be retracted dorsally and the peroneus longus retracted plantarly.

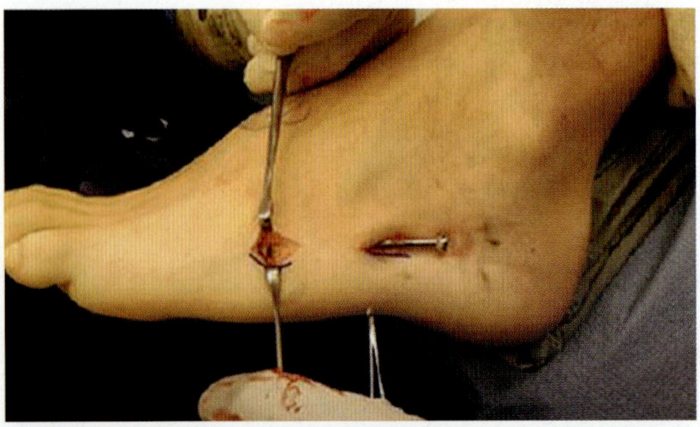

Figure 21-6. Exposure and preparation of the fracture site.

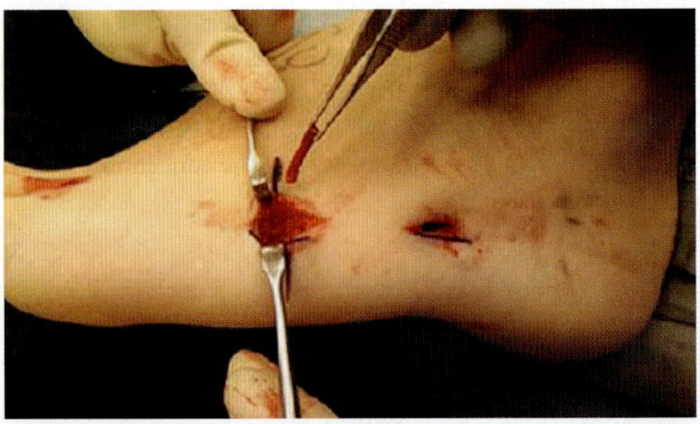

Figure 21-7. On-lay bone grafting of the fracture site after screw fixation is placed.

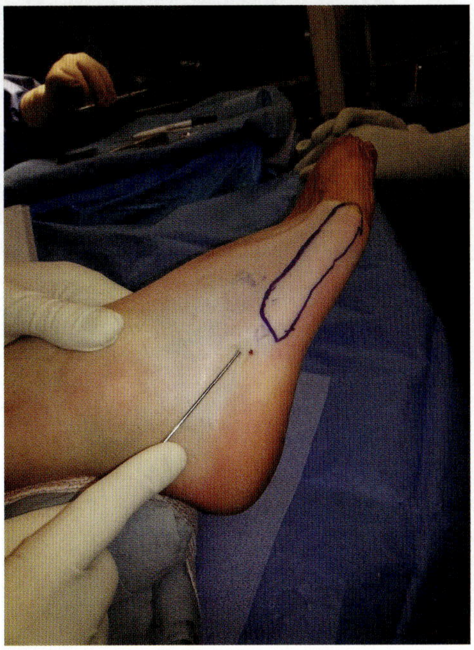

Figure 21-8. Guidewire placement for screw fixation.

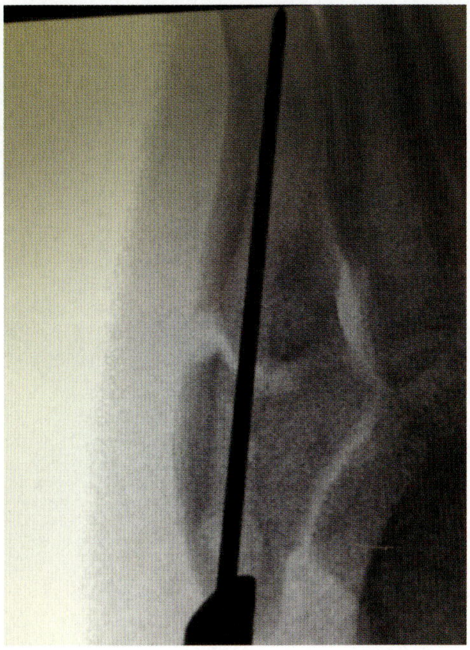

Figure 21-9. Proper guidewire placement as seen on XR.

- A guide wire is then placed down the metatarsal shaft on the "high and inside" position (Figure 21-8). The goal is to be in line with the shaft of the fifth metatarsal, which is usually dorsal and medial on an anteroposterior radiograph (Figure 21-9).
- With the wire in place, a 3.2-mm cannulated drill is advanced down the medullary canal and past the fracture site.
- Intramedullary taps are then used to determine optimal screw size. Taps sizes are increased until the forefoot begins to torque (Figure 21-10).
- The goal is to place the largest screw possible with threads just beyond the fracture site so that the screw does not straighten the curved fifth metatarsal bone and lead to gapping at the fracture site. A screw of estimated length can be imaged adjacent to the metatarsal to determine the appropriate size (Figure 21-11).

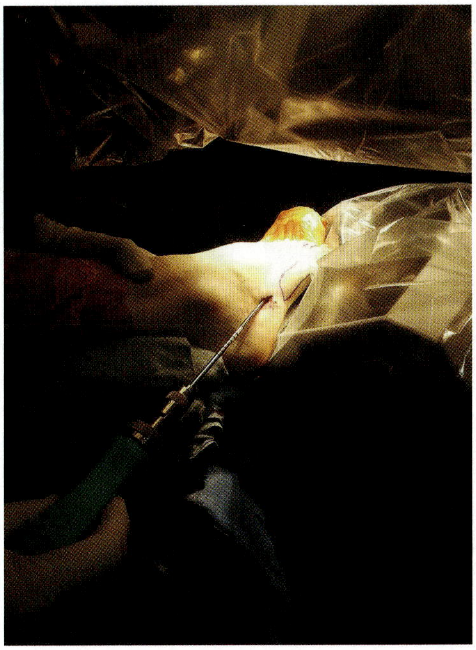

Figure 21-10. Use of intramedullary tap for canal preparation.

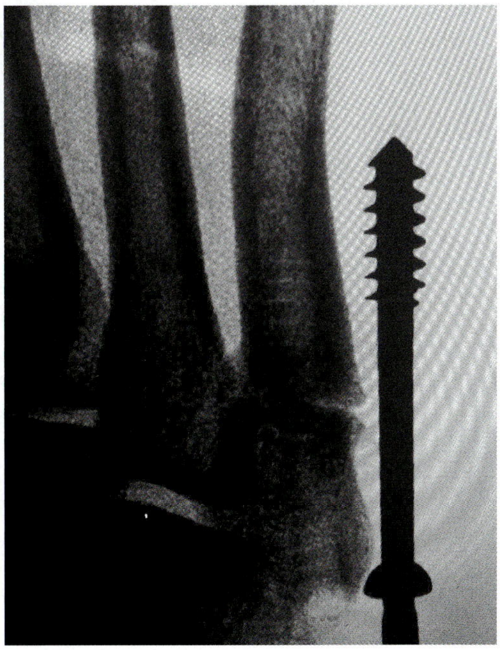

Figure 21-11. Determination of appropriate screw length.

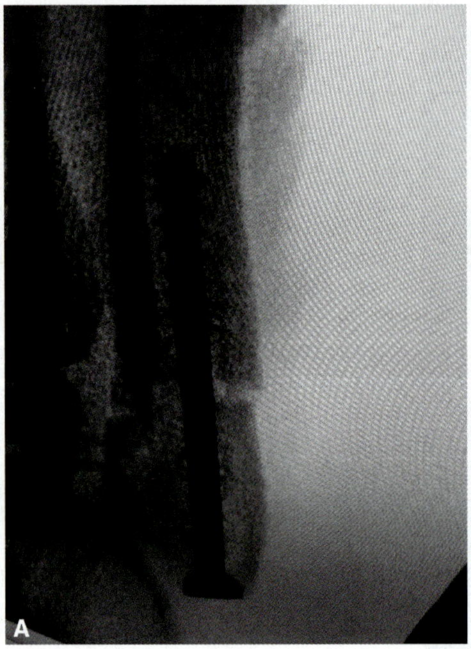

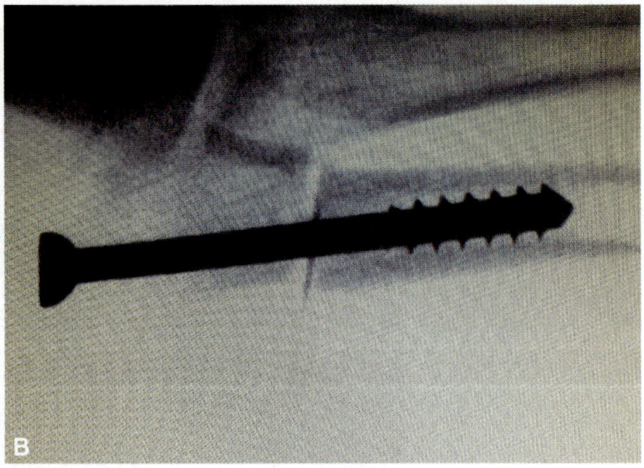

Figure 21-12. Anteroposterior (A) and lateral radiographs (B) demonstrating proper screw placement.

- Once the proper screw size is determined, the wire is removed and half of the BMAC is placed down the shaft of the bone.
- The appropriately sized screw is then placed into the intramedullary canal and advanced until compression is obtained. The screw should be sunk down enough such that prominence into the cubometatarsal joint is minimized (Figure 21-12).
- Once the wound is closed, a 22-gauge needle is used to place the rest of the BMAC at the fracture site percutaneously via fluoroscopy (Figure 21-13).
- Alternatively, headless compression screws may be used to minimize tarsometatarsal joint irritation from the screw heads (Figure 21-14).

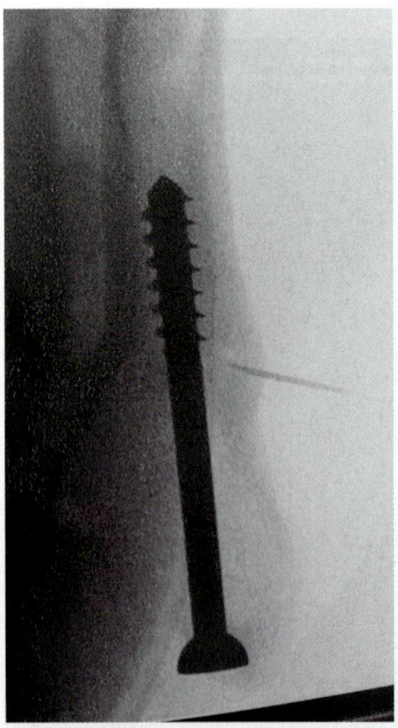

Figure 21-13. Injection of bone marrow aspirate concentrate at the fracture site.

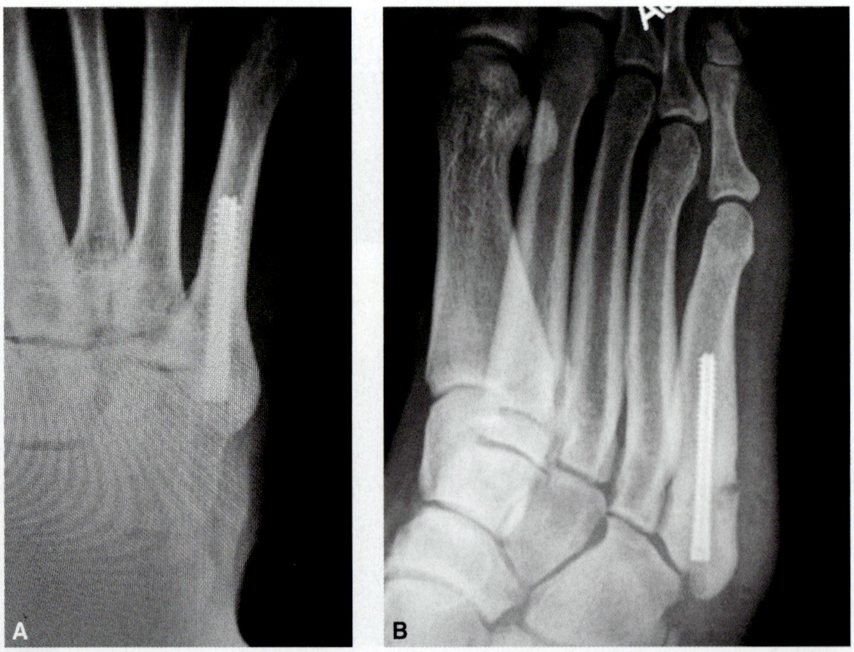

Figure 21-14. Example of headless screw fixation for a proximal fifth metatarsal fracture on AP (A) and oblique XRs.

References

1. Lee KT, Kim KC, Park YU, Kim TW, Lee YK. Radiographic evaluation of foot structure following fifth metatarsal stress fracture. *Foot Ankle Int*. 2011;32:796–801.
2. Aiyer AA, Shariff R, Ying L, Shub J, Myerson MS. Prevalence of metatarsus adductus in patients undergoing hallux valgus surgery. *Foot Ankle Int*. 2014;35:1292–1297.

Chapter 22
Navicular Stress Fractures

AKASH GUPTA
MARTIN O'MALLEY

Introduction

- Navicular stress fractures often present with vague complaints of pain on the dorsal foot and even pain in the ankle. The presentation is usually insidious in nature.
- Symptoms tend to improve with rest or immobilization but recur once activities are resumed.
- The findings from the physical examination are often impressive, and x-ray results are typically negative. As such, the diagnosis is often delayed.
- Patients with long second metatarsals and short first metatarsals are at particular risk.
- Patients with a cavus foot and metatarsus adductus are also at risk.
- Patients that have limited ankle dorsiflexion due to impingement have higher contact stresses with axial loading, which can predispose to stress fractures. Thus, athletes with repetitive axial loads, such as basketball and football players or track and field athletes, are at risk.
- These patients often have osteophytes over the dorsum of the talonavicular joint.

Classification

- Type I: fracture in the dorsal cortex (see Figure 22-1)
- Type II: fracture extends from dorsal cortex into navicular body (see Figure 22-2)
- Type III: complete fracture through both cortices (see Figure 22-3)

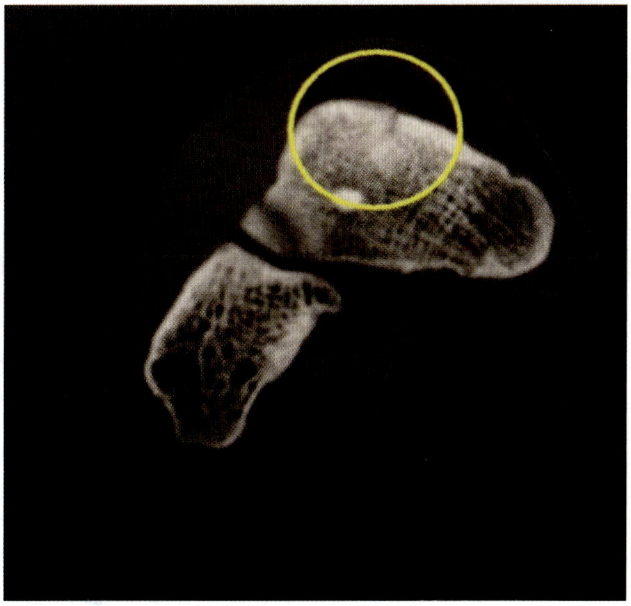

Figure 22-1. Type I navicular fracture.

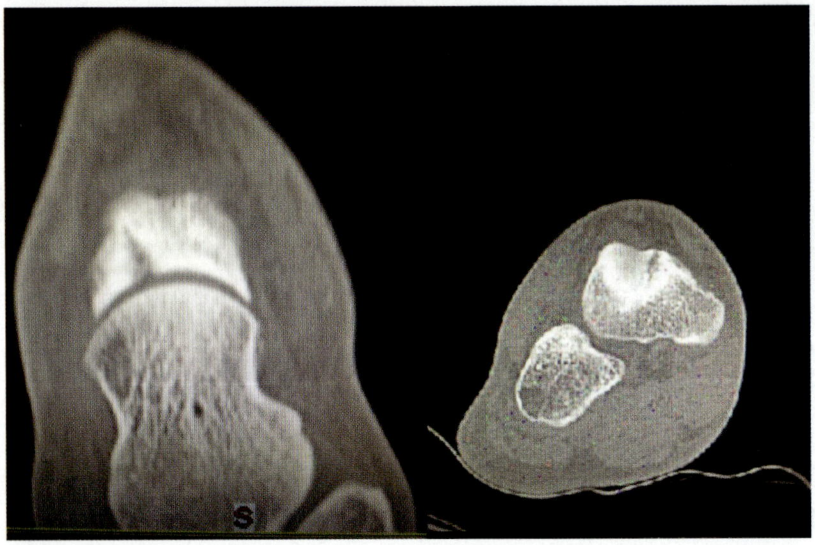

Figure 22-2. Type II navicular fracture.

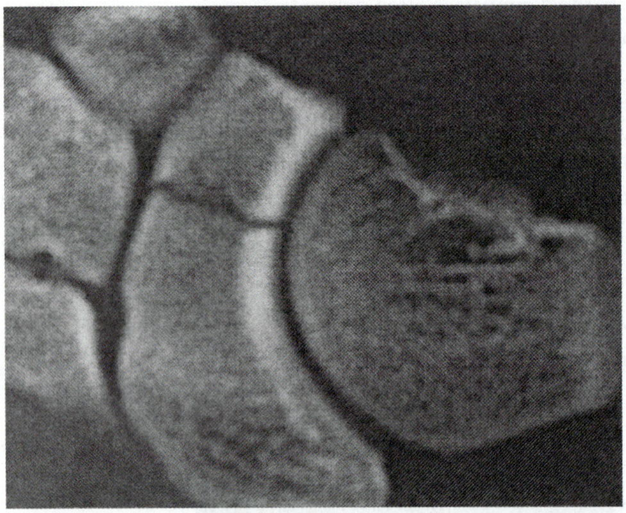

Figure 22-3. Type III navicular fracture.

Imaging

- X-rays: Routine weight-bearing radiographs (anteroposterior, lateral, and oblique) are typically the initial imaging modality of choice. However, these should not be used in isolation because radiographs have been shown to have very low sensitivity for navicular stress fractures. Moreover, most navicular fractures do not involve the plantar cortex, making them difficult to identify on radiographs until osteoclastic resorption has occurred. Rather, these images should be used to rule out other potential causes of medial foot and ankle pain, such as malalignment, talar neck spurring, or capsular avulsions (see Figure 22-4).
- Triple-phase bone scan: Given their high sensitivity and high positive predictive value in identifying these fractures, bone scans may be used to screen for navicular stress fractures. Despite the high sensitivity, a positive bone scan is not specific for this navicular stress fracture. Moreover, bone scans lack anatomic resolution and do not provide an accurate depiction of the specific fracture pattern. As such, this imaging modality has largely been replaced by magnetic resonance imaging (MRI).

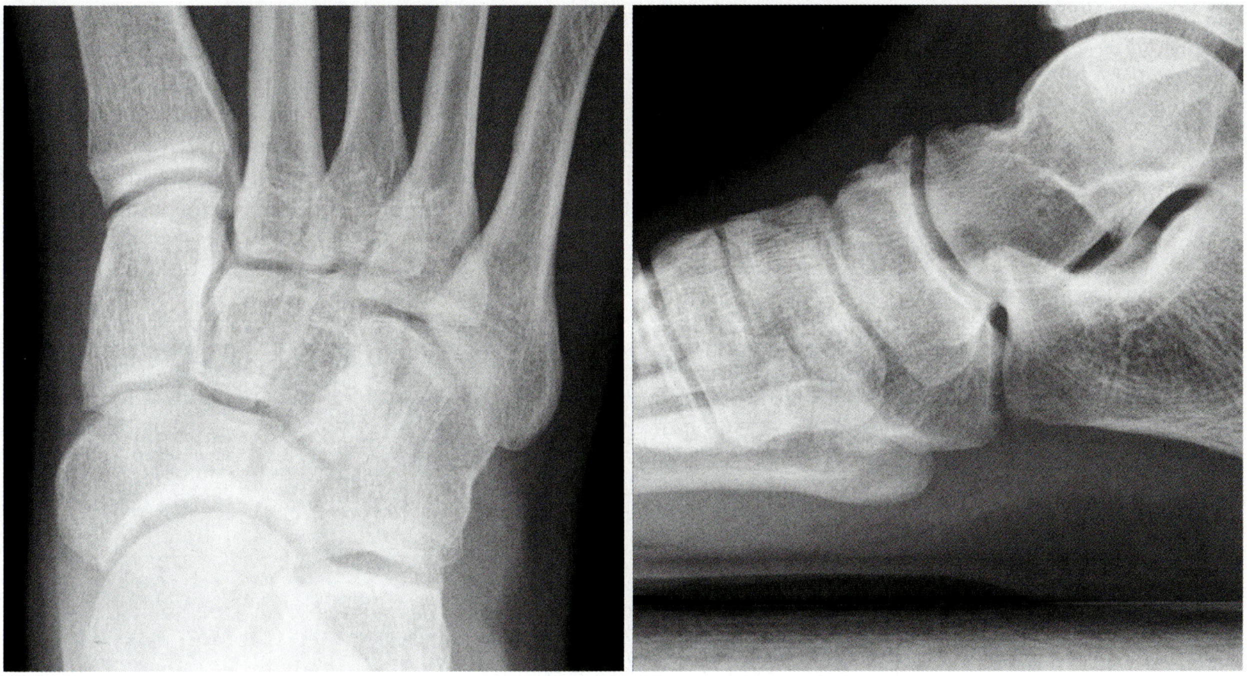

Figure 22-4. Anteroposterior and lateral radiographs demonstrating dorsal spurring of the talonavicular joint.

- MRI: MRI is considered the gold standard because it is the best at detecting bone edema and stress reaction, which may occur before a stress fracture. Navicular stress reactions present with similar symptoms as stress fractures, but lack an obvious fracture line on computed tomography (CT). By detecting such stress reactions early, steps may be taken to prevent the stress reaction from progressing into a full-blown stress fracture (see Figure 22-5). MRI has the additional advantage of avoiding radiation exposure.

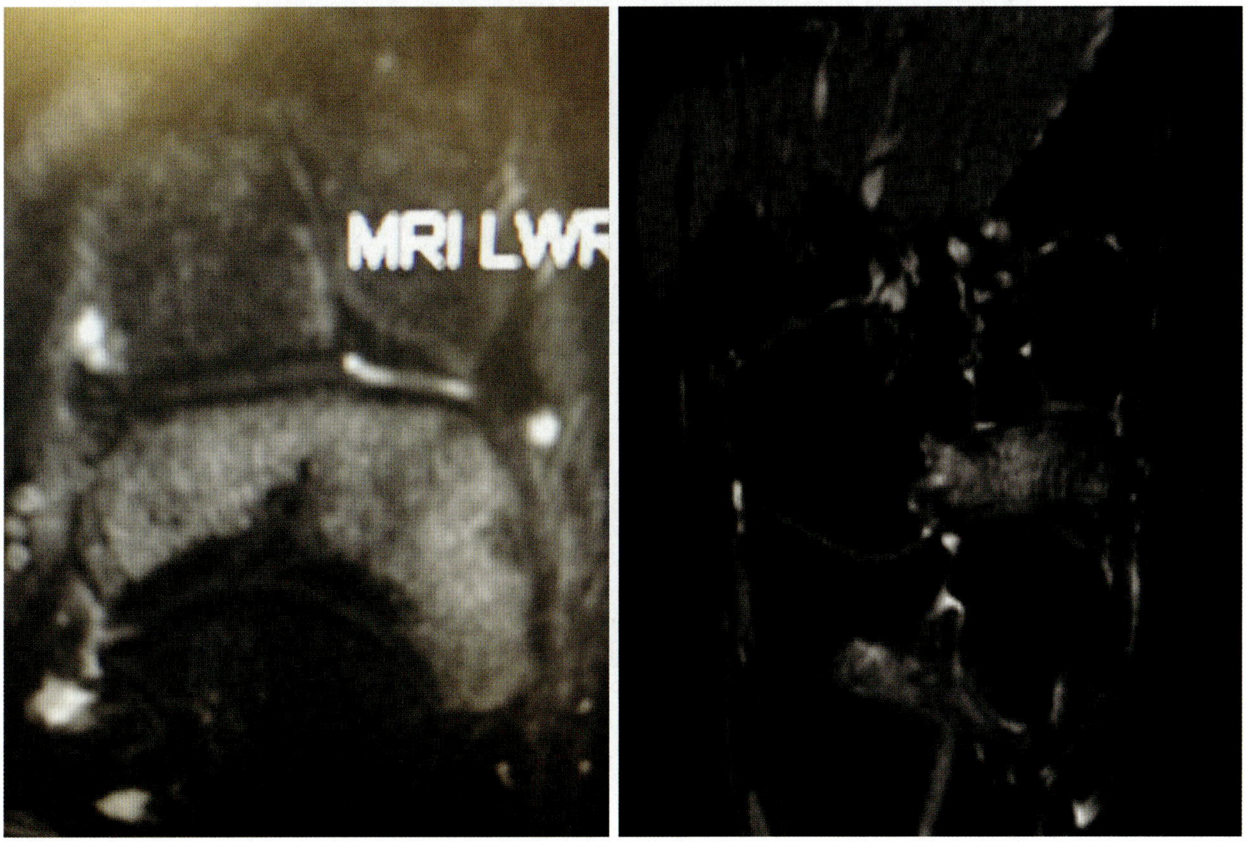

Figure 22-5. Magnetic resonance imaging demonstrating navicular stress fracture.

- CT: CT plays an important role in preoperative planning because it provides the best visualization of the fracture line (see Figure 22-6). Using the aforementioned CT-based classification system designed by Saxena et al,[1] navicular stress fractures can be divided into separate groups with associated treatment schemes. Furthermore, CT can also be used to monitor healing. Dorsal cortical proliferation, which is typically the first radiologic sign of healing, can be seen as early as 6 weeks following the injury using CT. Bony healing and consolidation is seen later, at around 3 to 4 months postinjury. Of note, repeat CT and MRI scans are often recommended to ensure positive signs of healing prior to return to sports.

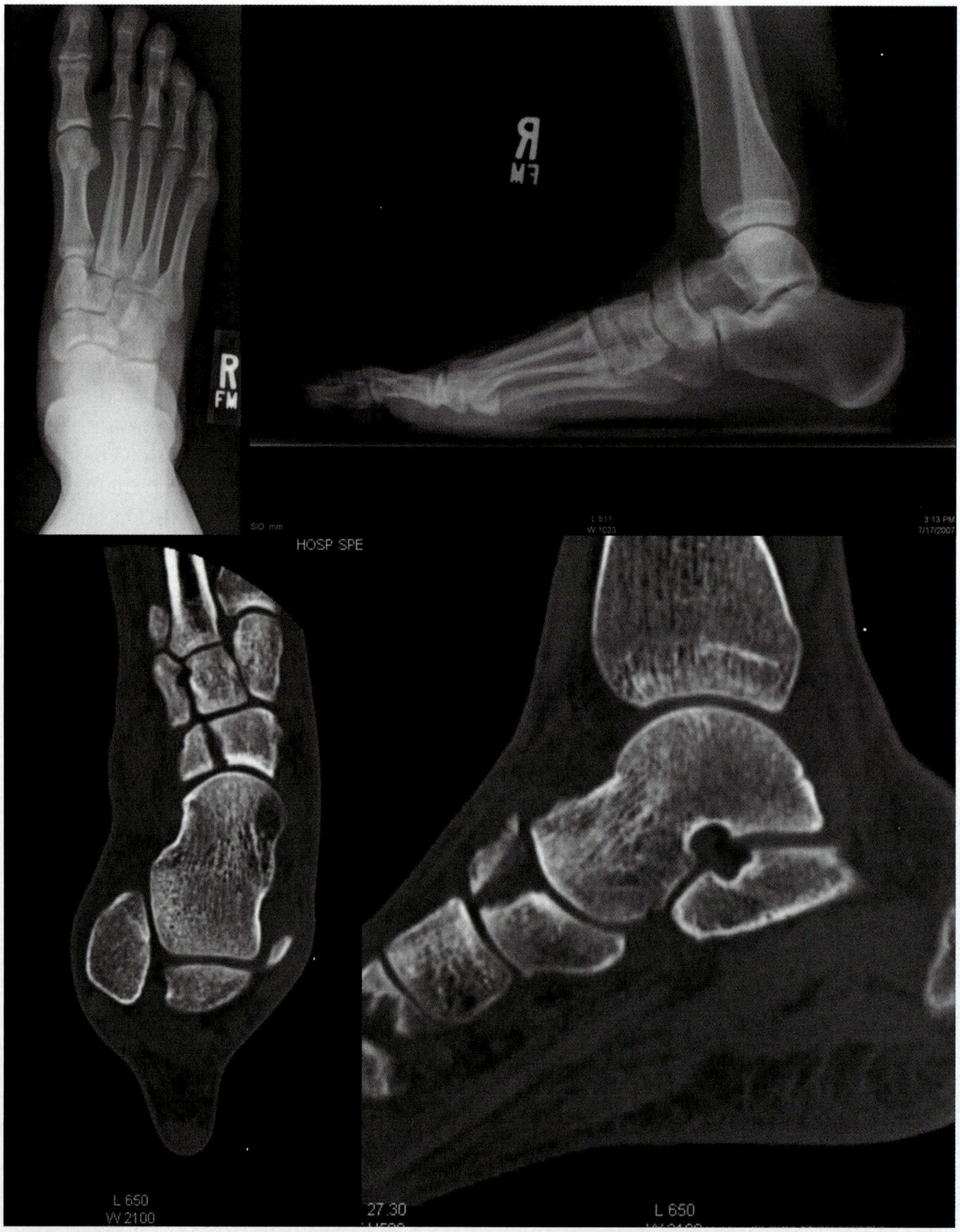

Figure 22-6. Radiographs and computed tomography depicting navicular body fracture.

Treatment Algorithm

- Type I: These can be treated nonoperatively with 6 weeks of strict non–weight-bearing or with a single percutaneous 3.5-mm screw and earlier gradual weight-bearing.
- Types II and III: These fractures are treated with open reduction internal fixation using one or two 3.5-mm screws, iliac crest bone marrow aspirate concentrate (BMAC), and autologous bone dowels obtained from the ipsilateral iliac crest.
- Anterior ankle impingement should be addressed at the time of surgery because this can limit ankle motion and increase stress in the area of the navicular fracture.
- Athletes may return to full activities when fracture healing is visualized on CT done at 10 weeks at the earliest.
- Postoperatively, patients are strict non–weight-bearing for 6 weeks but mobilize the ankle and the calf. If possible, bone stimulator and shockwave therapy are utilized and vitamin D supplementation is given to ensure a level over 50 ng/mL.
- CT scan is performed at 10 weeks with a goal of 100% union.

Relevant Anatomy

- The navicular's blood supply is derived from the dorsalis pedis (dorsal navicular) and posterior tibial (plantar navicular) arteries.
- This arterial network enters the navicular throughout its nonarticular surfaces and branches out medially and laterally, leaving the central third relatively avascular.
- A cadaver study identified this avascular region in a subset of specimens and suggested that perhaps patients with this anatomic variant are at increased risk for navicular stress fracture.
- The tarsal navicular's limited vascularity has important applications: without treatment, patients with navicular stress fractures may have difficulty healing because of the bone's limited vascular supply.
- As a result of this decreased blood flow, those with navicular stress fractures tend to experience delayed healing, high rates of nonunion, and prolonged time out of sport.

Equipment

- Tourniquet
- Headlight
- 18-Gauge and 22-gauge needles
- Dental pick and Freer elevator
- K-wires with wire driver
- Bone marrow aspirate set with trocar
- Implants
    - 3.5-mm small-fragment screws
- Mini C-arm

Positioning

- Supine with bump under ipsilateral hip so that foot is pointing straight up.
- Take care to pad all bony prominences.
- See Chapter 1 for a full description.

Technique

Bone Marrow Aspirate

- Bone marrow is aspirated from the ipsilateral iliac crest under local anesthesia and sedation if the patient had an ankle block or under spinal anesthesia.

- To extract the marrow, a hollow trocar needle is advanced into the cancellous bone of the anterior ilium, just posterior to the anterosuperior spine.
- Approximately 60 mL of bone marrow is removed with a standard syringe, prepared, and centrifuged using the Magellan system (Arteriocyte, Cleveland, OH) to produce BMAC.
- Concentrate of 3 to 4 mL is optimal.

Bone Grafting

- For patients that receive open bone grafting, the same entry point created by the aspirate stylet is used.
- The Magellan trocar needle is used to obtain five sleeves of tricortical bone graft from the iliac crest.

Fracture Fixation

- Dorsal approach to the navicular with a straight longitudinal incision centered over the fracture site with the aid of fluoroscopy.
- Take care to protect the superficial peroneal nerve and the deep neurovascular bundle while dissecting down to the capsule.
- The fracture site is identified using an 18-gauge needle (see Figure 22-7).
- Periosteum around fracture edges is elevated taking care not to strip the navicular.

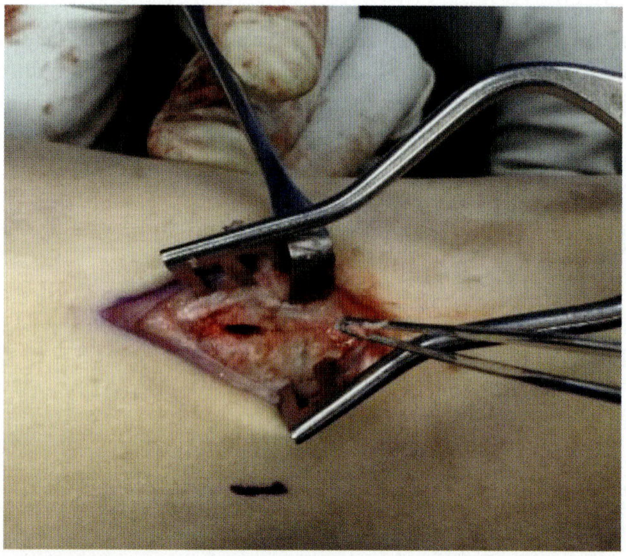

Figure 22-7. Use of an 18-gauge needle to identify the fracture site.

- The fibrous material at the fracture site is debrided using a scalpel and dental pick (see Figure 22-8).
- The sclerotic fracture edges can be drilled with a 0.045-in K-wire to expose healthy bone.
- After successful debridement, there is typically a gap of several millimeters so autograft with or without BMAC can be added to augment healing.
- Initially a guidewire is placed and the position is checked on fluoroscopy (see Figure 22-9).
- A single, 3.5-mm fully threaded cortical lag screw by technique can be placed percutaneously from lateral to medial (see Figure 22-10).

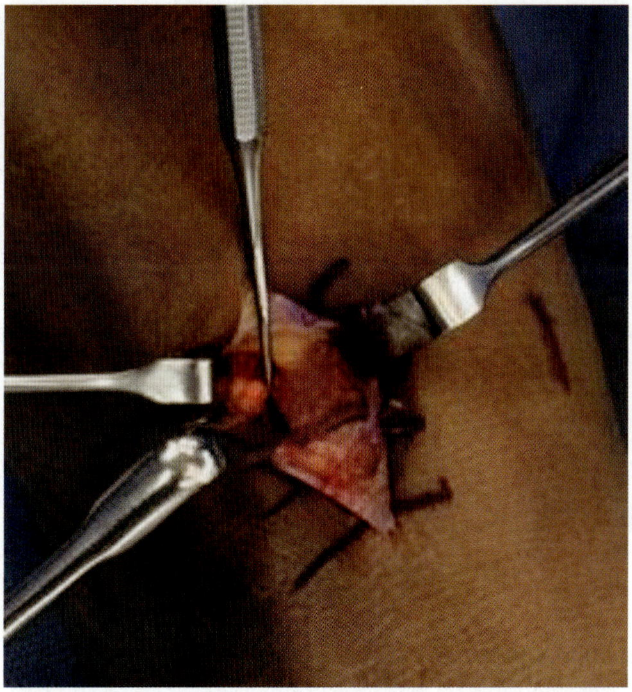

Figure 22-8. Debridement of interposed nonosseous tissue at the fracture site.

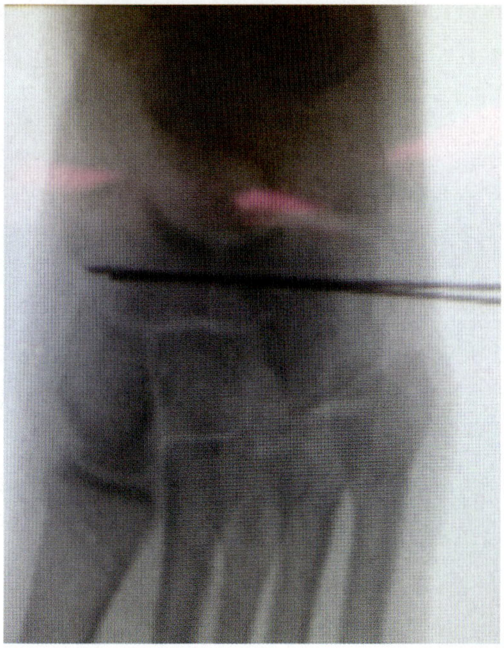

Figure 22-9. Guidewire placement across the fracture site.

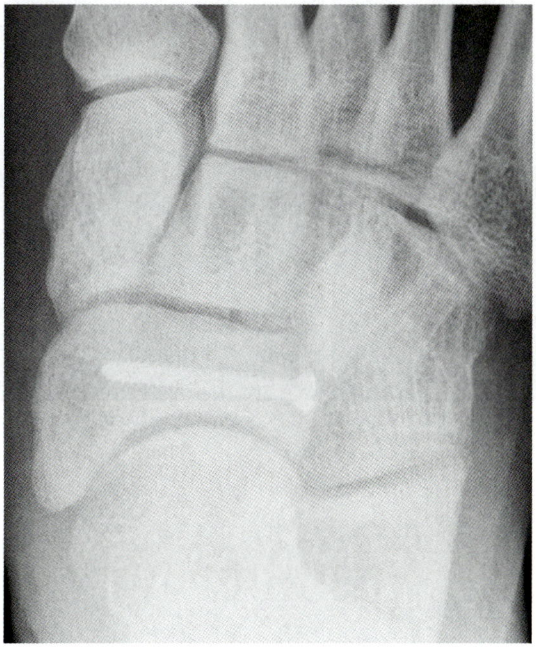

Figure 22-10. Radiograph demonstrating lag screw fixation across the fracture site.

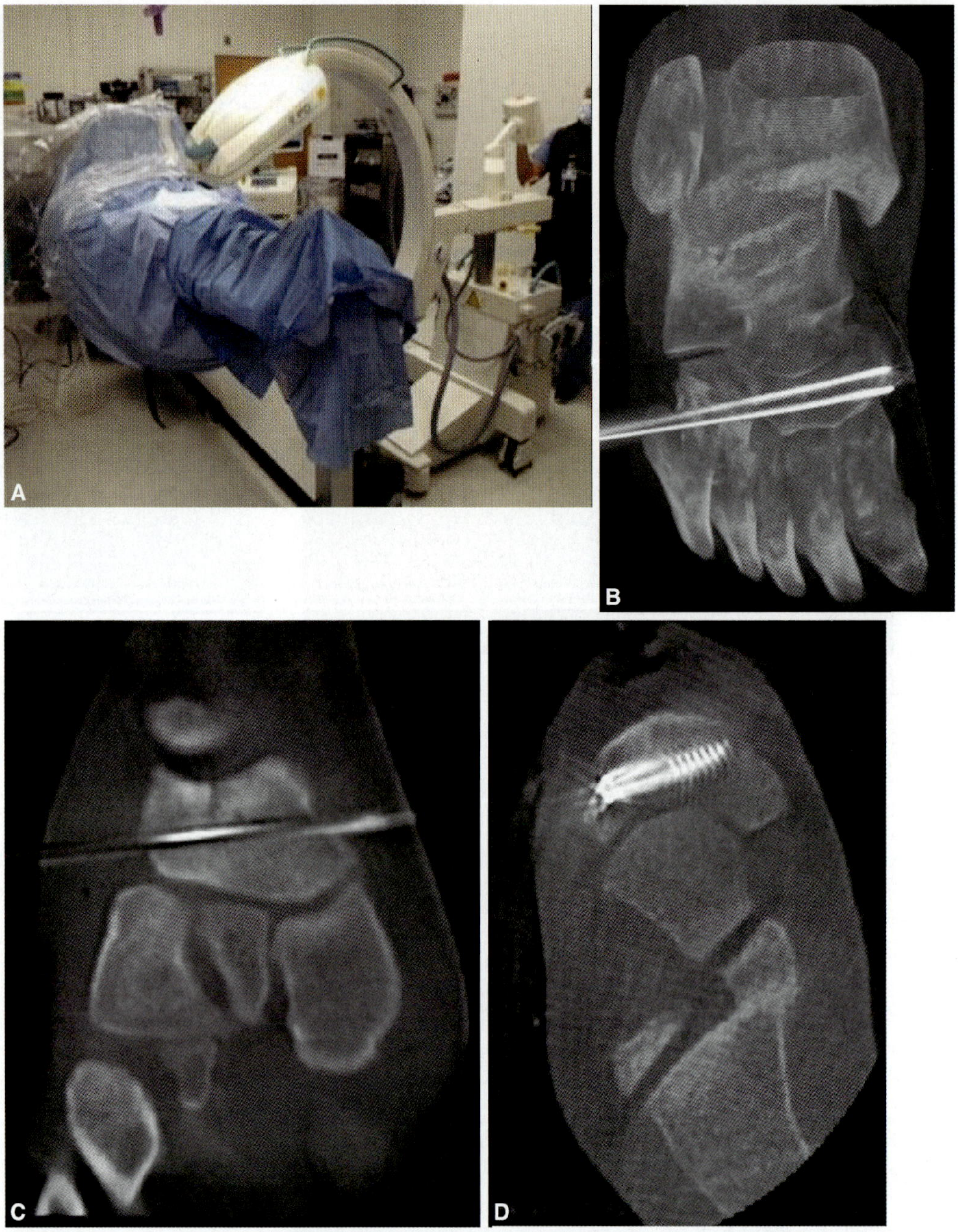

Figure 22-11. Use of intraoperative computed tomography to confirm appropriate placement of fixation.

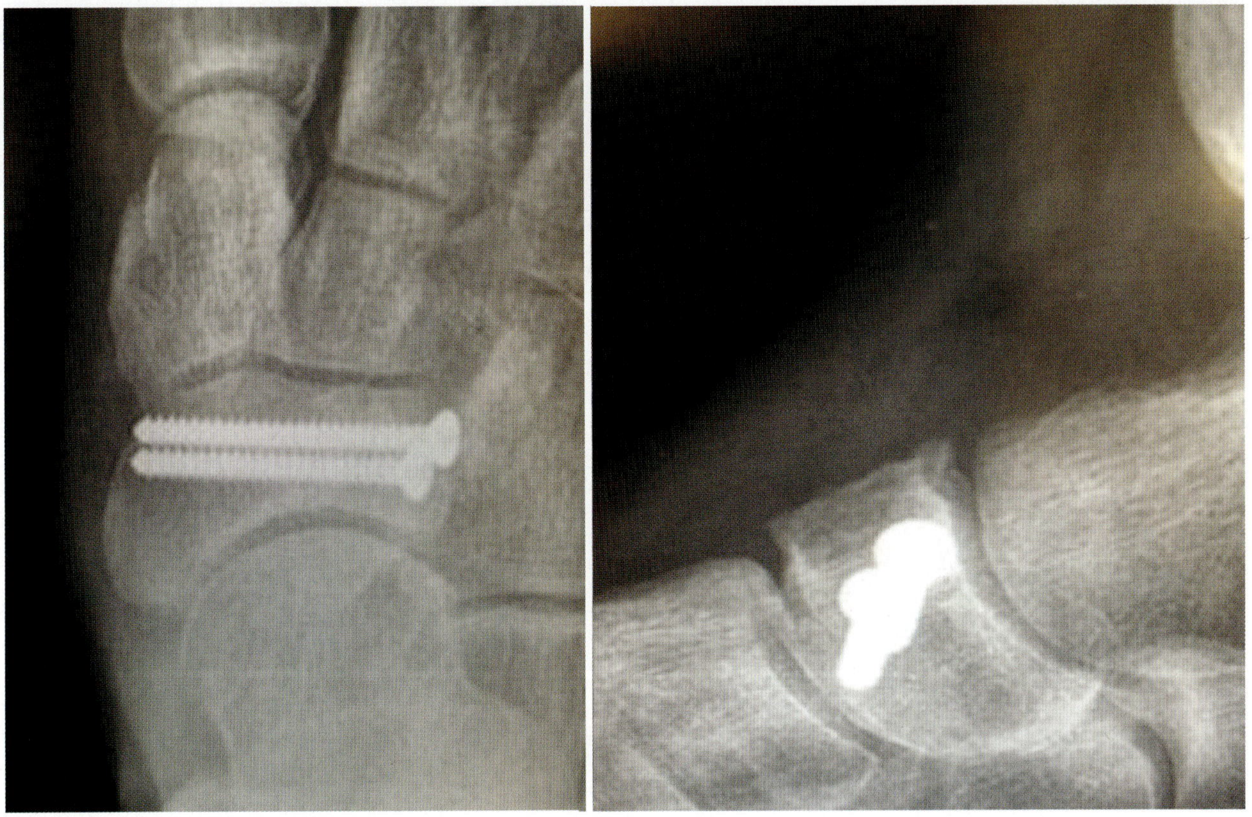

Figure 22-12. Additional screws are added for rotation control in unstable fractures.

- Given that the fracture line is often subtle and is difficult or impossible to see using standard fluoroscopy, intraoperative CT scan can be performed to confirm good position of the guidewire relative to the fracture line and within the anatomy of the navicular bone (see Figure 22-11).
- In cases of a complete fracture that is rotationally unstable, an additional 3.5-mm cortical screw can be placed (see Figure 22-12).

Reference

1. Saxena A, Fullem B, Hannaford D. Results of treatment of 22 navicular stress fractures: a new proposed radiographic classification system. *J Foot Ankle Surg*. 2000;39:96–103.

Section 7

Stress Fractures of the Foot and Ankle

Chapter 23

Medial Malleolar Stress Fractures

AKASH GUPTA
MARTIN O'MALLEY

Introduction

- Medial malleolar stress fractures are relatively rare injuries, accounting for only 0.6% to 4.1% of all lower extremity stress fractures.
- They occur in athletes who engage in repetitive jumping and running, such as basketball players and track and feel athletes.
- Athletes often present with nonspecific pain and normal radiographs.
- Surgical intervention ensures a quicker rate of healing and lower nonunion risk

Imaging

- X-rays: The majority of medial malleolar stress fractures are vertically oriented, and the fracture line typically extends proximally from the junction of the tibial plafond and medial malleolus. However, many athletes present with normal radiographs and nonspecific ankle pain. Clinicians should include this fracture in their differential diagnosis of ankle pain in the jumping athlete and consider advanced imaging.
- Magnetic resonance imaging (MRI): MRI can assist in detecting bone edema and stress reaction, which may occur before a stress fracture (Figure 23-1). Medial malleolar stress reactions present

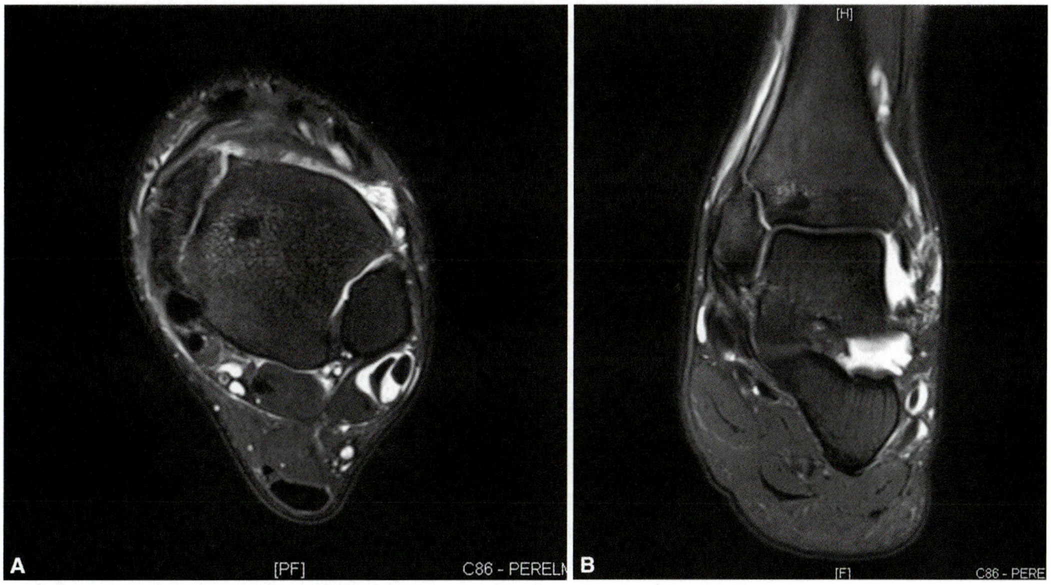

Figure 23-1. Axial (A) and coronal (B) T2-weighted magnetic resonance images demonstrating a medial malleolus stress reaction. Note the bone marrow edema.

with symptoms similar to those of stress fractures, but lack an obvious fracture line on computed tomography (CT). By detecting such stress reactions early, steps may be taken to prevent the stress reaction from progressing into a full-blown stress fracture. Obtained preoperatively, MRIs can also assist in detecting osteochondral defects. MRI has the additional advantage of avoiding radiation exposure.

- CT: CT scans are critical to the understanding of fracture geometry and should be obtained preoperatively on all patients. Most often, the fracture line is vertical, originating anteriorly and inferiorly at the junction of the medial malleolus and tibial plafond with an intact posterior cortex (Figure 23-2). In addition to these stress fractures, CT scans can help identify tibial and talar osteophytes.

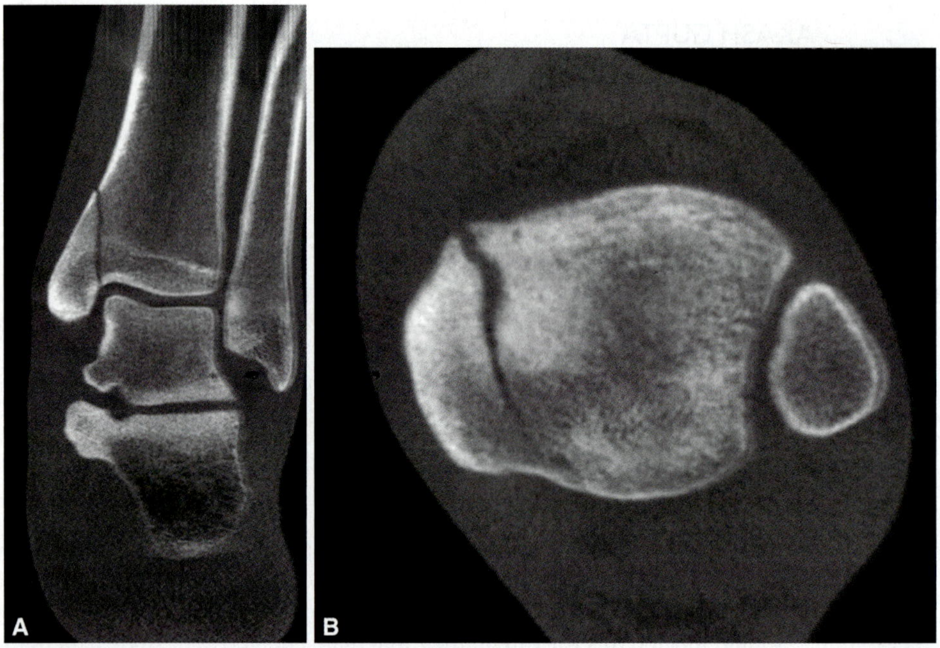

Figure 23-2. Anteroposterior radiograph (A) demonstrating a traditional medial malleolus stress fracture. Axial (B) computed tomography image demonstrating a traditional medial malleolus stress fracture with an intact posterior cortex.

Treatment Algorithm

- Malleolar stress fractures can be treated either conservatively with immobilization and reduction in weight-bearing activities or with surgery. However, conservative treatment has been associated with prolonged healing rates and tendency toward nonunion. With conservative treatment, fracture union and return to full activity can take as long as 6 to 8 months.
- With operative treatment, return to play can be expected as early as 3 months following surgery. Given the upper limit of how long nonoperative treatment can take, surgery is the preferred method of treatment for these fractures.
- Historically, the reported operative treatment of medial malleolar stress fractures had been the use of two partially threaded cancellous screws placed obliquely to the fracture similar to a standard transverse medial malleolus fracture. Biomechanical studies then showed the superiority of perpendicular screw placement across fracture lines compared to oblique placement with regard to maximizing fracture compression.
- Placing screws perpendicularly across the fracture is preferred because oblique fixation can cause superior fracture displacement.
- With regard to vertical fractures, medial malleoli repaired with a combination of screws and a stabilization plate have been shown to be more capable of withstanding offset axial load than are medial malleoli repaired with screws alone. Plate fixation at the apex of the fracture line prevents superior migration and provides a more stable construct to prevent micromotion (Figure 23-3).

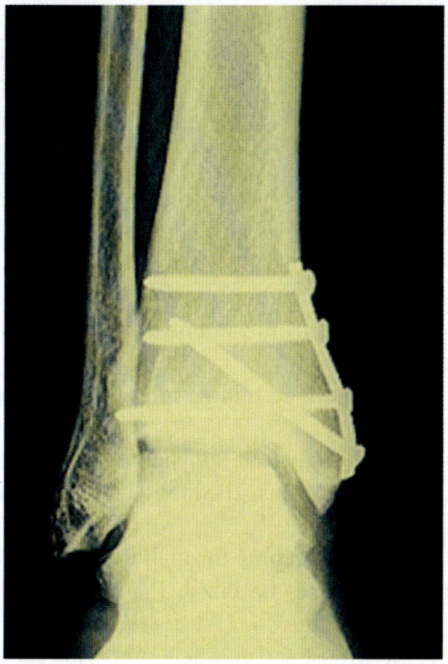

Figure 23-3. Plate fixation used to treat a medial malleolus stress fracture.

- Therefore, open reduction and internal fixation with both screws and a plate is most likely to ensure a relatively quick and successful recovery compared to other surgical and nonsurgical alternatives.
- Address anteromedial impingement at the time of surgery.

Equipment

- Tourniquet
- Headlight
- K-wires with wire driver
- Bone marrow aspirate set with trocar
- Implants
  - 1/3 tubular plate
  - 3.5-mm cancellous screws
  - 4.0-mm cannulated screws
- 1/4 and 1/2 in osteotomes
- Narrow rongeurs
- Mini C-arm
- 22-Gauge needle

Positioning

- Supine, with bump under ipsilateral hip so that foot is pointing straight up
- Take care to pad all bony prominences.
- See Chapter 1 for full description.

Technique

Bone Marrow Aspirate

- Bone marrow is aspirated from the ipsilateral iliac crest under local anesthesia and sedation if the patient had an ankle block, or under spinal anesthesia.
- To extract the marrow, a hollow trocar needle is advanced into the cancellous bone of the anterior ilium, just posterior to the anterosuperior spine.

- Approximately 60 mL of bone marrow is removed with a standard syringe, prepared, and centrifuged using the Magellan system (Arteriocyte, Cleveland, OH) to produce the bone marrow aspirate concentrate (BMAC).
- 3 to 4 mL of the concentrate is optimal.

Fracture Fixation

- Mark out the medial malleolus including the anterior and posterior aspects, as well as the tip.
- An incision is made halfway between the anterior and posterior aspects of the medial malleolus. The incision is approximately 8 cm and extends from 1 cm proximal to the apex of the fracture to just short of the tip of the medial malleolus.
- If impingement lesions or osteophytes are identified radiographically, then the distal extent of the incision should curve more anteriorly.
- Skin flaps are mobilized and care is taken to protect the subcutaneous long saphenous vein, usually running just anterior to the medial malleolus. The long saphenous nerve accompanies the vein.
- If anteromedial osteophytes are present, an arthrotomy through the capsule can be made anteriorly and the anteromedial shoulder of the joint can be visualized. The osteophytes can then be removed with a rongeur or 1/4- to 1/2-in curved osteotome.
- Sharply dissect down onto the medial malleolus, and elevate a subperiosteal layer and the split fibers of the deltoid to create room for the plate directly medial. Care is taken not to dissect too far posteriorly and violate the posterior tibial tendon.
- The fracture site should not be opened.
- Contour a 1/3 tubular plate such that the top hole is proximal to the apex of the fracture and the distal hole extends close to the tip of the medial malleolus.
- Place bicortical 3.5-mm cortical screws through the plate, with one screw being proximal to the apex of the fracture and two screws crossing perpendicular to the fracture site (Figure 23-4).
- Ensure the screws crossing the fracture site are not prominent into the incisura, which could cause widening of the syndesmosis.
- The distal hole of the plate can be filled with a short screw into the medial malleolus, taking care not to violate the far cortex and have a screw prominent into the medial gutter.

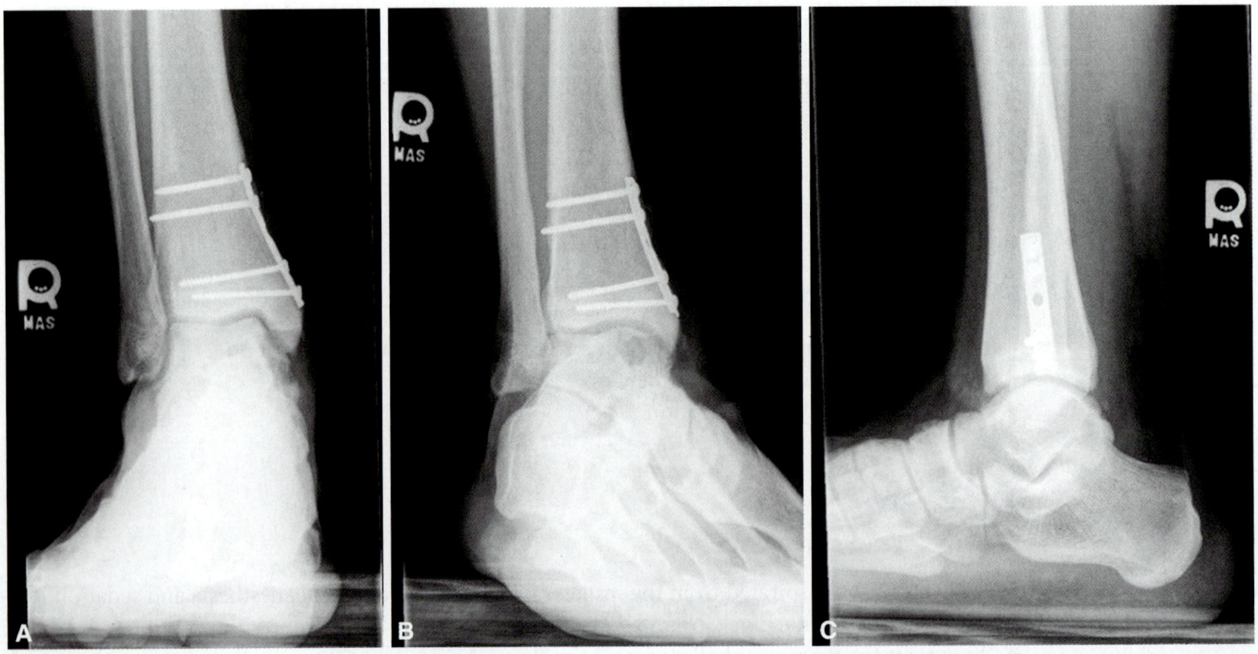

Figure 23-4. Anteroposterior (A), mortise (B), and lateral radiographs (C) demonstrating antiglide plate fixation with distal screws perpendicular to the fracture line.

- Alternatively, the distal hole can be filled with a screw directed proximal to the medial shoulder of the joint and across the fracture (Figure 23-5).
- If additional fixation is needed, 4.0-mm cannulated cancellous screws can be inserted anteriorly and posteriorly into the medial malleolus. Guidewires are placed into the anterior and posterior

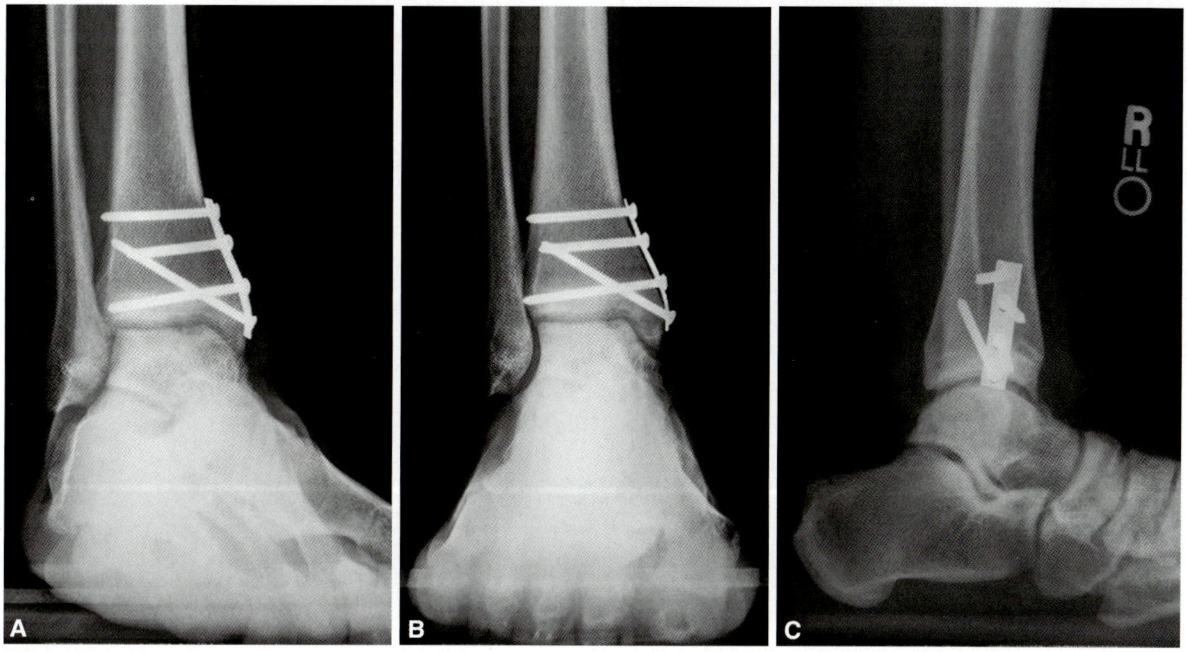

Figure 23-5. Alternative screw orientation for fixation, as seen on AP (A), Mortise (B), and Lateral (C) radiographs.

colliculus of the medial malleolus. The wires should be parallel or slightly divergent. Ensure that the screws are not violating the medial shoulder of the joint. Unicortical cancellous screws are then placed after drilling over the top of the guidewires (Figure 23-6).
- Once the wound is closed, BMAC can be injected into the fracture site using a 22-gauge needle.

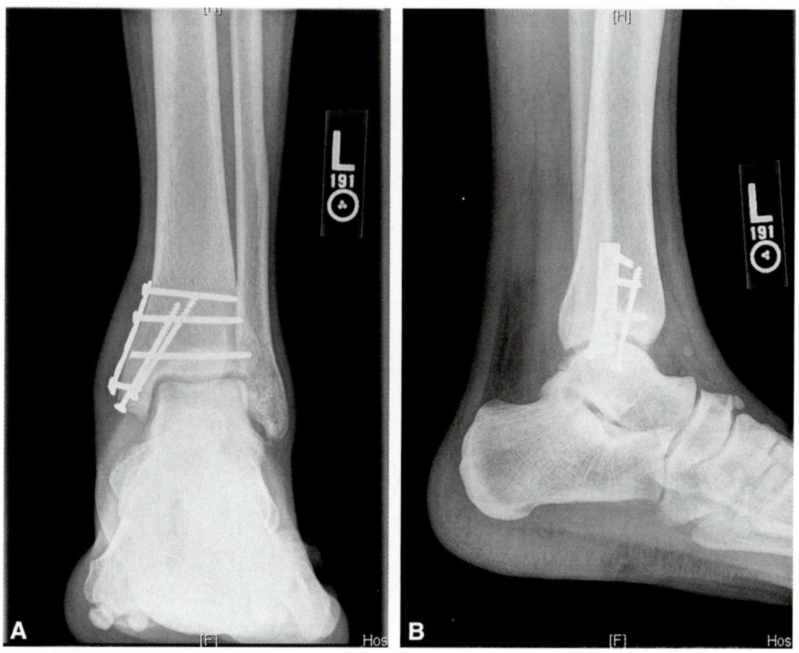

Figure 23-6. Anteroposterior (A) and lateral (B) radiographs depicting the placement of partially threaded cancellous screws in addition to plate fixation to provide an enhanced construct and stability.

Postoperative Care

- Patients are kept non–weight-bearing for 2 weeks.
- At 2 weeks, patients are transitioned to weight-bearing as tolerated in a CAM boot.
- Patients can be allowed to use stationary bicycles at 4 weeks postoperatively and begin to wean out of the CAM boot.

Section 8
Ankle Trauma

Chapter 24
Pilon Fractures

MATTHEW ANDERSON
STEFANOS HADDAD
ANDREW J. ROSENBAUM

Sterile Instruments/Equipment

- Tourniquet
- Implants
  - Distal tibia periarticular plating system locking and nonlocking
  - Tubular plates
  - Small fragment plates and screws
  - Mini-fragment plates and screws
  - Plan for bone graft—autograft, allograft, DBX, or other substitutes
- Large external fixator
- Small-caliber Kirschner wires
- Wire driver/drill
- Large universal distractor
- Pointed and serrated bone clamps
- Small and large bone picks and hooks
- Bone foam or other radiolucent support for injured leg
- Bulky Jones splint materials
- Intraoperative fluoroscopy

Positioning/Preparation

- Preoperative computed tomography (CT) for planning
- Discuss pain management with anesthesia; regional nerve block is recommended.
- Supine positioning with a towel bump under the hip on operative side to make foot neutral. Lateral positioning may be necessary to access the posterior malleolus.
- Use bone foam or padding to elevate surgical leg above contralateral.
- Pad bony prominences (eg, contralateral heel).
- Place distal thigh tourniquet and secure with silk tape.
- Administer prophylactic antibiotics (1-2 g cefazolin or a similar antibiotic).
- The operative limb should be prepped in the usual sterile fashion. The external fixator pins are also prepped so that they can be included in the sterile field.
- Drape with 1 to 2 U-drapes and an extremity drape, leaving proximal leg to calf on sterile field.

Surgical Approach

The surgical approach for definitive fixation depends on the fracture pattern. The anterior approaches provide access to the plafond for adequate restoration of the articular surface, but the choice is usually determined by the site of comminution.

Direct Anterior Approach

- Mark out incision starting 10 cm proximal to the joint and 2 cm lateral to the anterior crest of the tibia, passing between malleoli and ending 5 cm distal to the joint (Figure 24-1).
- Stay superficial on initial dissection to avoid injuring superficial peroneal nerve branches. Identify the superficial peroneal nerve, release along its length, and protect.
- Incise the deep fascia in line with the skin incision. Identify the plan between the tibialis anterior (TA) and extensor hallucis longus (EHL) proximally.
- Identify the neurovascular bundle of the anterior tibial artery and deep peroneal nerve.
- The nerve can then be retracted medially with the TA or laterally with the EHL (Figure 24-2).
- Incise the joint capsule in line with the skin incision.
- Expose the entire width of the ankle joint by subcapsular dissection (Figure 24-3).

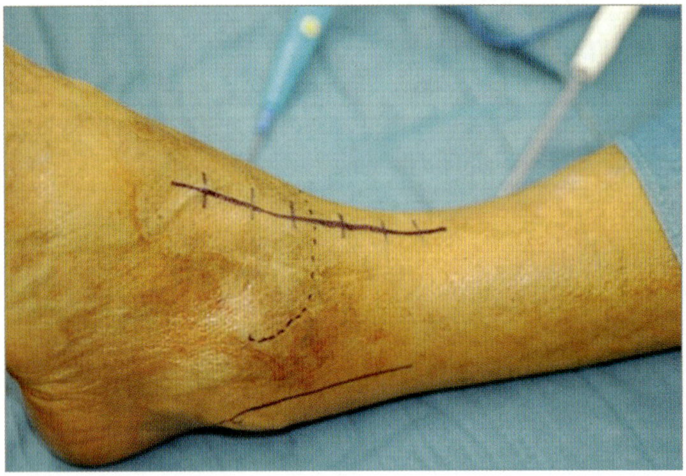

Figure 24-1. Anterior approach—a 10-cm longitudinal skin incision is performed lateral to the tibialis anterior tendon. Reprinted with permission from Kristen KH, Trnka HJ, Wien F. Ankle arthrodesis with an anterior approach. *Tech Foot Ankle Surg*. 2007;6(4):243-248. doi:10.1097/BTF.0b013e31815bc388.

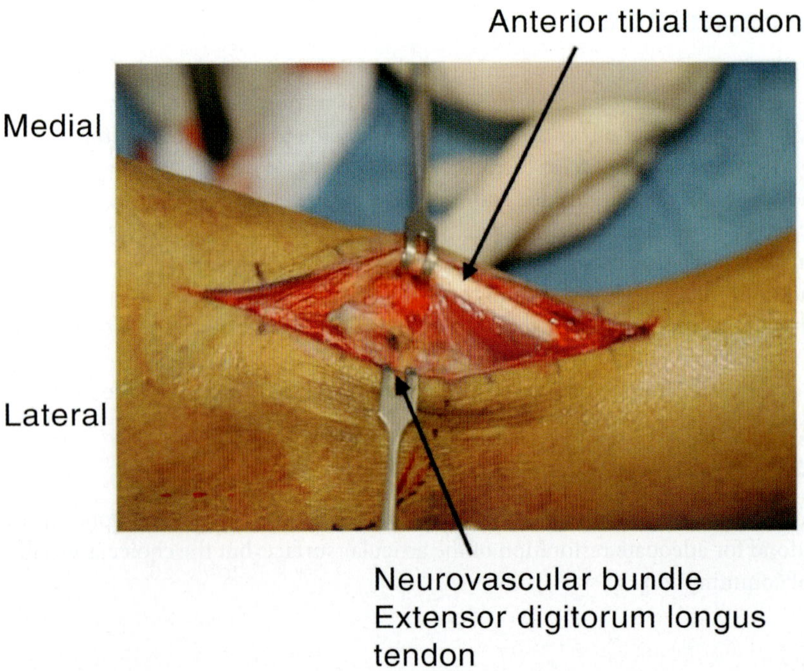

Figure 24-2. The neurovascular bundle is gently mobilized; the tibialis anterior tendon is retracted medially and the extensor digitorum longus tendon laterally. Reprinted with permission from Kristen KH, Trnka HJ, Wien F. Ankle arthrodesis with an anterior approach. *Tech Foot Ankle Surg*. 2007;6(4):243-248. doi:10.1097/BTF.0b013e31815bc388.

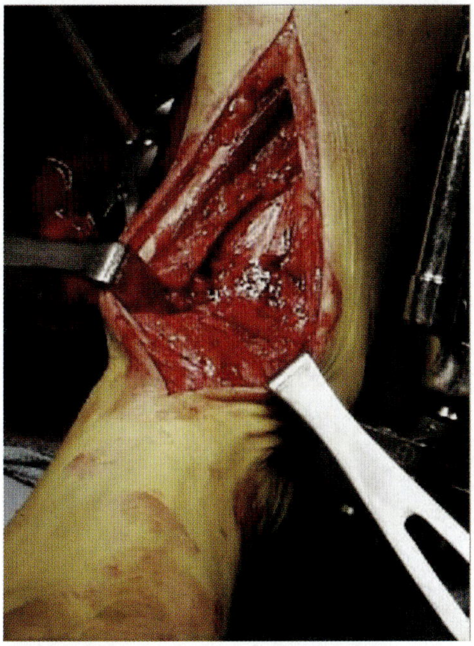

Figure 24-3. Anterior approach and exposure of the ankle joint. Reprinted with permission from Vienne P. Agility total ankle replacement. *Tech Foot Ankle Surg*. 2005;4(1):62-68. doi:10.1097/01.btf.0000153685.03182.a8.

Modified Anteromedial Approach

The modified anteromedial approach makes a turn at the level of the ankle joint, providing greater access to the joint. It is helpful when significant medial comminution is present.

- Mark out an incision starting 1 cm lateral to the anterior crest of the tibia following the course of the TA to the level of the joint, make a 110° turn medially, and end 1 cm distal to the medial malleolus.
- Identify the medial aspect of the TA tendon. Ideally, the paratenon should not be violated.
- Incise down to bone just medial to the TA, creating full-thickness flaps to minimize risk of subsequent necrosis (Figure 24-4).
- Incise the joint capsule in line with the skin incision and subcapsullarly dissect to expose the plafond.

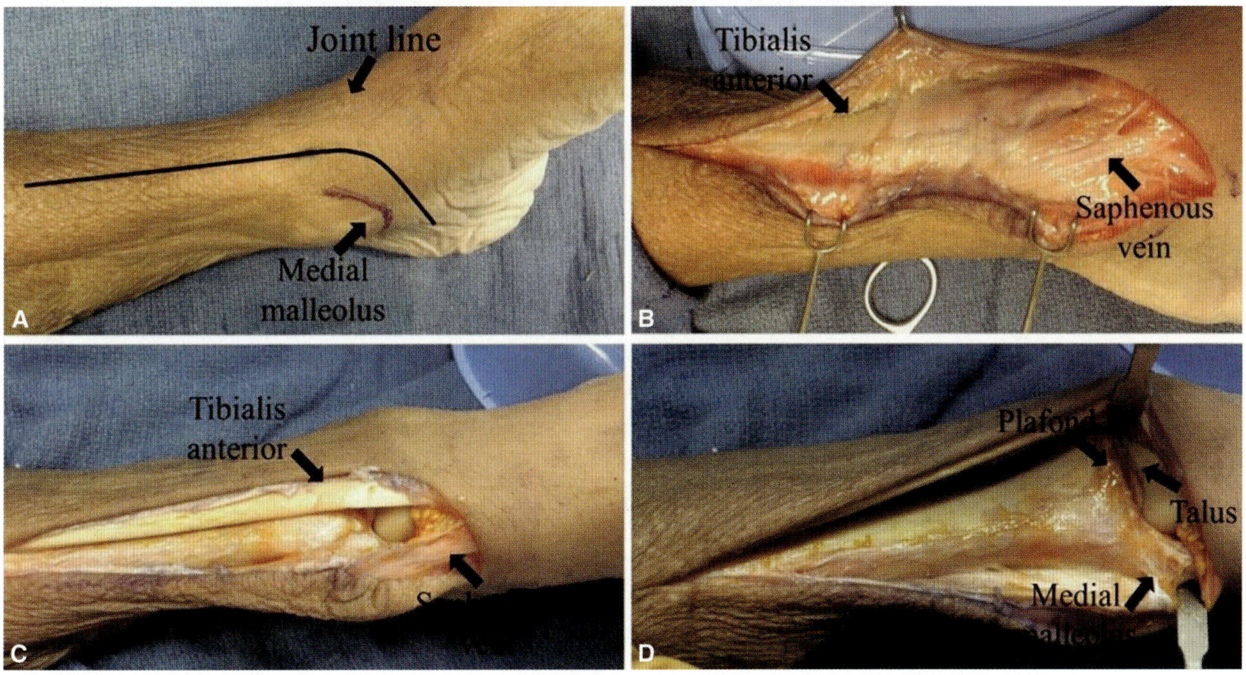

Figure 24-4. Extensile anteromedial approach. A, The skin incision is 1 cm lateral to the tibial crest proximally and then turns at a 110° angle at the ankle joint to end 1 cm distal to the medial malleolus. B, Full-thickness skin flaps are created to reveal the tibialis anterior tendon and extensor retinaculum. The saphenous vein and nerve should be protected. C, The extensor retinaculum is incised longitudinally, preserving the sheath of the tibialis anterior. D, Retraction of tibialis anterior laterally and the full-thickness skin flap medially provides a wide exposure of the anterior plafond from the medial malleolus to the anterolateral edge. Reprinted with permission from Warner SJ, Lorich DG. Surgical approach options for pilon fractures. *Tech Foot Ankle Surg*. 2016;15(4):169-174. doi:10.1097/BTF.0000000000000124.

Anterolateral Approach

The anterolateral approach avoids making a dissection of the medial soft tissue and aids in reduction of the anterolateral fragment, but does not provide access if there is significant medial comminution.

- Mark out incision longitudinally oriented in line with the fourth ray and proximally centered between the tibia and fibula, no more than 7 cm from the joint line and distal over the fourth ray (Figure 24-5).

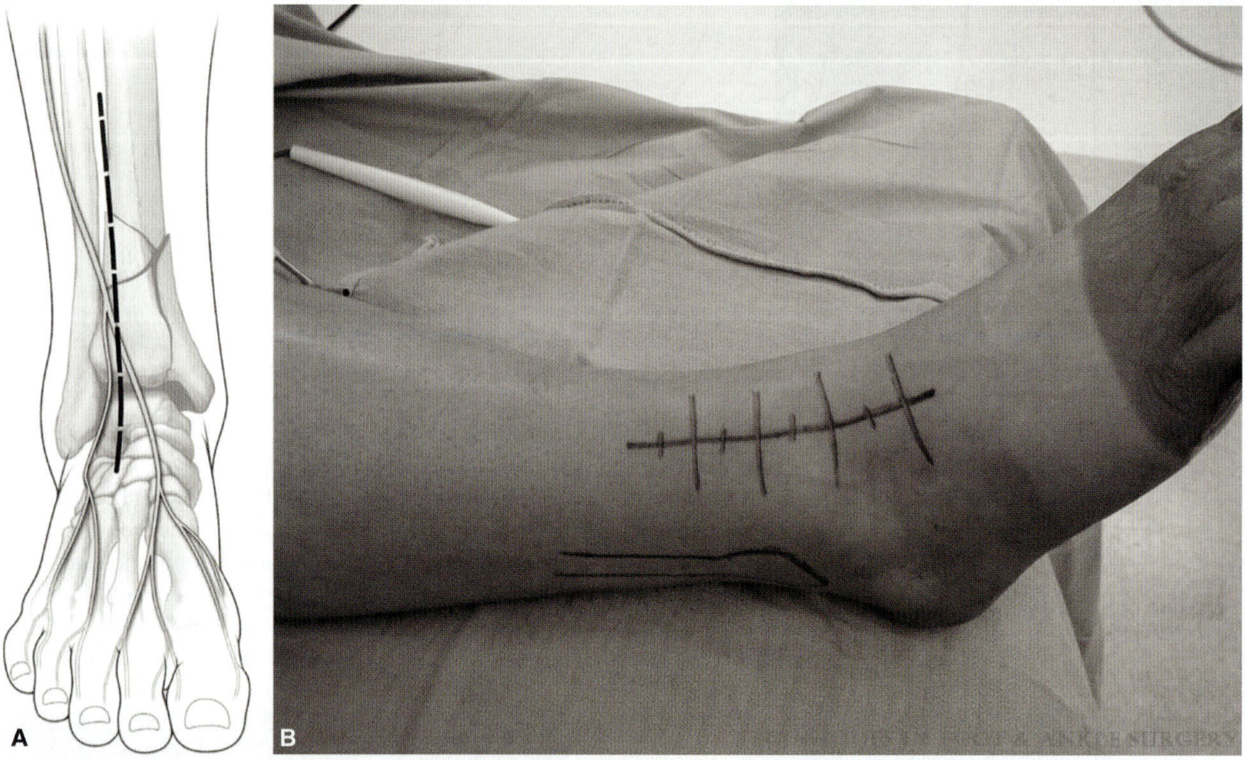

Figure 24-5. A, This schematic demonstrates the location of the anterolateral surgical incision. The incision is typically placed in line with the fourth metatarsal and centered at the ankle joint. The proximal extension is usually limited by the origin of the anterior compartment musculature. B, A typical incision location and length. This allows for the exposure of the articular surface for reduction and placement of plates at the distal tibial metaphysis. Proximal plate placement and fixation typically requires an additional approach more proximally or, more frequently, multiple small incisions for lateral to medial screw placements. Distally, the talar neck is exposed to allow for the placement of a distractor across the ankle joint. Reprinted with permission from Nork SE, Barei DP, Gardner MJ, Mehta S, Benirsche SK. Anterolateral approach for pilon fractures. *Tech Foot Ankle Surg*. 2009;8(2):53-59. doi:10.1097/BTF.0b013e3181a77e45.

- Care must be taken to identify superficial peroneal nerve and its branches, which can be mobilized and retracted medially or laterally (Figure 24-6).
- The superior and inferior extensor retinacula are incised in line with the skin just lateral to the extensor digitorum longus (EDL) and peroneus tertius tendons. This incision is continued proximally through the anterior compartment fascia.
- The entire anterior compartment is retracted medially (Figure 24-7).
- The joint capsule is incised longitudinally. Transversally oriented vessels are often encountered and require cauterization.

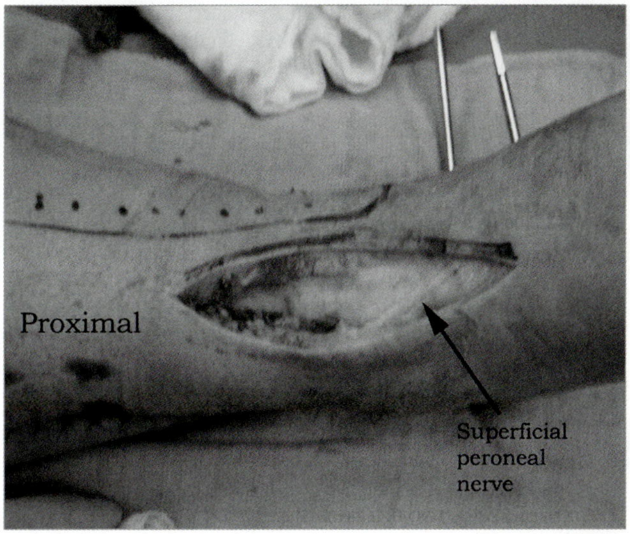

Figure 24-6. The superficial peroneal nerve invariably crosses the surgical incision and must be protected throughout the operative procedure. Reprinted with permission from Nork SE, Barei DP, Gardner MJ, Mehta S, Benirsche SK. Anterolateral approach for pilon fractures. *Tech Foot Ankle Surg*. 2009;8(2):53-59. doi:10.1097/BTF.0b013e3181a77e45.

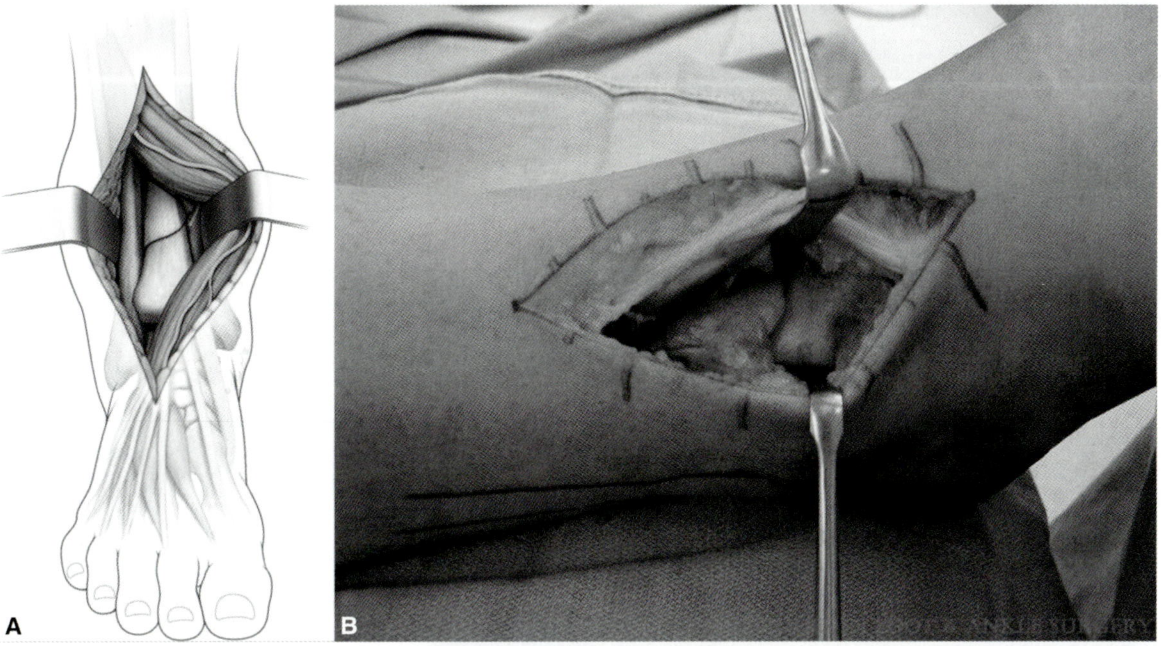

Figure 24-7. A, The deep dissection allows for the exposure of the distal tibial metaphysis after medial retraction of the entire anterior compartment. B, After an arthrotomy of the ankle joint, the distal tibia and the talar neck are exposed. The anterior tibiofibular ligaments are left attached to the anterolateral articular segment. Reprinted with permission from Nork SE, Barei DP, Gardner MJ, Mehta S, Benirsche SK. Anterolateral approach for pilon fractures. *Tech Foot Ankle Surg*. 2009;8(2):53-59. doi:10.1097/BTF.0b013e3181a77e45.

Posterolateral Approach

Particularly useful if there is posterior comminution; reduction of the Volkmann fragment and the fibula (Figure 24-8)

- Mark out incision midway between the posterior border of the fibula and the Achilles tendon.
- During superficial dissection, take care to protect the sural nerve.
- Incise the deep fascia longitudinally.
- Access the posterior lateral surface of the fibula by retracting the peroneus longus and brevis medially and releasing from the fibula.

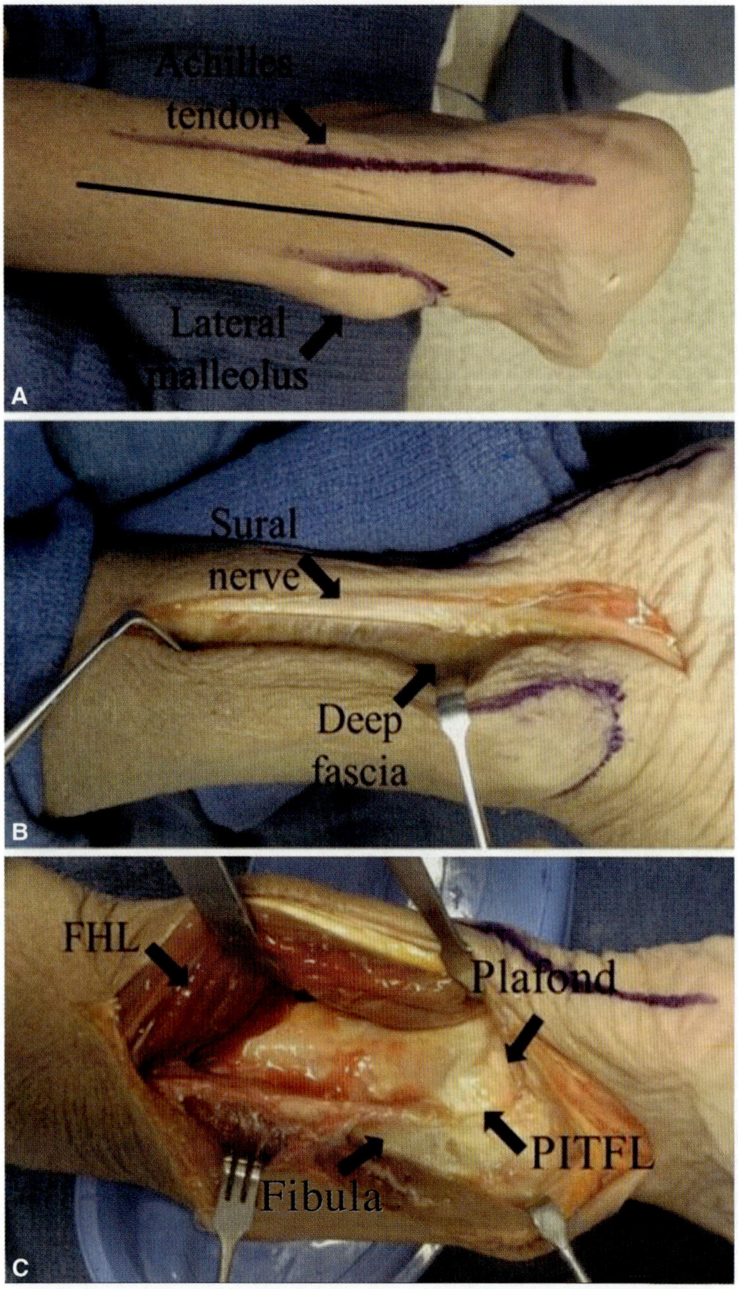

Figure 24-8. Posterolateral approach. The incision is centered between the lateral border of the Achilles tendon and the medial border of the lateral malleolus (A). Dissection through subcutaneous tissue reveals the sural nerve and deep fascia (B). An interval between the flexor hallucis longus (FHL) and peroneals is developed to expose the posterior fibula and posterolateral plafond (C). PITFL, posterior inferior tibiofibular ligament. Reprinted with permission from Warner SJ, Lorich DG. Surgical approach options for pilon fractures. *Tech Foot Ankle Surg*. 2016;15(4):169-174. doi:10.1097/BTF.0000000000000124.

- To access the Volkmann fragment, bluntly dissect between the flexor hallucis longus (FHL) and peroneal tendons and retract the FHL medially to expose the posterior malleolus. Care must be taken to not release the posterior–inferior tibiofibular ligament (PITFL), which will devitalize the posterior malleolar fragment.

Reduction and Fixation Techniques

The treatment goal of pilon fractures is restoration of the articular surface while avoiding significant damage to the soft tissues. This is most often achieved in a staged manner, initially with external fixation with or without open reduction internal fixation (ORIF) of the fibula, until soft-tissue swelling resolves, followed by definitive ORIF.

External Fixation

The goals of external fixation are restoration of length with the talus under the plafond and the foot in a neutral anatomic position (Figure 24-9).

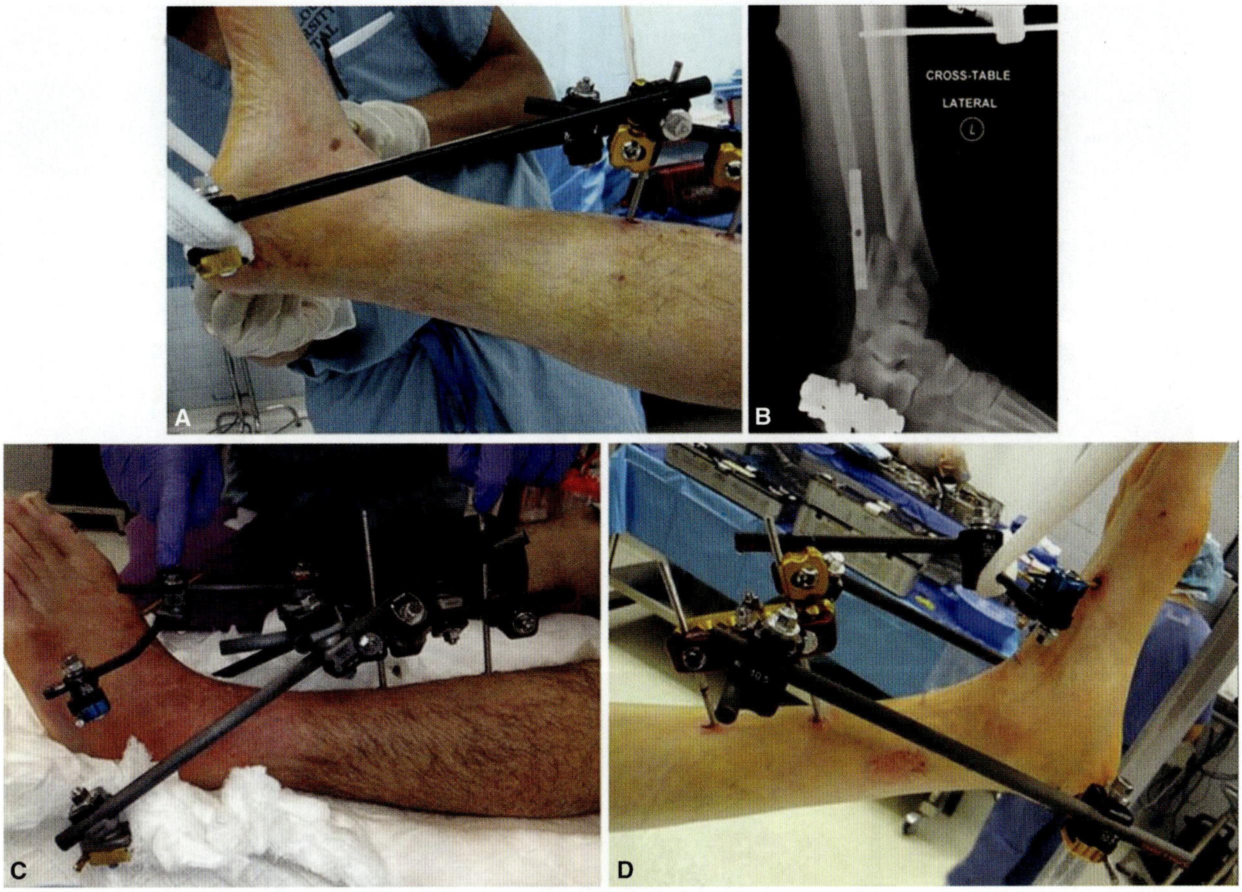

Figure 24-9. A, Ankle-spanning fixator with solitary connecting bars and no forefoot stabilization. B, As the fixator clamps "creep," gravity will cause the foot/fracture fragment to slowly displace posteriorly, placing additional pressure on the anterior soft tissues, and may actually delay their recovery. X-ray demonstrating the posterior translation of the distal fracture segment, rotating around the calcaneal pin, despite the fibular plate and connecting bars. Note anterior skin tethering against proximal fracture line. C, Spanning fixator with forefoot support keeping fracture aligned and soft tissues at rest. D, Note skin wrinkles now amenable to surgical intervention. Reprinted with permission from Watson JT. Complications in tibial pilon fractures: avoiding errors in judgment. *Tech Foot Ankle Surg*. 2016;15(4):175-187. doi:10.1097/BTF.0000000000000131.

- Application of a spanning biplanar external fixator starts by identifying the proximal extent of the tibial fracture.
- Insert tibial 5-mm Schanz pin out of the anticipated area for definitive fixation.
- Insert centrally threaded 5-mm Schanz pin into the calcaneus.
- Insert 4-mm Schanz pin into midfoot through the medial, middle, and lateral cuneiforms.
- Securing the transcalcaneus pin to the tibial pin should restore the majority of length and reduce the talus under the plafond. Restoration of the dime sign is helpful to ensure adequate distraction. Securing the midfoot pin to the tibial pin aids in maintaining a plantigrade foot.

Open Reduction Internal Fixation

Anatomic restoration of the tibial plafond is the goal of ORIF of the tibia. Restoring the articular surface will not matter without restoring the ability to transfer load from the plafond to the diaphysis of the tibia. These goals must be accomplished while maintaining soft-tissue viability. This makes preoperative planning utilizing radiographs and axial CT scan vital to proper fixation of pilon fractures (Figure 24-10).

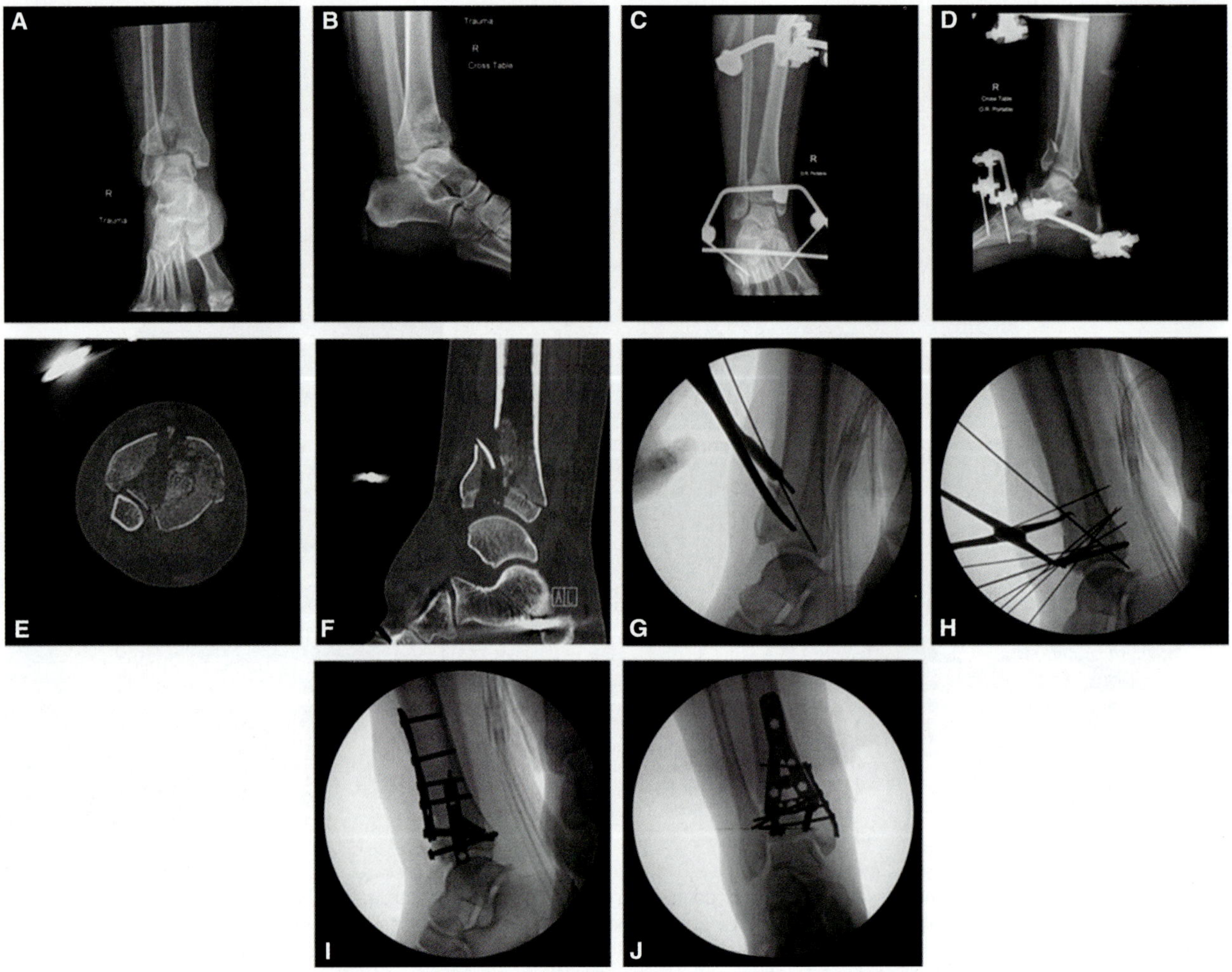

Figure 24-10. Anteroposterior (A) and lateral (B) x-rays of a high-energy tibial pilon fracture. An ankle spanning external fixator was applied initially and traction x-rays (C) and a computed tomography (D) scan were obtained for definitive surgical planning. The fibula is intact. The primary deforming forces are shortening and anterior displacement. E, The main fracture line exits anteromedially that was used to access the posterior malleolus fragment and the central impaction. F, The sagittal reconstruction shows the posterior joint surface flexed and the amount of subchondral bone available to assist with the reduction. G, Working from back to front through an anteromedial approach, the posterior joint surface was reduced and K-wired. Then the central impaction was reduced and bone grafted. H-J, Finally the anterolateral joint and the medial malleolus fragment were reduced and stabilized. Reprinted with permission from Siegel J, Tornetta P III. Fracture pattern assessment of tibial pilon fractures. *Tech Foot Ankle Surg*. 2016;15(4):162-168. doi:10.1097/BTF.0000000000000137.

ORIF of Fibula

ORIF of the fibula can be performed at the time of application of the external fixator and can provide indirect reduction of associated anterolateral and Volkmann fragments. In the high energy imparted to generate pilon fractures, the associated fibula fractures often have compressive components, resulting in comminution not typically seen in rotation injuries and requiring more robust fixation (Figure 24-11).

- Utilize the posterolateral approach.
- Avoid extension deformity by bumping the entire leg.
- Reduce the fibula using direct and indirect techniques.
- Use pinpointed reduction clamps or K-wires to hold reduction. Application of external fixator before fibula fixation can restore fibula length and aid in reduction.
- Apply precontoured distal fibular plates or 3.7- or 3.5-mm dynamic compression plates to the lateral malleolus and held with K-wires and a small bone holding clamp.
- Ensure restoration of length and secure plate to proximal fibula using another bone holding clamp.
- Continue to adjust the position until anatomic alignment of the fibula is confirmed under fluoroscopy and fix the plate with screws.
- Close incision using the Allgower–Donati suture technique with nylon sutures.

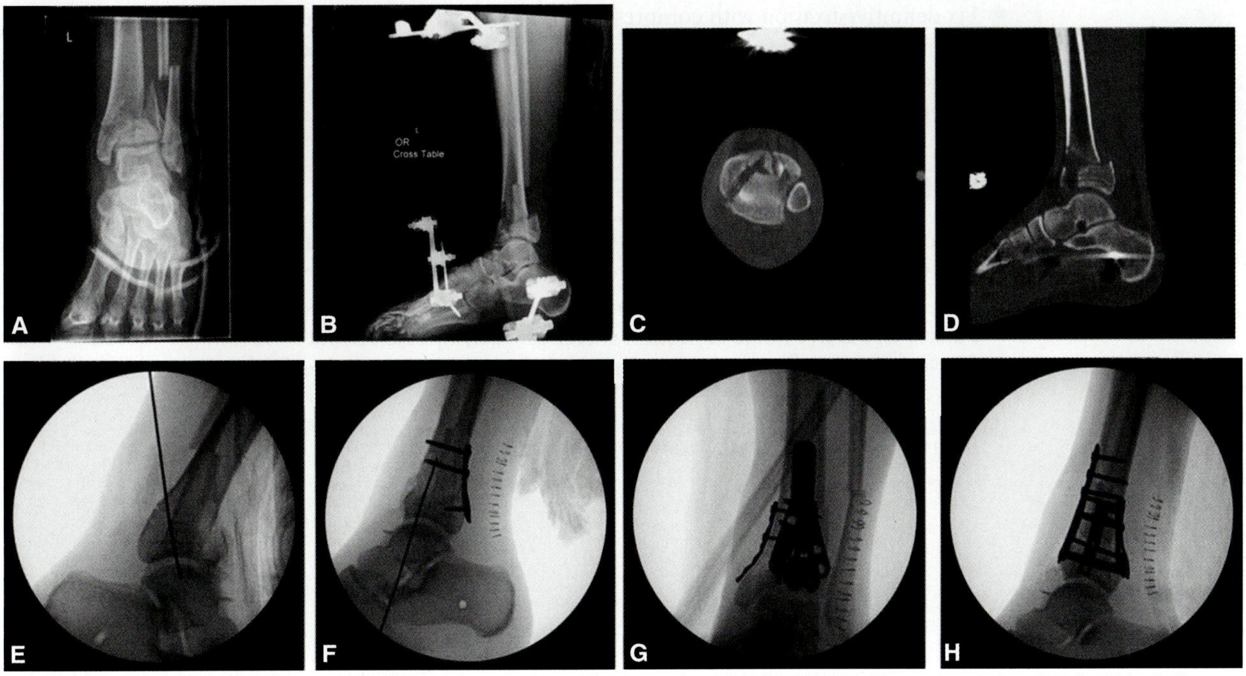

Figure 24-11. A, Anteroposterior injury radiograph of a high-energy tibial pilon fracture. The articular surface is impacted and both the tibia and fibula are short. B, After ankle-spanning external fixation, both the fractures are out to length. C, D, There is an obvious large posterior malleolus fracture. Given the available cortical evaluation of the fracture lines and the reduction posteriorly, the posterior malleolus was first reduced to the talus and the posterior shaft through a prone, posterolateral approach (E) and then stabilized taking care not to interfere with anterior fixation (F). G, H, The patient was then flipped and an anteromedial approach was used to reconstruct the anterior joint injury. The medial malleolus fracture fragment was also buttressed. Reprinted with permission from Siegel J, Tornetta P III. Fracture pattern assessment of tibial pilon fractures. *Tech Foot Ankle Surg*. 2016;15(4):162-168. doi:10.1097/BTF.0000000000000137.

ORIF of Tibia

The goal of ORIF of pilon fractures is restoration of the articular surface with a stable platform. Proximal plate screws may be placed percutaneously.

Preoperative planning should comprise the following:

- Identify the main articular fragments.
- Identify the best area or areas to buttress the epimetaphyseal region.
- Determine the approach or approaches necessary to provide articular fragment fixation and metaphyseal buttressing.
- Determine the number of implants necessary to provide adequate fixation.
- Choose exposures based on fixation needs and soft-tissue constraints.
- Expose distal tibia utilizing appropriate approach.
- Apply joint distraction using external fixator or universal distractor.
- Reduction should occur in a stepwise manner building upon the most anatomic fragments with typical order:
    - Reduce the posterolateral Volkmann fragment relative to the fibula.
    - Reduce the posteromedial fragment to the Volkmann fragment.
    - Reduce/tamp down central plafond comminution.
    - Reduce medial malleolar/anterior plafond fragments.
    - Reduce anterolateral fragment.
- Each reduction is provisionally held with K-wires, avoiding anticipated placement of definitive fixation implants.
- Confirm articular reduction via fluoroscopy.
- Reduce metaphyseal fragments to restore anatomic alignment in all planes.
- Apply definitive plate fixation, periarticular plate plus additional plates to adequately retain reduction, and provisionally hold with bone holding clamps and K-wires.
- Confirm reduction and placement with fluoroscopy.

- Fix definitive fixation with compression, if possible. Proximal screws can be placed percutaneously.
- Confirm accuracy of reduction.
- Remove all provisional fixation.
- Careful layered closure and application of bulky splint with foot in neutral plantigrade position

Postoperative Care

- Postoperative pain management—femoral and popliteal nerve catheters as needed
- Bulky dressing reduced when sutures out in 2 to 3 weeks
- Non–weight-bearing until radiographic healing is noted, approximately 12 weeks
- Passive and active range of motion exercises when sutures are out
- Ankle foot orthosis as needed to maintain plantigrade foot while non–weight-bearing

Chapter 25
Ankle Fractures

KEEGAN COLE
HAMZA MURTAZA

Sterile Instruments/Equipment

- Tourniquet, if desired, unless contraindicated
- Small self-retaining retractors (Weitlaner)
- Small Hohmann retractors
- Small pointed bone reduction clamps (Weber clamps)
- Small serrated bone reduction clamps
- Dental pick
- Freer, Cobb, and/or periosteal elevators
- Implants: anatomically contoured locking or nonlocking periarticular fibular plates (lateral or posterolateral), one-third tubular plates; small and mini-fragment plates/screws
- Long 3.5- or 4.0-mm cortical screws for syndesmosis
- Long 3.0-, 3.5-, or 4.0-mm cortical, cancellous, or cannulated screws for medial malleolus/anterior colliculus
- Mini-fragment screws and mini-fragment plates for fibular lag screws and for posterior or medial malleolar comminution
- K-wires and wire driver/drill

Positioning

- Patient positioning is variable depending on fracture pattern and operative plan.
- Supine positioning with ipsilateral hip bolster for most lateral malleolar, bimalleolar, and trimalleolar fractures
- Abstaining from using a hip bolster allows more external rotation for posteromedial exposure.
- Figure-of-four positioning increases ability to expose posteromedially.
- Lateral or prone position may be necessary for access to the posterior malleolus.
- Prone position allows open reduction internal fixation (ORIF) of medial and lateral malleolus, albeit from an unusual perspective.
- Lateral position may allow fixation of medial malleolus with sufficient external rotation of the hip.

Approaches

- Direct lateral and posterolateral approach
  - Skin incision directly over, or on the posterior aspect of, the fibula
  - Requires protection of superficial peroneal nerve (Figure 25-1)
  - Plane between posterior border of fibula and peroneal tendons
  - May be preferable for:
    - Access to the fibula for lateral or posterolateral plating
    - Access to the posterior malleolus in the interval between flexor hallucis longus (FHL) and peroneal tendons
    - Allowing a separate anterolateral approach for pilon fractures

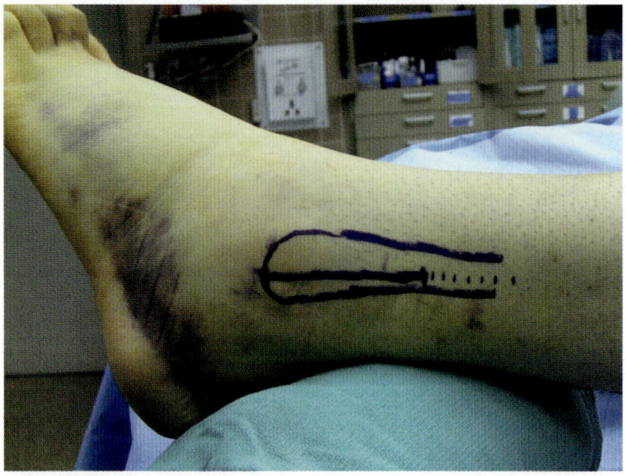

Figure 25-1. Incision for the lateral approach to the fibula, which can be used for direct lateral and posterolateral plating. Reprinted with permission from Easley ME, Wiesel SW. *Operative Techniques in Foot and Ankle Surgery*. 1st ed. Philadelphia, PA: Wolters Kluwer Health/Lippincott Williams & Wilkins; 2010. Chapter 135 Figure 7A.

- Posteromedial approach
  - Access the posterior portion of the medial malleolus, and the posterior malleolus can be achieved anterior to the posterior tibial (PT) tendon or posterior to the PT/flexor digitorum longus (FDL) tendons.
  - The FHL is retracted posteriorly and laterally with the PT neurovascular bundle.
- Anteromedial approach
  - Gently curved skin incision parallel to saphenous vein and nerve
  - Access to the medial malleolus and medial gutter

Reduction and Fixation Tips

Fibula Fractures—Rotational Mechanism

K-wires

- K-wires are used after reduction for provisional fixation and should be driven anterior to posterior to avoid obstruction of the lateral or posterolateral plate (Figure 25-2).

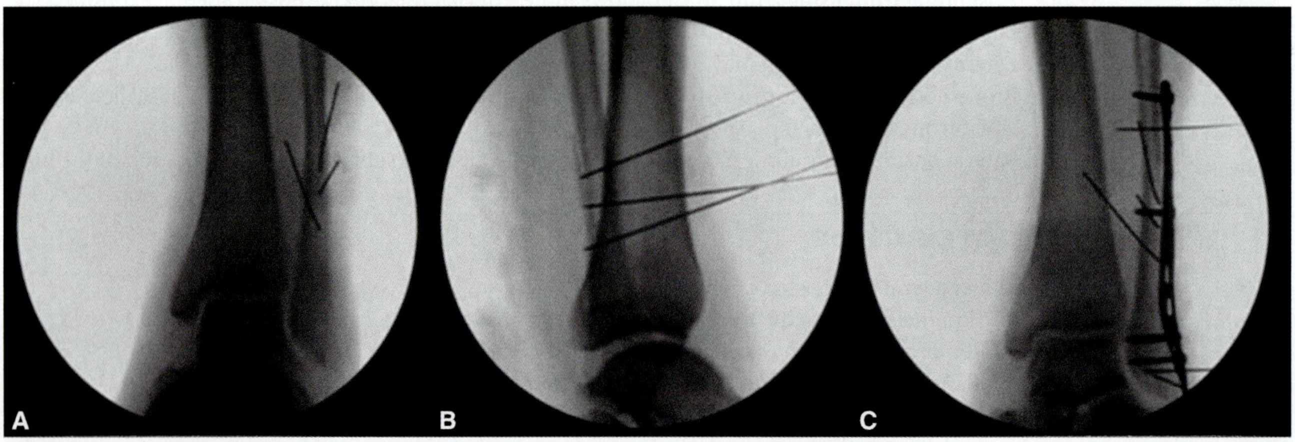

Figure 25-2. Obtain provisional fixation with K-wires in the sagittal plane to avoid plate interference.

Lag Screws

- In addition to plate fixation, most spiral fibular fractures benefit from lag screw fixation.
- Lag screws may be placed before lateral plate placement or through a posterolateral plate after antiglide positioning and distal/proximal fixation to augment compressive fixation force at fracture (Figure 25-3).

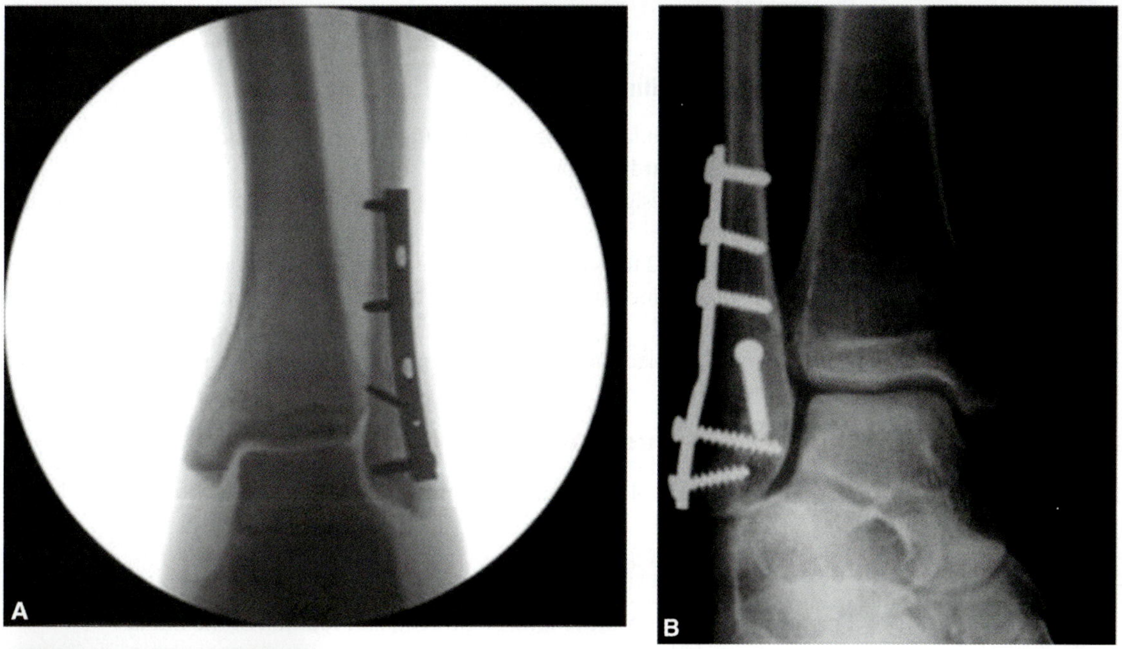

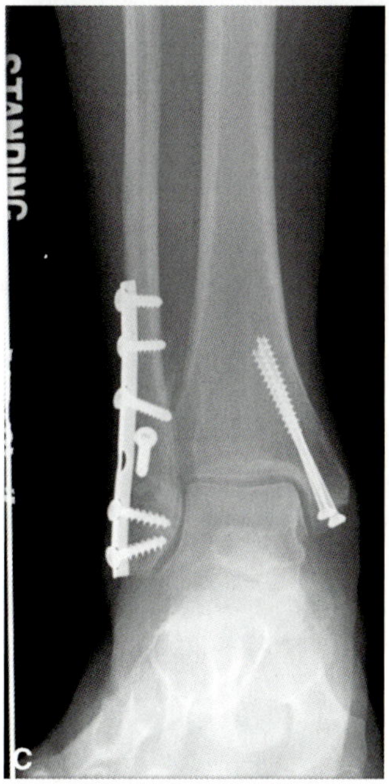

Figure 25-3. Anteroposterior radiograph demonstrating lag screw fixation with a neutralization plate for fibular stabilization. Reprinted with permission from Easley ME, Wiesel SW. *Operative Techniques in Foot and Ankle Surgery*. 1st ed. Philadelphia, PA: Wolters Kluwer Health/Lippincott Williams & Wilkins; 2010. Chapter 135 Tech Figure 7A and B.

- Posterior-to-anterior placement avoids soft-tissue stripping anteriorly.
- 2.0-, 2.4-, or 2.7-mm screws provide adequate fixation, with small heads less likely to interfere with plate application or cause peroneal irritation.
- Use of a mini-fragment lag screw allows to upsize to a slightly larger small-fragment screw if fixation is inadequate.

Plating

- Posterolateral plating allows posterior-to-anterior distal screws in the lateral malleolus that may provide better distal fixation because they are longer and bicortical.

- Antiglide plate position on fracture apex is biomechanically favorable.
- Reduced implant prominence with posterior placement decreases removal rates.
- In osteoporotic bone, consider converging distal screw tips to improve fixation by creating a thread interference fit or use a locking plate.
- Unicortical cancellous screws should be utilized distally in lateral plating to avoid impingement of the incisura.

Intramedullary Nailing

- The technique of fibular nailing is increasing in popularity and offers a minimally invasive approach with little hardware prominence.
- Improvements in design have decreased backout and allow placement of syndesmotic screws through the nail.
- Cortical step-off of 2 to 3 mm is acceptable so long as the mortise is reduced.
- Significant displacement may require percutaneous manipulation or a minimal access incision to obtain reduction.
- Correct guidewire placement along the longitudinal fibular access is critical to prevent malreduction.

Fibula Fractures—Abduction Mechanism

- Abduction produces a transverse comminuted fibular fracture above the level of the syndesmosis.

Fibular Length

- Fragments help determine length, alignment, and rotation of the fibula.
- Contralateral ankle x-rays can be used for comparison.
- Fibular lengths and fibulotalar articulation should also be compared for symmetry.
- The dime sign and the fibular Shenton line can be utilized as an additional aid.

Direct Reduction of the Fibula

- If comminuted fragments are present, mini-fragment screws can be used for fixation.
- To increase fixation stiffness across comminution, stacked one-third tubular plates can be utilized (Figure 25-4).
- If significant comminution is present, a mini-fragment anterior fibular plate can be used to supplement fixation.

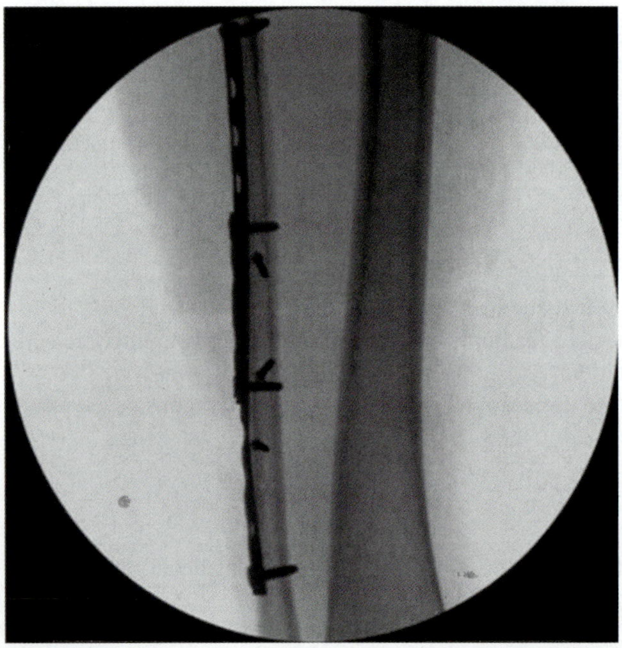

Figure 25-4. In the presence of comminution, stacking one-third tubular plates allows for a stiffer fixation construct across the fracture site.

Indirect Restoration of Fibular Length

- Initially, stabilize the plate distally via multiple K-wires and/or screws.
- Proximal to the plate, insert a bicortical fibular screw as a push screw.
- A laminar spreader applies a distraction force between the push screw and proximal end of the plate to restore its length (Figure 25-5).
- A serrated clamp controls the plate and maintains proximal plate–bone apposition.
- In osteoporotic bone, distracting across screws alone can potentially compromise definitive distal screw fixation because distraction forces may result in cavitation of metaphyseal bone.

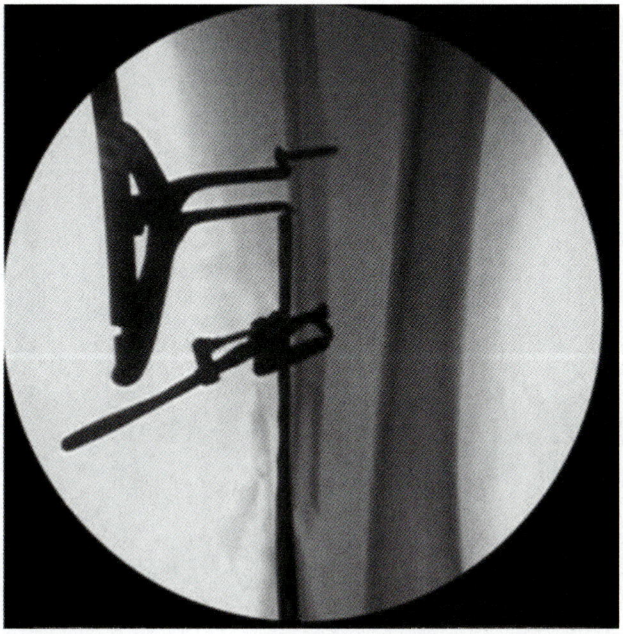

Figure 25-5. Indirect restoration of fibular length via a push screw proximal to the plate and distraction across the fracture site applied with a laminar spreader.

Fibula Fracture—Adduction Mechanism

- This mechanism produces a transverse or short oblique fracture of the distal fibula at or below the level of the syndesmosis.
- A tensioned plate can provide adequate rotational stability for small avulsion fractures (Figure 25-6).

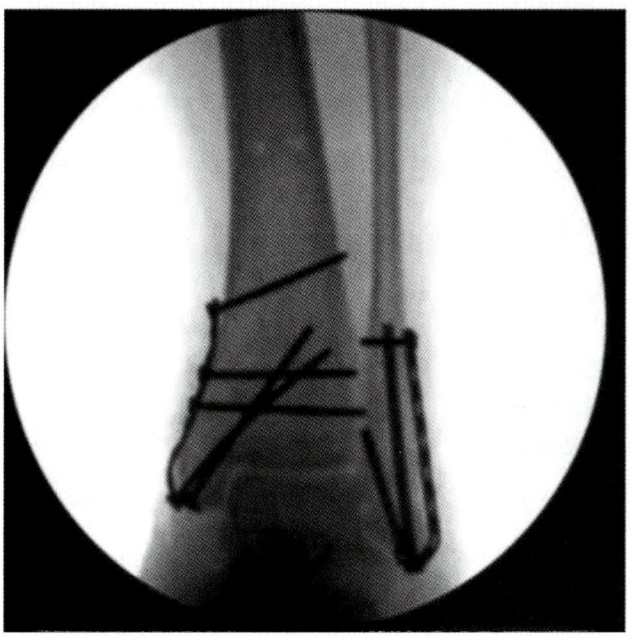

Figure 25-6. Tension plate application for an avulsion fracture of the fibula.

Medullary Screw Fixation

- For this method of fixation to be successful, a rotationally stable fracture pattern is required.
- Of critical technical necessity, the starting point must be centered anteroposterior and lateral and be collinear with the canal of the fibula.
- The starting hole is overdrilled using a larger 3.2- or 3.5-mm drill.
- The medullary canal of the fibula is prepared using a long 2.5-mm calibrated drill bit.
- If marginal articular impaction of the medial plafond exists, it is imperative to diagnose and treat it by elevating the plafond and supporting it with bone graft (Figure 25-7).

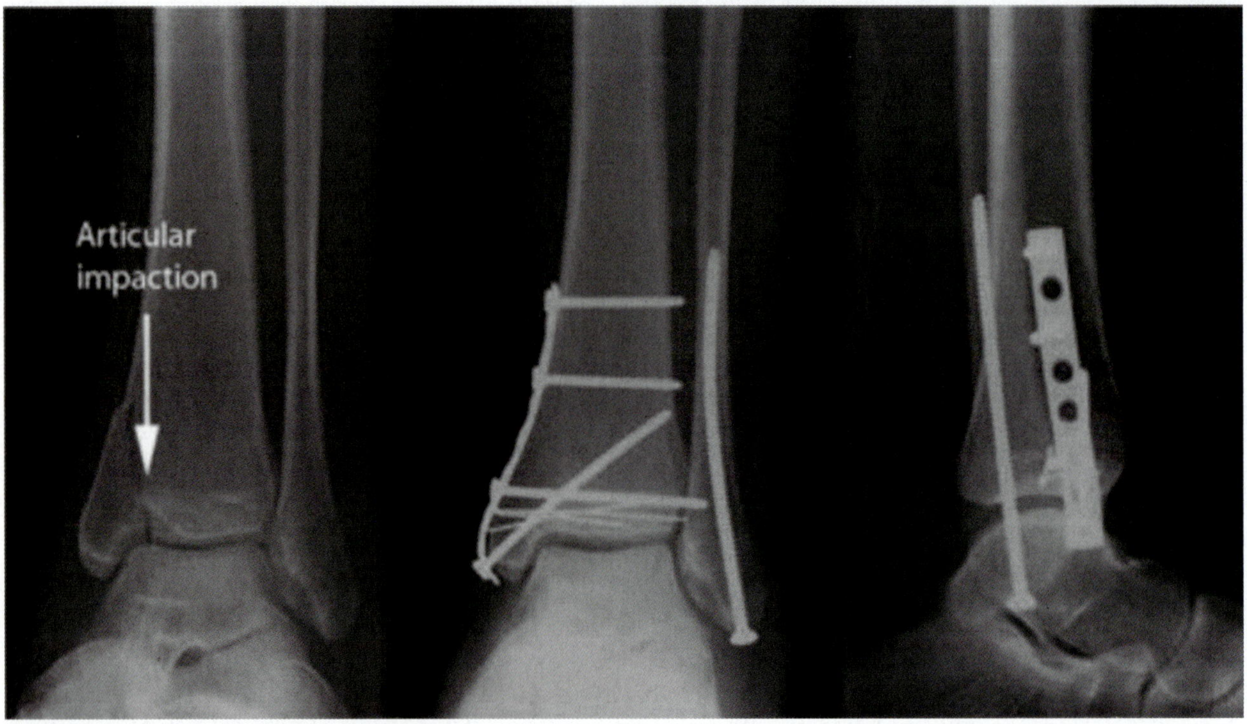

Figure 25-7. Articular impaction of the plafond must be suspected in supination adduction mechanism injuries. The defect should be bone grafted, and fixation can be achieved via wires.

Medial Malleolar Fractures

- Regardless of the fixation method chosen, visualization of the medial malleolus from the anterior ankle joint to the PT tendon including the cortical surface ensures anatomic reduction.
- For comminuted or collicular avulsion fractures, consider mini-fragment plate/screws.
- Two 3.5- or 4.0-mm cancellous lag screws or cortical screws are used for larger fracture fragments (Figure 25-8).
- In osteoporotic bone, bicortical medial malleolar lag screws enhance fixation strength, but over-compression must be avoided.
- Preliminary K-wires are inserted parallel to the screw trajectory, but away from the anticipated start point, and serve as an external visual guide.
- Alternatively, cannulated screws can be placed via guidewires.

The Chaput (or Tillaux-Chaput) Fracture Fragment and/or the Wagstaf-Lefort Avulsion Fracture Fragment

- If the fibular approach is sufficiently posterior for an adequate skin bridge, approach through a separate anterolateral approach.
- A mini-fragment straight plate, or a small hook plate, placed anteriorly is used for fixation (Figure 25-9).

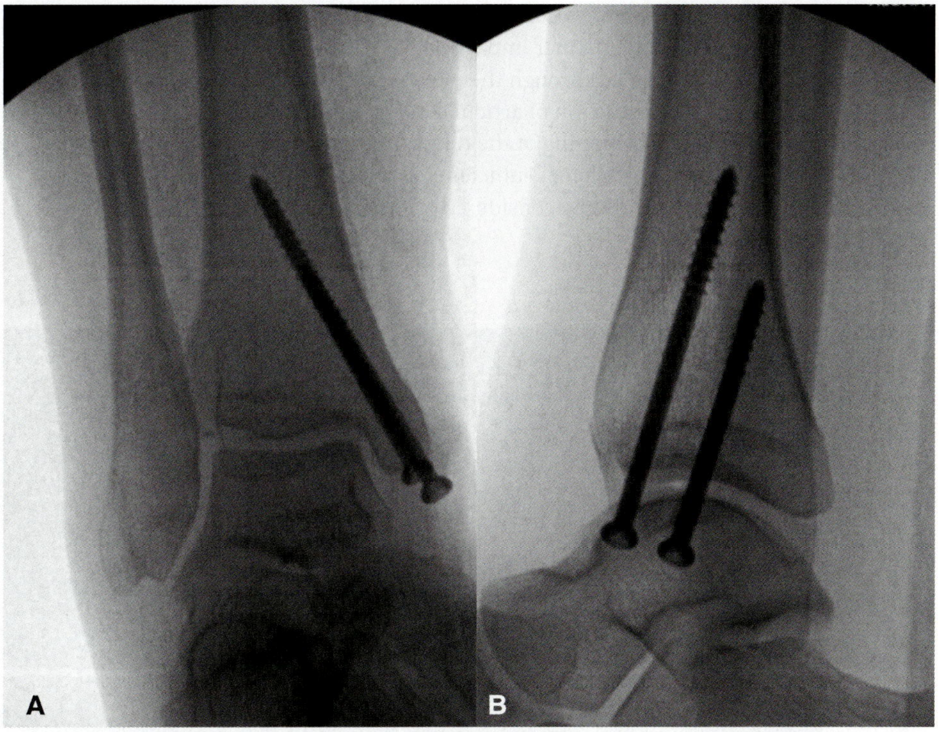

Figure 25-8. AP (A) and lateral (B) intra-operative images demonstrating medial malleolar fixation with partially threaded cancellous screws.

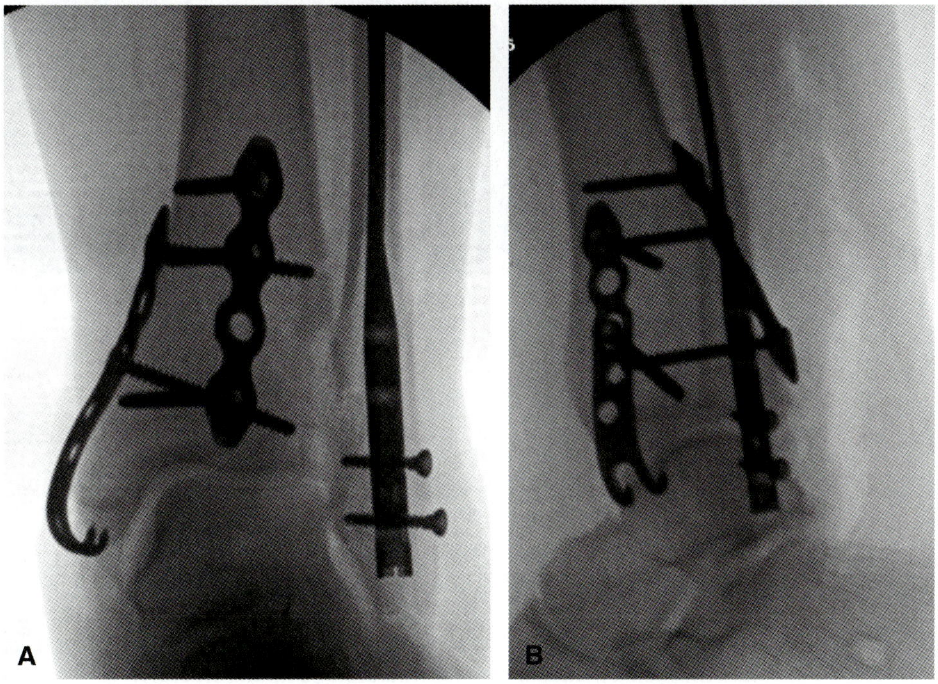

Figure 25-9. A, AP and lateral (B) radiographs demonstrating an anti-glide plate construct for posterior malleolar fixation. Reprinted with permission from Gardner MJ, Dunbar R, Henley MB, et al. *Harborview Illustrated Tips and Tricks in Fracture Surgery*. 1st ed. Philadelphia, PA: Wolters Kluwer Health/Lippincott Williams & Wilkins; 2010. Figure 22-15.

The Posterior Malleolus

- Lateral x-ray underestimates the size of the posterior malleolar fracture fragment and the articular involvement.
- A 30° external limb rotation provides a plain film view tangential to the fracture line.

- Consider preoperative computed tomography to identify interfragmentary fragments, fracture line orientation, and articular impaction.
- ORIF is performed through the posterolateral or posteromedial approach.
  - Anatomic reduction of articular surface is required.
  - Antiglide positioning of the one-third tubular or smaller plate with or without supplemental lag screw fixation is often sufficient (Figure 25-9).
  - T-plates can also be considered for buttressing (Figure 25-10).

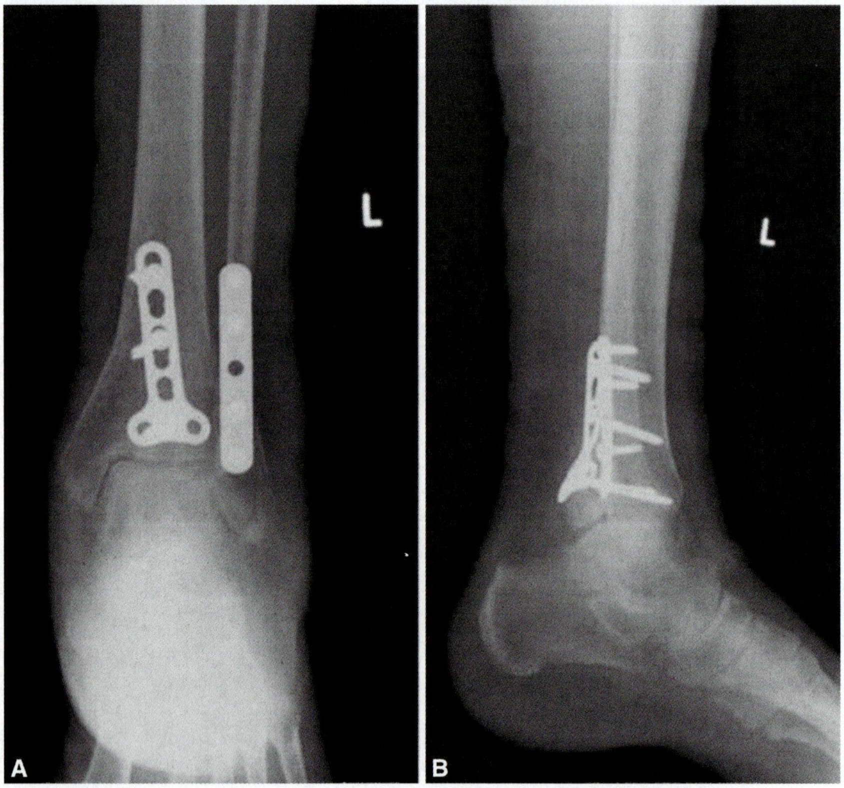

Figure 25-10. A, AP and lateral (B) radiographs demonstrating T-plate fixation of a posterior malleolus fracture.

- Posterolateral Approach
  - Provides exposure to the fracture superiorly and posteromedially, but not laterally because of the posterior tibiofibular ligament (PTFL).
  - Positioning and approach as described earlier
  - Care must be taken not to damage the PTFL or the peroneal artery deep to the FHL muscle belly.
  - Portions of the posterior malleolar fragment can sometimes be accessed for cleaning and reduction through a medial malleolar fracture or a fibular fracture.
- Posteromedial Approach
  - Position and approach as described earlier with prone or figure-of-four supine positioning
  - Provides unobstructed access to the fracture plane compared to the posterolateral approach.
- Indirect Reduction and Percutaneous Fixation
  - Allows supine positioning of patient in trimalleolar fracture patterns.
  - Anatomic reduction of the fibula may reduce the posterior malleolus indirectly.
  - A large bone reduction clamp or dental pick may assist in the reduction.

- Plate fixation of the fibula can obscure radiographic assessment of the posterior malleolus reduction.
- Provisional K-wire stabilization or lag screw fixation of the fibula prevents this obstruction.
- Anterior-to-posterior cannulated lag screws secure the posterior malleolar fragment (Figure 25-11).

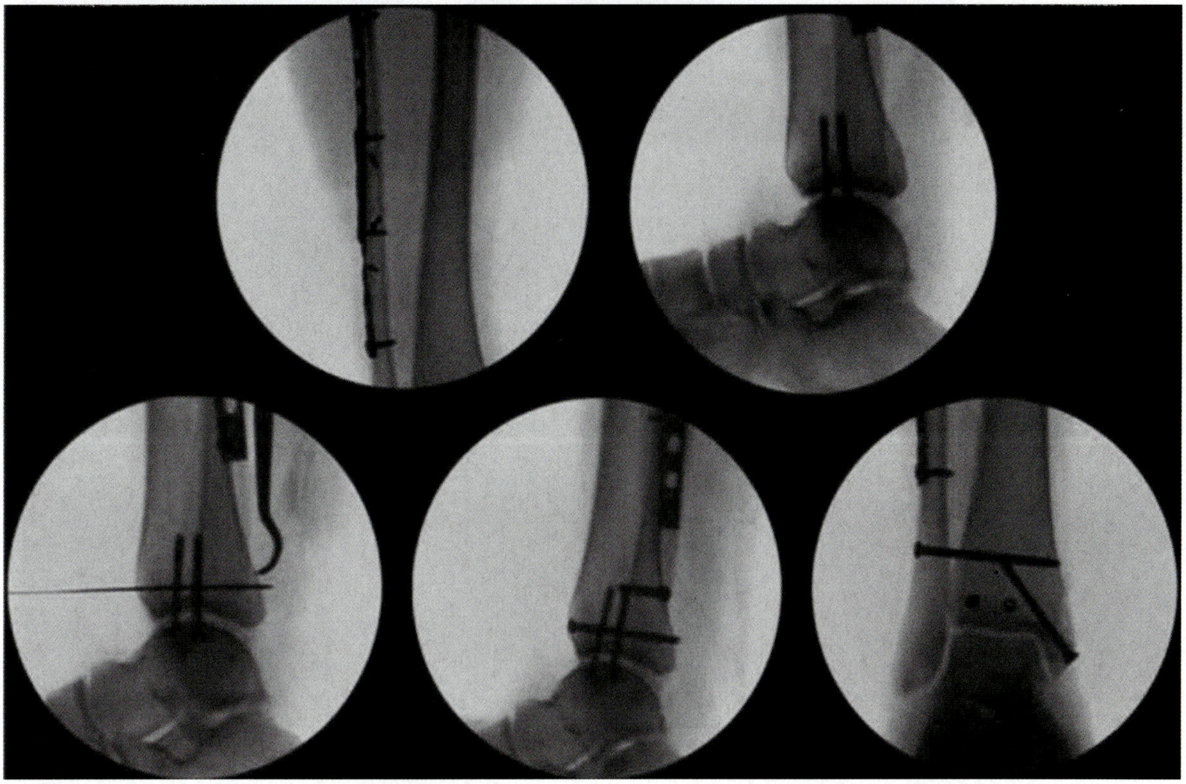

Figure 25-11. Flouroscopic images demonstrating a posterior malleolar fracture near completely reduced after fibular and medial malleolar fixation. A pick is used posteriorly to maintain reduction, whereas percutaneous anterior-to-posterior K-wires provisionally stabilize the fragment followed by cannulated screw fixation. Note that a more distal fibular plate would make radiographic assessment of the posterior malleolus fracture difficult.

Syndesmosis

- Reduction
  - Regardless of fixation method, malreduction is common, and, as such, the threshold for open reduction should be low.
  - Open reduction can be obtained through the lateral approach by mobilizing soft tissues anteriorly or through a separate anterolateral approach if the skin bridge is adequate.
  - Provisional fixation is obtained with periarticular forceps and K-wires.
- Stabilization
  - Stabilization of the syndesmosis can be achieved with screw, suture, staples, or bolt fixation.
  - Fixation should be perpendicular to the incisura and, therefore, can be placed through a laterally based fibula plate (Figure 25-12).
  - Fixation placed through posterolateral or posterior fibular plates can result in anterior displacement of the fibula if provisional fixation is inadequate.
  - Malreduction can be caused by prominent screws in the incisura from the fibular construct.
  - Syndesmosis screws are positional, and overtightening should be avoided (Figure 25-13).
  - For avulsion fractures of the tibia involving the syndesmosis, the Chaput fragment, open reduction, and internal fixation, as described earlier, are necessary.

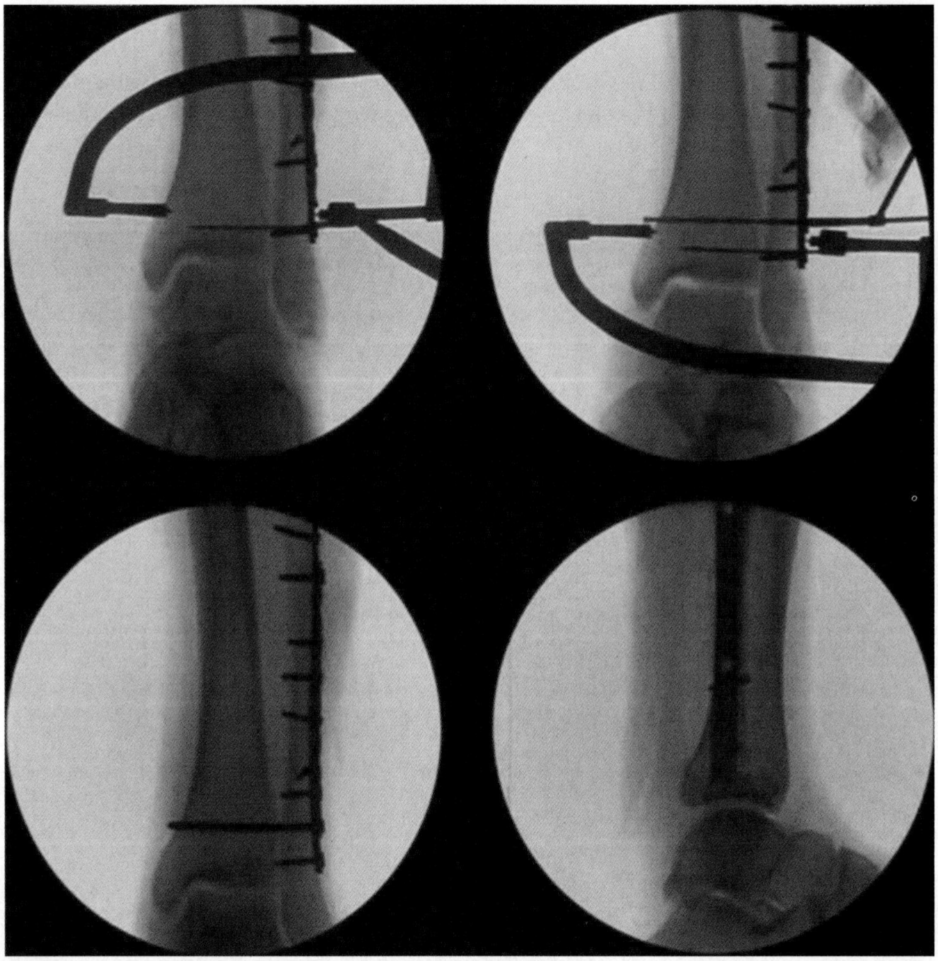

Figure 25-12. Fluoroscopic images demonstrating reduction of the syndesmosis with a periarticular clamp followed by definitive posi- tional screw fixation parallel to the plafond. Provisional K-wire fixation separate from the planned screw helps prevent displacement of fibula during screw application.

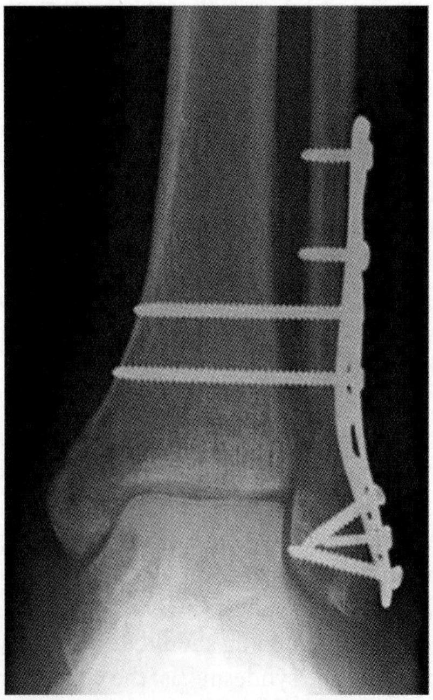

Figure 25-13. Syndesmotic screws are position screws, not lag screws; therefore, care must be taken not to overcompress the syndesmosis.

Chapter 26
Talus Fractures

KHUSDEEP S. VIG
CURTIS T. ADAMS
ANDREW J. ROSENBAUM

Sterile Instruments/Equipment

- Radiolucent table
- Periosteal elevators (dental probe, Cobb elevator, freer elevator, etc)
- Small and medium bone reduction forceps
- Mini-/small lamina spreaders
- Small distractors
- Ex-fix equipment
- Small interfragmentary (3.5 mm) cortical screw fixation
- Mini-fragment (2.7 or 2.0 mm) screw/plate instrumentation
  - Extra-long mini-screw (2.7 or 2.0 mm) with screw lengths up to 60 mm in length
- Titanium constructs to allow for postoperative magnetic resonance imaging (MRI) to assess for osteonecrosis
- Bioabsorbable pegs
- Headless articular screws
- Headlamp, if desired

Positioning

- Radiolucent table without attachments at the foot (Figure 26.1)
- Supine positioning with a bump under the ipsilateral hip until ankle malleoli on operative side are horizontal
- Prone position for posteromedial or posterolateral approaches
- Lateral recumbent effective for posterior-to-anterior fixation
- Position patient with foot at end of table.
- Drape with U-drape (one or two), and extremity drape.
- Place C-armor, if desired.
- Position C-arm machine perpendicular to foot/ankle from contralateral side.
  - Anteroposterior (AP), mortise, and lateral of the ankle
  - AP and oblique of the foot
  - Canale view of the heel with maximum dorsiflexion and x-ray 15° caudad

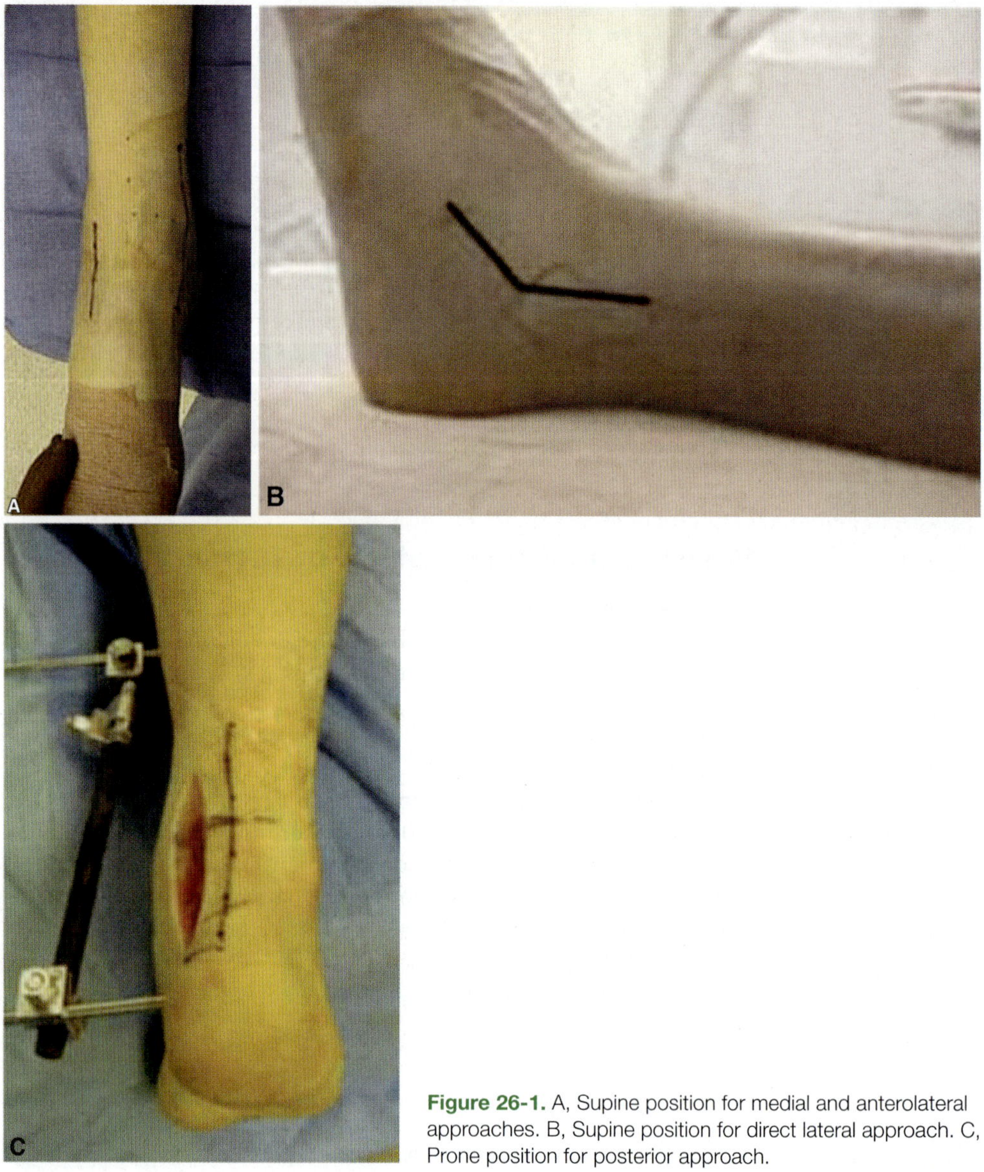

Figure 26-1. A, Supine position for medial and anterolateral approaches. B, Supine position for direct lateral approach. C, Prone position for posterior approach.

Surgical Approaches

- Medial and anterolateral approach via dual incision technique (Figure 26-2)
  - Medial incision
    - Landmarks: dorsomedial tip of the medial malleolus extending in line with the axis of the foot to the tarsal navicular
      - 5 mm dorsal to axis of posterior tibial tendon
      - Extension distal to navicular tuberosity
  - Anterolateral incision
    - Landmarks: parallel and 5 to 6 cm lateral to medial incision
- Medial or in line with syndesmosis for lateral neck of talus
- Shift more lateral to syndesmosis for comminution of the lateral process.
  - Deep dissection
    - Dangers: lateral branch of the superficial peroneal nerve
    - Incise the lateral retinaculum.
    - Retract extensor digitorum tendons medially, exposing extensor digitorum brevis.

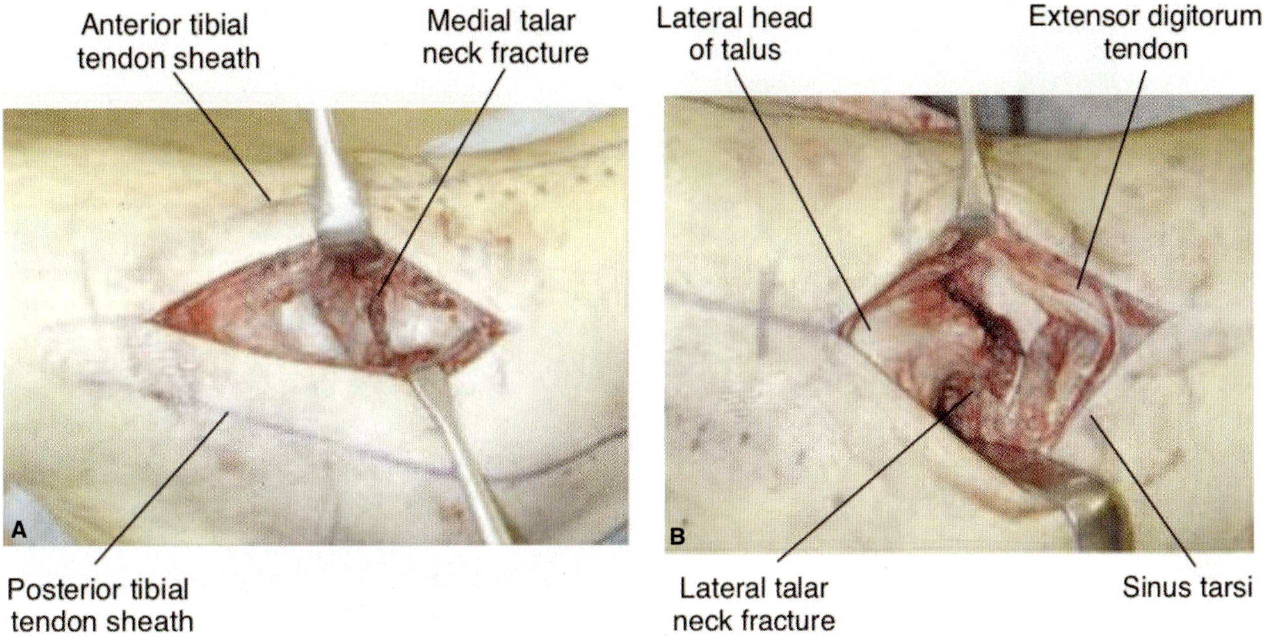

Figure 26-2. A, Medial approach. B, Anterolateral approach.

- Reflect brevis distally hinging on its proximal origin, allowing access to lateral capsule of the talus.
- Lateral capsulotomy in line with the axis of the talar neck

- Transmalleolar Approach
  - Indications: displaced body or complex talar neck fractures
  - Skin incision
    - Landmarks: dorsomedial tip of the medial malleolus extending in line with the axis of the foot to the tarsal navicular
      - 5 mm dorsal to axis of posterior tibial tendon
      - Extension distal to navicular tuberosity
      - Extend longitudinally in line with axis of medial malleolus just proximal to the supramalleolar region.
  - Medial malleolar osteotomy (Figure 26-3)
    - Expose the medial malleolus; keep the periosteum intact.
    - Retrograde drill and tap distal tip of malleolus.
    - Use very thin oscillating saw blade to make an oblique osteotomy directed toward shoulder of medial ankle mortise.
      - Advance only to the level of the medial subchondral bone.
    - Complete the osteotomy by gentle levering of a thin-wide osteotome on the inner cortical bone.
    - Perform an anterior and partial posterior capsulotomy of the medial malleolus (allows mobilization of the medial malleolar fragment).
    - Gently retract to protect deltoid vessels perfusing medial body of talus.
    - Reduce and internally fix malleolus with two parallel 3.5- or 4.0-mm partially threaded cancellous screws.
- Posterior approach (Figure 26-4)
  - Indications: isolated posterior talar body fracture, displaced Hawkins III fracture
  - Skin incision
    - Landmarks: midpoint of the calcaneus one fingerbreadth medial or lateral to the Achilles tendon, extending 6 to 8 cm superiorly

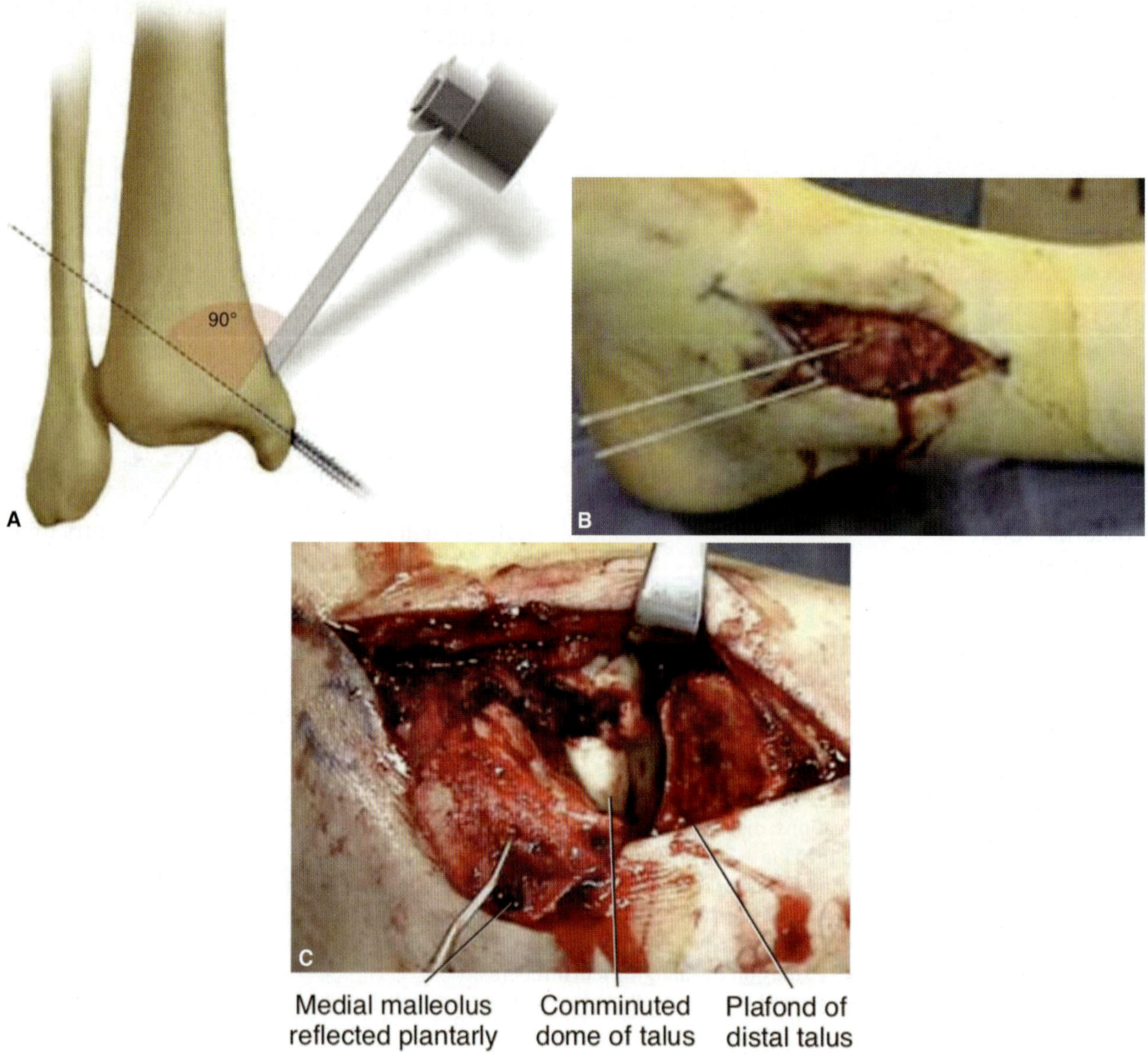

Figure 26-3. A, Transtectal medial malleolar osteotomy. B, Predrilling medial malleolus. C, Completed malleolar osteotomy.

- Deep dissection
  - Incise the deep posterior compartment fascia.
  - Safely retract posterior tibial artery and nerve.
  - Reflect the flexor hallucis longus laterally (landmark for posterior body of talus).
- Lateral approach (Figure 26-5)
  - Indications: lateral process talar fractures
  - Skin incision
    - Landmarks: 3 cm proximal to the distal tip of the lateral malleolus extending 6 to 8 cm longitudinally and anteriorly in a curvilinear shape in line with the axis of the foot
  - Deep dissection
    - Longitudinal incision of the lateral retinaculum and subtalar capsule

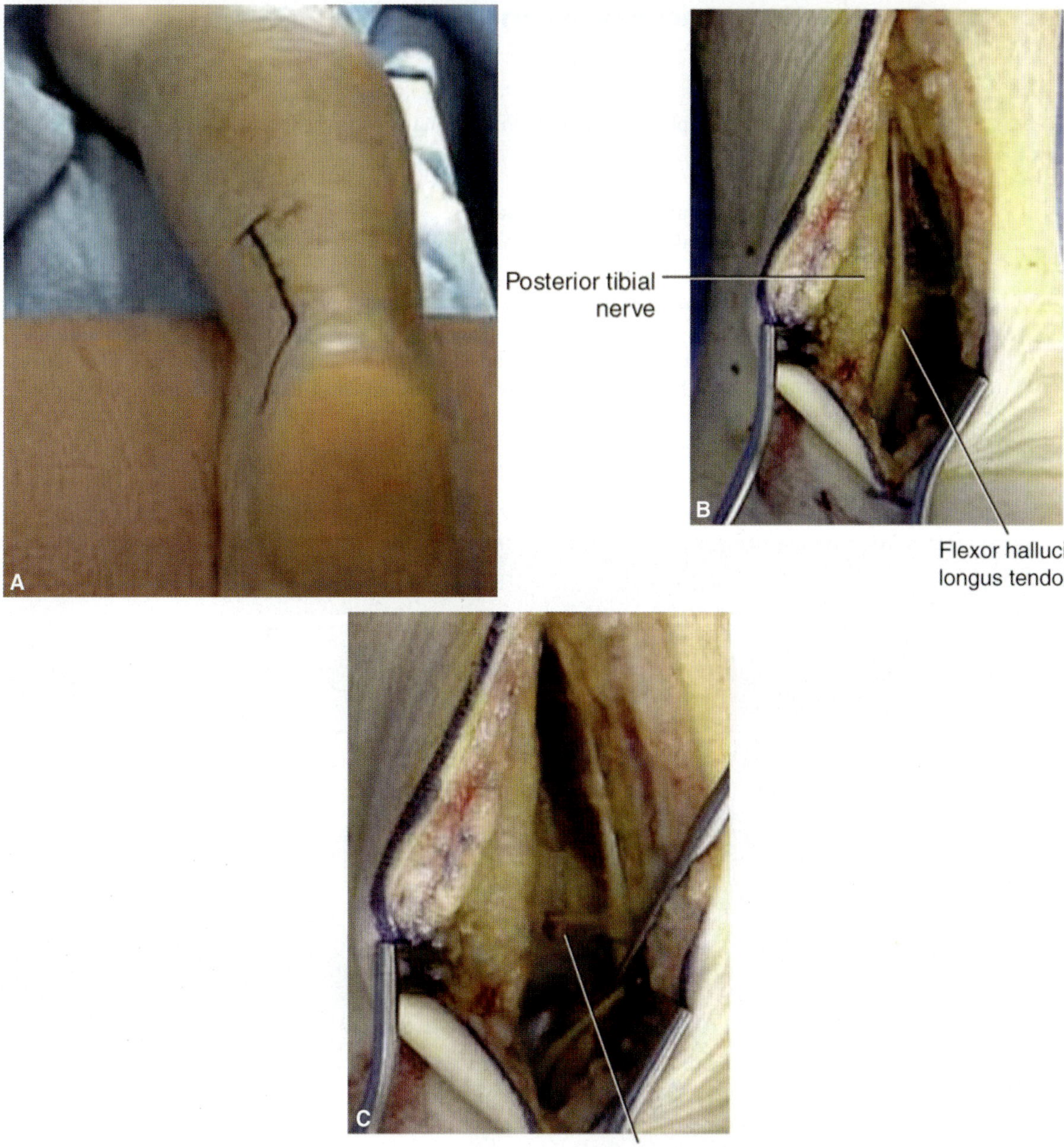

Figure 26-4. A, Posteromedial incision. B, Flexor hallucis longus concealing posterior talus. C, Hemarthrosis of posterior capsule.

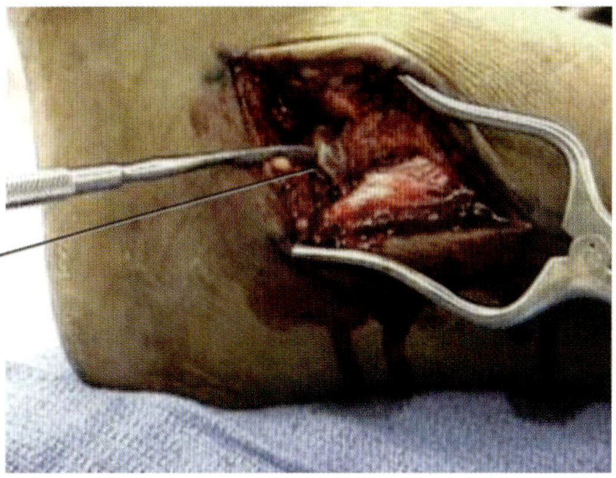

Figure 26-5. Using a Freer elevator to reduce the lateral process of the talus fragment.

Reduction and Fixation (Figures 26-6 and 26-7)

- Talar neck fractures
  - Closed reduction
    - Apply dorsal to plantar pressure while plantarflexing the forefoot, with application of longitudinal traction.
  - Open reduction
    - Use medial and anterolateral approach.
    - Sharply dissect along medial neck and head to expose body, neck, head, and talonavicular joint.
    - Disimpact medial talar neck with lamina spreader, restoring length and alignment of medial/dorsal neck.
    - Derotate body fragment (typically flexed and malrotated) with percutaneous, posterolateral 4.0-mm external fixator pin in body fragment. Ensure anatomic reduction of intra-articular subtalar fracture extension.

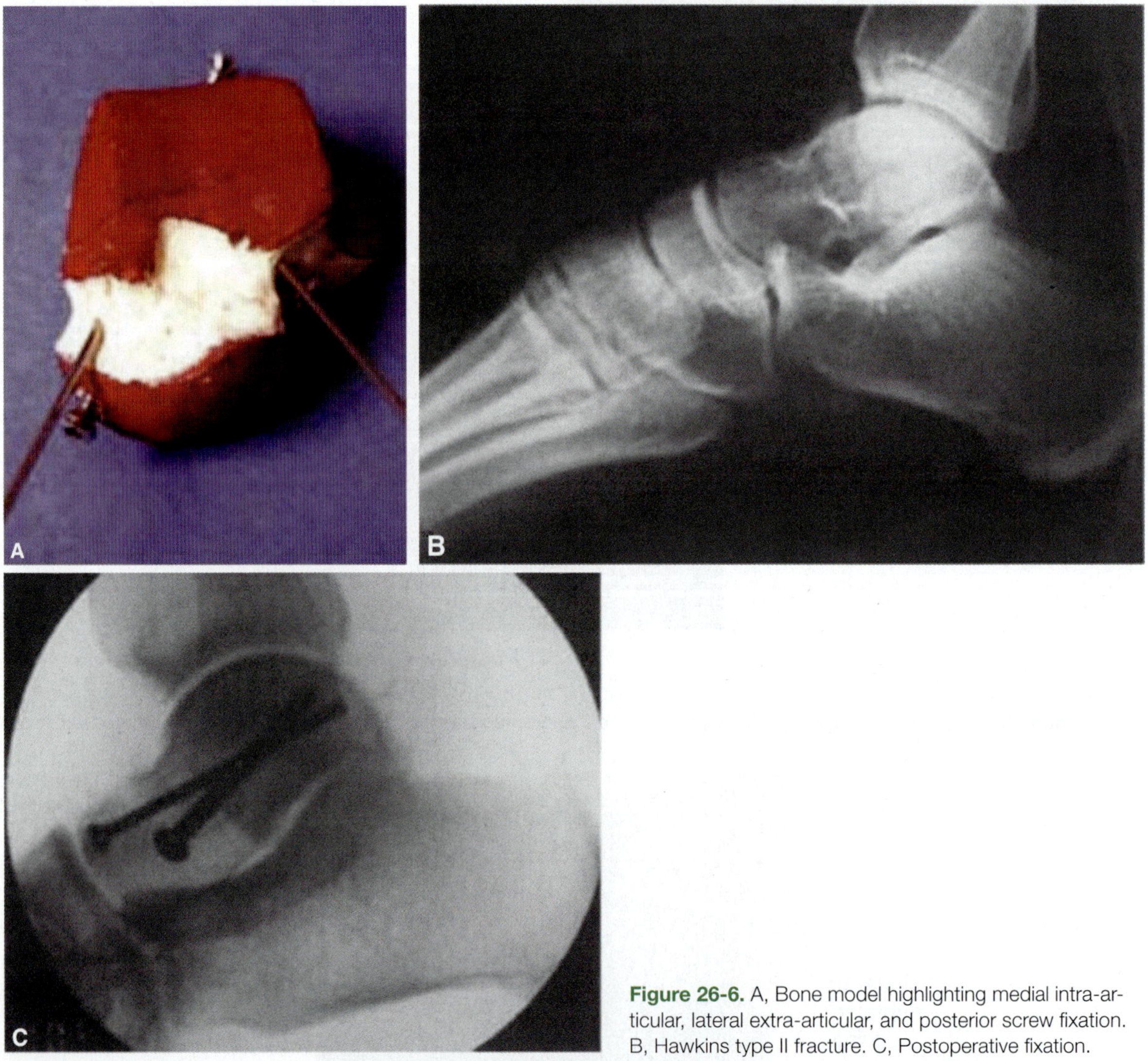

Figure 26-6. A, Bone model highlighting medial intra-articular, lateral extra-articular, and posterior screw fixation. B, Hawkins type II fracture. C, Postoperative fixation.

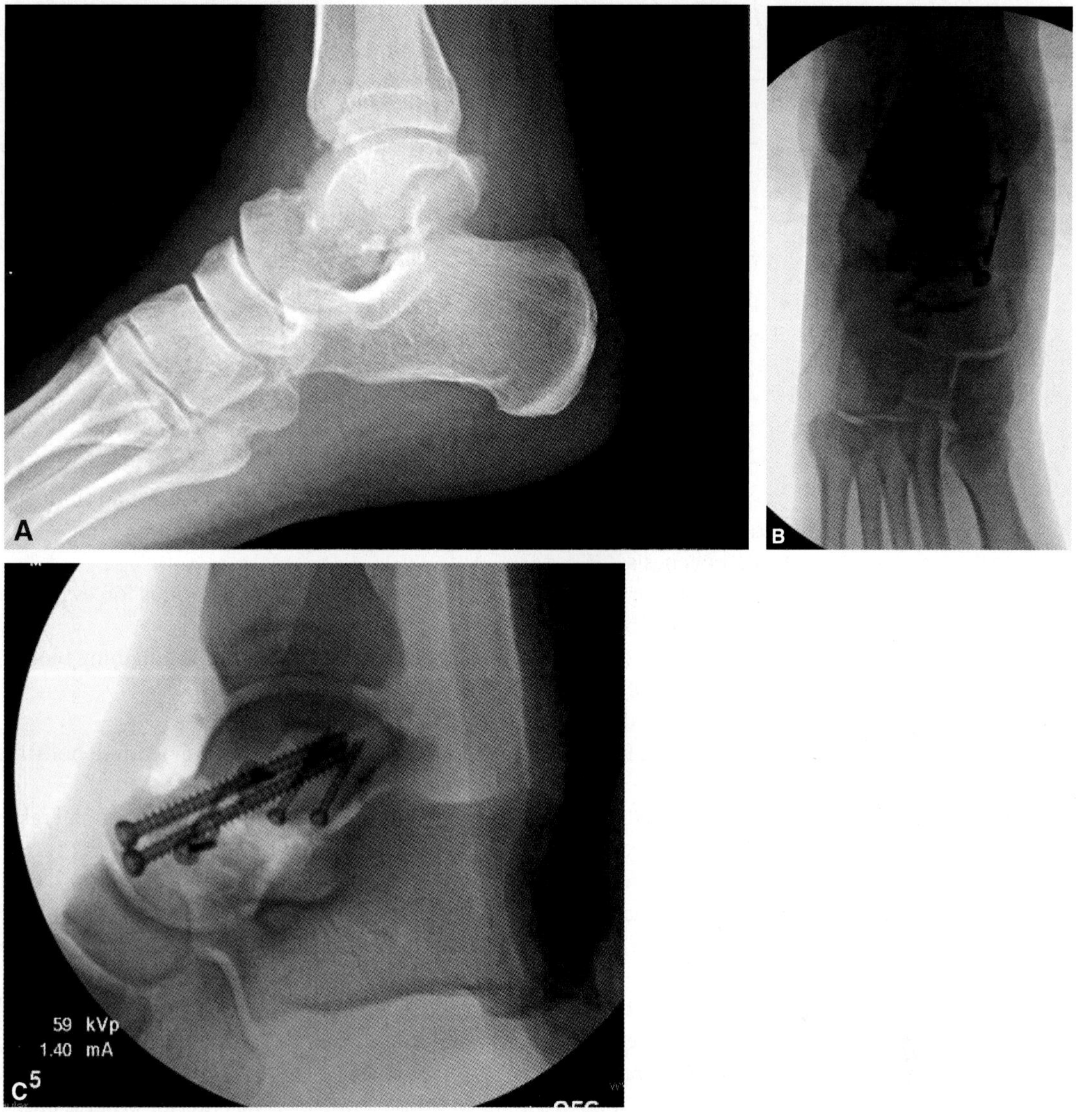

Figure 26-7. A, Lateral radiograph demonstrating a displaced talar neck fracture. B, C, Anteroposterior and lateral radiographs of the foot demonstrating fixation. A 2.4-mm plate (Arthrex, Naples, FL, USA) was placed medially to bridge the comminution and prevent shortening of the fracture and varus collapse. Two fully threaded 4.5-mm screws (Arthrex, Naples, FL, USA) were then placed as well to stabilize the fracture. Two cannulated partially threaded 3.0-mm screws (Arthrex, Naples, FL, USA) were placed into the lateral process, which was also broken. Images courtesy of Andrew Rosenbaum, MD.

- Temporary fixation
  - Secure reduction with a Kirschner wire, inserted retrograde through the talar head, across the fracture, and into the posterior body.
  - If there is medial fracture comminution, insert a lamina spreader into the fracture gap before securing reduction with a K-wire.
  - Use fluoroscopy to ensure restoration of length and anatomy of medial talar neck.
  - Expose lateral talar neck fracture line, typically located at the lateral shoulder of the talar dome.
  - Reduce by rotating fragments around medial K-wire.
  - Obtain Canale image of talar neck to view final reduction.

- Permanent fixation
  - Expose articular surface of talar head via subluxation of medial talonavicular joint.
  - Countersink an interfragmentary 3.5-mm screw retrograde through talar head and advance posterolaterally to posterior body of the talus.
  - Laterally, advance second interfragmentary screw along the proximal neck, directed posteromedially.
  - If talar neck is comminuted (especially lateral neck), may span with bridging plate, via four- or five-hole 2.0-mm mini-plates. May contour plates to achieve anatomic reduction and fixation.
- Provisional external fixation of talar neck
  - Indications: open fractures, talar body extrusion, gross contamination, extensive local soft-tissue injury
  - Used to maintain length of the talus, facilitate soft-tissue management, restore general alignment
  - Pins placed in calcaneus, first metatarsal, and, if necessary, in body of talus. Lateral bar may be added with pin crossing fourth and fifth metatarsals for additional stability.

- Extruded talar body
  - Pathogenesis
    - Hyperdorsiflexion with axial load to the body of the talus forces posteromedial dislocation of the talar body.
      - Tethered by the deep deltoid ligament (often only remaining blood supply to body)
  - Reduction of the body fragment
    - Skin incision
      - Open fracture dislocations, often with large medial wound; body fragment may be accessed through wound.
      - Closed dislocations addressed via posteromedial or posterolateral incision
    - Closed reduction
      - Place hindfoot in equinus to open tibiotalar interval.
      - Distract subtalar joint via axial traction through heel of foot.
      - Apply manual, anterior-to-posterior pressure on dislocated talar body, anterior to posterior.
      - May be blocked by intact deep deltoid ligament, acting as tether on body
    - Percutaneous reduction
      - Advance 4-mm pin through posterior tuberosity of the calcaneus in line with the long axis of the bone to the subchondral surface of the anterior process of the calcaneus.
    - Allows traction to the torn posterior capsule of the ankle
      - Place medial-to-lateral 4-mm pin bicortically across distal tibia.
      - Place 4-mm pin deep into body of talus through 1.5-cm longitudinal incision.
      - Distract hindfoot joints through distal tibial and calcaneal pins, either manually or with distractor. Talar body is reduced via joystick pin.
    - Open reduction
      - Medial approach in addition to percutaneous 4-mm pins as described
      - Maintain distraction through tibial and calcaneal pins.
      - Distract tibiotalar and talocalcaneal joints via lamina spreader, using medial incision.
      - Reduce talar body fragment with joystick pin.
      - Secure the reduction with temporary spanning K-wires before converting to permanent screws or mini-plates.
- Talar body fractures
  - Pathogenesis
    - Up to 23% of talus fractures involve the talar body.
    - Fracture patterns: coronal, sagittal, horizontal shear, and crush fractures of the weight-bearing surface
  - Reduction and fixation
    - Approach: medial transmalleolar
    - Reduce the posterior portion of the body to the anterior body fragment.
    - Provisionally fix the body using K-wires from medial and lateral portals.
    - Secure the provisional fixation using countersunk interfragmentary 2.0- or 2.7-mm screws.

- Posterior talar body fractures
  - Pathogenesis
    - Displaced, intra-articular posterior talar body fractures are commonly in the coronal plane.
  - Approach: posteromedial
    - Femoral distractor via 4-mm pins placed in medial calcaneus and distal third of medial tibia
      - Allows for distraction of the ankle and subtalar joint
    - Use Hohmann retractors for gentle retraction of the posterior tibial nerve and artery medially and the flexor hallucis longus tendon laterally.
      - Reduce the fracture using dental probes.
      - Provisionally fix with smooth K-wires posteriorly and anteriorly.
      - Secure the fixation with a posterior mini-plate contoured in a curvilinear manner to securely buttress posterior talus.
- Lateral process fractures
  - Pathogenesis
    - Forced inversion
    - May occur via avulsion mechanism, or as isolated or comminuted fractures
  - Approach: lateral
    - Distract fracture fragments to inspect subtalar joint.
    - Remove small fragments and utilize large fragments to restore anatomy of lateral process.
    - Provisionally fix anterior or posterior osteochondral fragments using smooth K-wires.
    - Provisionally fix the direct lateral fragments of the lateral process with K-wires.
    - Secure isolated lateral process fractures with interfragmentary mini-screws and utilize screw and plate fixation to buttress comminuted lateral process fractures.
      - Buttress plate will allow resistance to displacement against axial loads to the lateral process.

Postoperative Care

- Place sterile dressing with Xeroform, 4 × 4 gauze, and Mini Kerlix.
- Immobilize in padded bulky Jones splint, with absolute restriction on weight-bearing.
- Leave splint in place until follow-up in 2 weeks.
- Repeat radiographic imaging (AP and lateral of ankle and foot, and Canale view of talus).
- Immobilize in splint or Controlled Ankle Motion boot, with no weight-bearing for a total of 6 to 8 weeks.
- May begin passive range of motion exercises once wound is sufficiently healed and fracture fixation is deemed adequately secure.
- Once radiographs demonstrate callous formation and bony healing, may transition patient to graduated weight-bearing with physical therapy.

Section 9
Foot Trauma

Chapter 27
Metatarsal Neck Fractures

CURTIS T. ADAMS
STEFANOS HADDAD
ANDREW J. ROSENBAUM

Sterile Instruments/Equipment

- Tourniquet
- Implants
  - Mini-fragment screws and plates
  - Consider having available autograft, cancellous allograft, and demineralized bone matrix (DBM).
- 0.062-in K-wires
- Wire driver/drill
- Small pointed reduction forceps or towel clips
- Oscillating saw
- Bulky Jones splint materials
- Intraoperative fluoroscopy

Positioning/Preparation

- Discuss pain management with anesthesia; regional nerve block recommended.
- Place in supine position with a towel bump under the hip on operative side to make foot neutral with operating table.
- Place operative foot at end of operating table.
- Pad bony prominences (eg, contralateral heel).
- Place distal thigh or proximal calf tourniquet and secure with silk tape.
- Surgeon and assistants may stand or sit on provided stools.
- Administer prophylactic antibiotics (1-2 g cefazolin or a similar antibiotic).
- Drape with one to two U-drapes and an extremity drape, leaving entire foot on sterile field; toes should be prepped into field.

Surgical Approach

Varies depending on metatarsal fracture. There are three generally accepted rays or longitudinal segments of the metatarsals, with corresponding surgical approaches and fixation techniques: first metatarsal, second to fourth metatarsals, and fifth metatarsal.

First Metatarsal

- Requires anatomic reduction because of importance in weight-bearing during gait cycle
- Center a longitudinal incision along dorsal or medial aspect of first metatarsal, from medial cuneiform to first proximal phalanx. Avoid areas of soft-tissue injury if possible, or extend skin defect into necessary surgical incision.
- *Dorsal incision* (Figures 27-1 to 27-3)

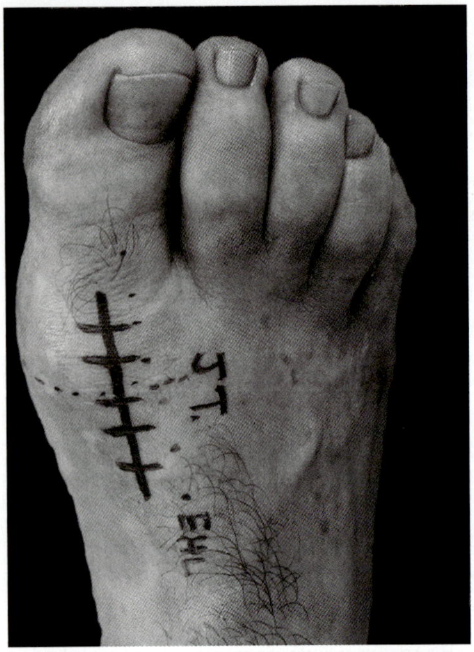

Figure 27-1. Incision runs medial to extensor hallucis longus tendon; beware of the dorsomedial cutaneous nerve. Capsular incision is medial to the skin incision, along the medial border of the bone and joint. From Miller SD. Interposition resection arthroplasty for hallux rigidus. *Tech Foot Ankle Surg*. 2004;3(3):158-164. doi:10.1097/01.btf.0000135271.60598.d5.

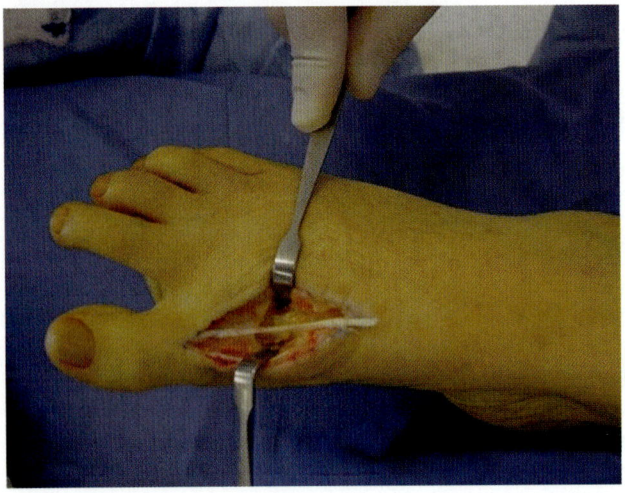

Figure 27-2. Dorsal view of metatarsophalangeal exposure, with the extensor hallucis brevis identified and already retrieved distally. From Ortiz C, Wagner E. Hallux varus and plantar plate repair. *Tech Foot Ankle Surg*. 2017;16(3):99-107. doi:10.1097/BTF.0000000000000151.

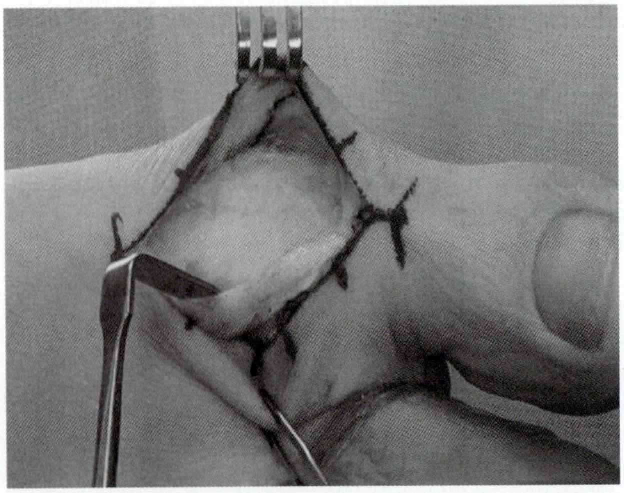

Figure 27-3. Intraoperative photograph showing incision placement, capsular exposure, and retraction of the extensor hallucis longus. From Hasselman CT, Shields N. Resurfacing of the first metatarsal head in the treatment of hallux rigidus. *Tech Foot Ankle Surg*. 2008;7(1):31-40. doi:10.1097/BTF.0b013e318165c356.

  - Sharply dissect, creating full-thickness skin flaps.
  - May ligate dorsal superficial vein as it crosses first metatarsal; protect and retract longitudinal vessels.
  - Identify the extensor hallucis longus and retract medially; retract the extensor hallucis brevis laterally.
  - Protect dorsomedial and dorsolateral cutaneous nerves lying on either side of metatarsal shaft; laterally protect the deep peroneal nerve and digital nerve branch to second metatarsal (branching in first dorsal web space).
  - Proximally, identify and protect the dorsalis pedis vessels.
- *Medial incision* (Figures 27-4 to 27-6)
  - Recommended for isolated first metatarsal fractures
  - Incision should be the length of the metatarsal and similar to the dorsal approach, centered over medial border of the first ray.
  - Angle incision dorsally along dorsal plane of foot to remain centered over the metatarsal; extend to distal prominence.
  - Identify and retract dorsal margin of the abductor hallucis muscle.
  - If first tarsometatarsal joint must be exposed, may elevate distal fibers of tibialis anterior tendon along proximal metatarsal shaft.

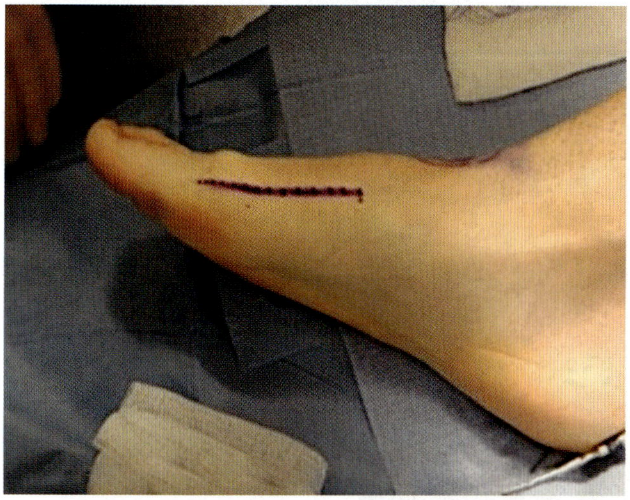

Figure 27-4. Medial incision over the first metatarsal extending over the distal prominence. From Klein J, Zachwieja E, Donnally C III, Aiyer A, Baitner A. A modified technique for the treatment of severe adolescent hallux valgus: a modification of the first metatarsal double osteotomy. *Tech Foot Ankle Surg*. 2018;17(2):90-102. doi:10.1097/BTF.0000000000000169.

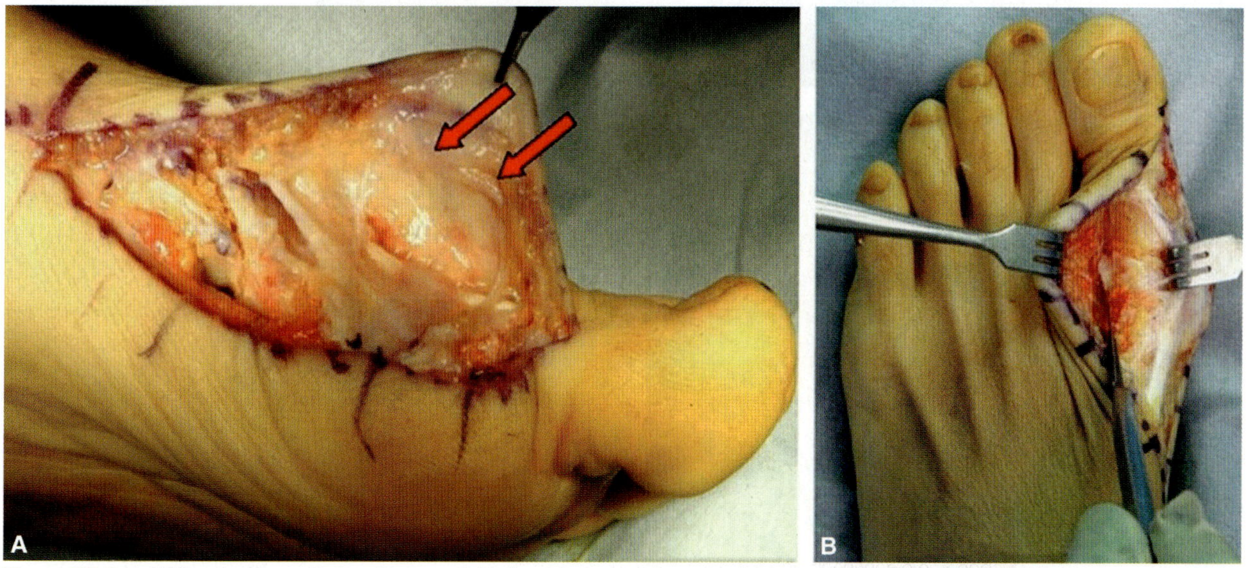

Figure 27-5. A, Midline incision with the dorsomedial hallucal branch of the superficial peroneal nerve embedded within the skin flap (red arrows). B, Exposure and release of lateral contracted soft tissues including the transverse head of the adductor hallucis tendon. From Jung H-G, Lopez RGL, Lee S-H, Shin M-H, Eom J-S. Proximal reverse chevron metatarsal osteotomy and lateral release through 1 medial incision for hallux valgus correction. *Tech Foot Ankle Surg*. 2014;13(3):145-149. doi:10.1097/BTF.0000000000000050.

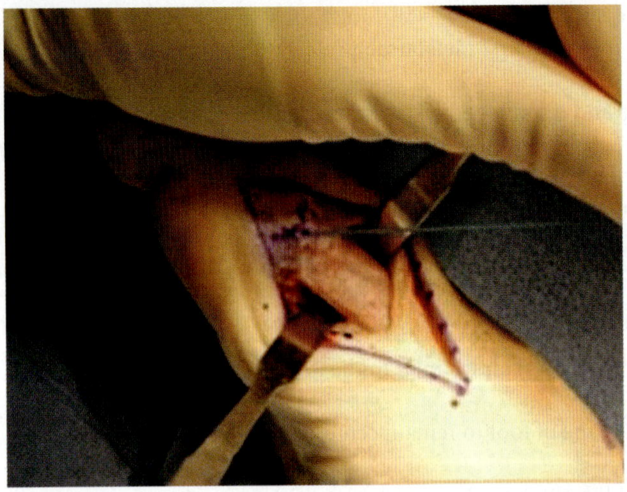

Figure 27-6. Subperiosteal dissection allowing visualization of first metatarsal. From Klein J, Zachwieja E, Donnally C III, Aiyer A, Baitner A. A modified technique for the treatment of severe adolescent hallux valgus: a modification of the first metatarsal double osteotomy. *Tech Foot Ankle Surg*. 2018;17(2):90-102. doi:10.1097/BTF.0000000000000169.

Second to Fourth Metatarsals (Figures 27-7 to 27-9)

The approach to the middle three metatarsals differs depending on number and location of fractures, as well as soft-tissue injury which may constrain incision sites. Preservation of venous drainage is critical,

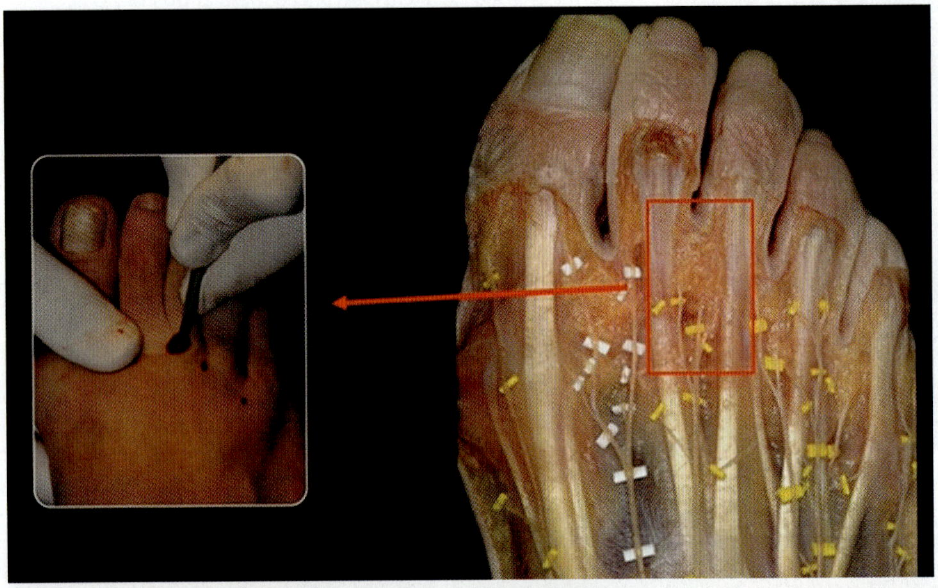

Figure 27-7. Anatomic relationship in the surgical approach. From De Prado M, Cuervas-Mons M, Golanó P, Vaquero J. Distal metatarsal minimal invasive osteotomy (DMMO) for the treatment of metatarsalgia. *Tech Foot Ankle Surg*. 2016;15(1):12-18. doi:10.1097/BTF.0000000000000093.

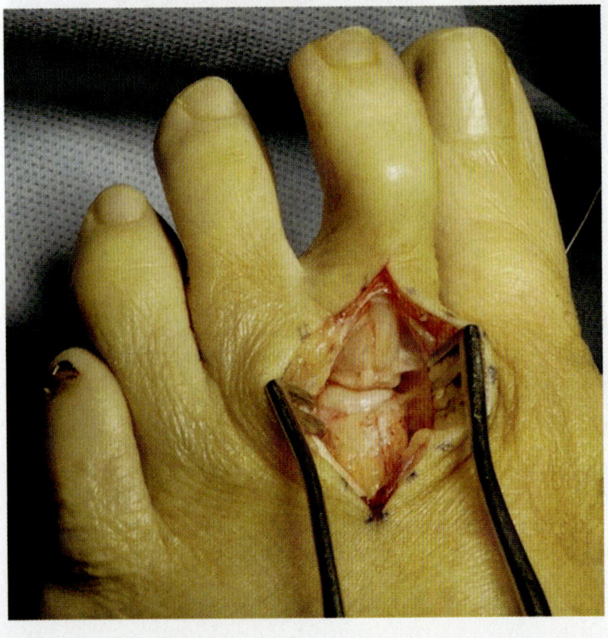

Figure 27-8. A self-retractor is positioned and secured between the extensor tendons. From Weil L Jr, Sung W, Weil LS Sr, Glover J. Corrections of second MTP joint instability using a Weil osteotomy and dorsal approach plantar plate repair: a new technique. *Tech Foot Ankle Surg*. 2011;10(1):33-39. doi:10.1097/BTF.0b013e31820b4b3c.

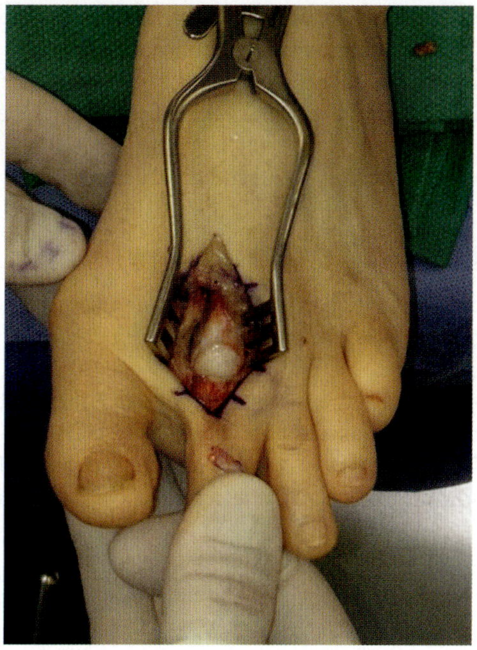

Figure 27-9. Self-retaining retractors used to expose the metatarsal head and to protect the extensor tendon laterally. From DeCarbo WT, Dial, DK. The Weil osteotomy: a refresher. *Tech Foot Ankle Surg*. 2014;13(4):191-198. doi:10.1097/BTF.0000000000000061.

especially of longitudinal veins. Where multiple metatarsals are fractured, incisions may be made between metatarsals 2 and 3, 3 and 4, and 4 and 5 to grant optimal access for reduction and fixation.

- Extend incision over appropriate metatarsals from tarsometatarsal to metatarsophalangeal joints.
- Identify the optimal surgical interval between the long extensor tendon superficially and short extensor tendon deeply.
- Protect superficial veins and medial/lateral digital nervovascular bundles on either side of the metatarsal shaft.

Fifth Metatarsal (Figure 27-10)

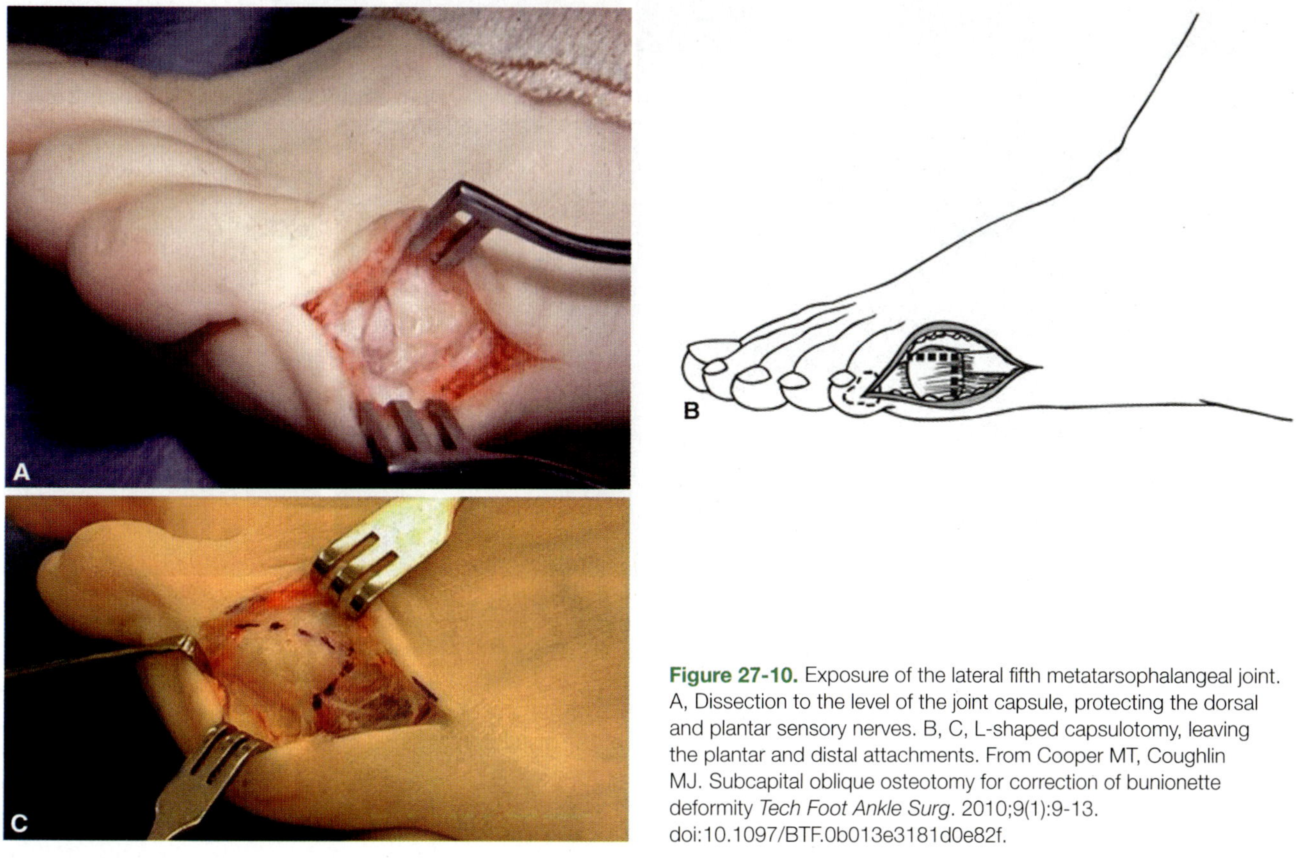

Figure 27-10. Exposure of the lateral fifth metatarsophalangeal joint. A, Dissection to the level of the joint capsule, protecting the dorsal and plantar sensory nerves. B, C, L-shaped capsulotomy, leaving the plantar and distal attachments. From Cooper MT, Coughlin MJ. Subcapital oblique osteotomy for correction of bunionette deformity *Tech Foot Ankle Surg*. 2010;9(1):9-13. doi:10.1097/BTF.0b013e3181d0e82f.

May be approached via incision between fourth and fifth metatarsals, or via a separate, lateral approach

- Make incision over length of fifth metatarsal along lateral border.
- Protect laterally located branches of the sural nerve.
- Identify and retract the short saphenous vein subcutaneously to expose deeper fascia overlying the abductor digiti minimi muscle.
- Incise fascia and retract muscle fibers plantarly to expose the fracture site.

Reduction and Fixation Techniques

All fracture reduction should follow standard goals of achieving length, alignment, and rotation, with attention paid to restoring the anatomic cascade or parabola of metatarsal heads. Compare with contralateral extremity to assess symmetry.

- Malalignment of metatarsals in the axial plane will disrupt the cascade of metatarsal heads, and may lead to overloading of more plantar metatarsal heads, causing metatarsalgia.

Fracture fixation utilizes standard principles of stability and compression. Highly comminuted fractures may be bridged with mesh plates or longer bridging plates, with the addition of bone graft, DBX, or similar products.

First Metatarsal (Figure 27-11)

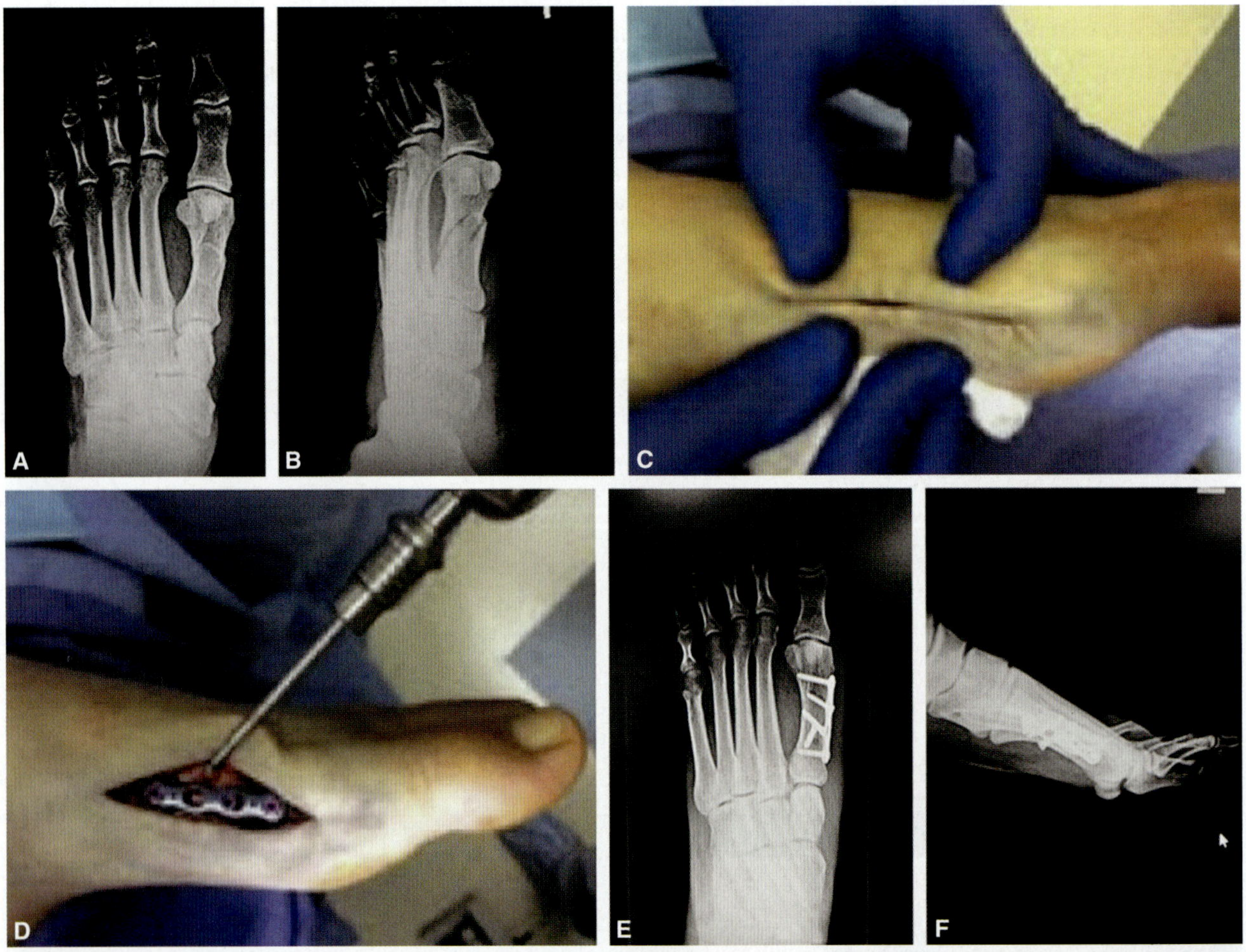

Figure 27-11. A, B, Preoperative radiographs revealing first metatarsal diaphyseal fracture. C, Incision is placed along medial aspect of first metatarsal. D, Lag screw and plate fixation of first metatarsal. E, F, Postoperative radiographs after open reduction and internal fixation of first metatarsal. From Cuttica DJ, Putnam RM. Metatarsal fractures: what should be fixed and how to fix it. *Tech Foot Ankle Surg*. 2014;13(4):177-183. doi:10.1097/BTF.0000000000000043.

- Sesamoids are weight-bearing portions of the distal first ray, and must align with the parabola of lateral metatarsal heads.

- Using a small rongeur and dental pick, clean soft-tissue and bony fragments interposed between fracture ends.
- Elevate periosteum adjacent to fracture ends to visualize anatomic reduction.
- Reduce manually or with the aid of pointed reduction clamps, and secure with clamps placed perpendicular to fracture plane.
- In amenable oblique fractures, place lag screw perpendicularly across adequate sized fracture fragments to achieve maximal compression. Position screw to allow for medial or dorsal plate. For longer or spiral fracture patterns, multiple lag screws may be placed where possible. Secure lagged fracture with a neutralization plate.
- For transverse fractures, achieve reduction with pointed reduction forceps, and provisionally stabilize with 0.062 K-wires. Ensure anatomic alignment in rotational and flexion/extension planes via fluoroscopy and manipulation of great toe.
- Fix transverse fracture with a mini-plate, small T-plate, 0.3-mm tubular plate, or a similar mini-fragment compression plate. Achieve axial compression across fracture site via eccentrically placed cortical screws, with two or more screws proximal and distal to the fracture.

Second to Fourth Metatarsals (Figures 27-12 to 27-15)

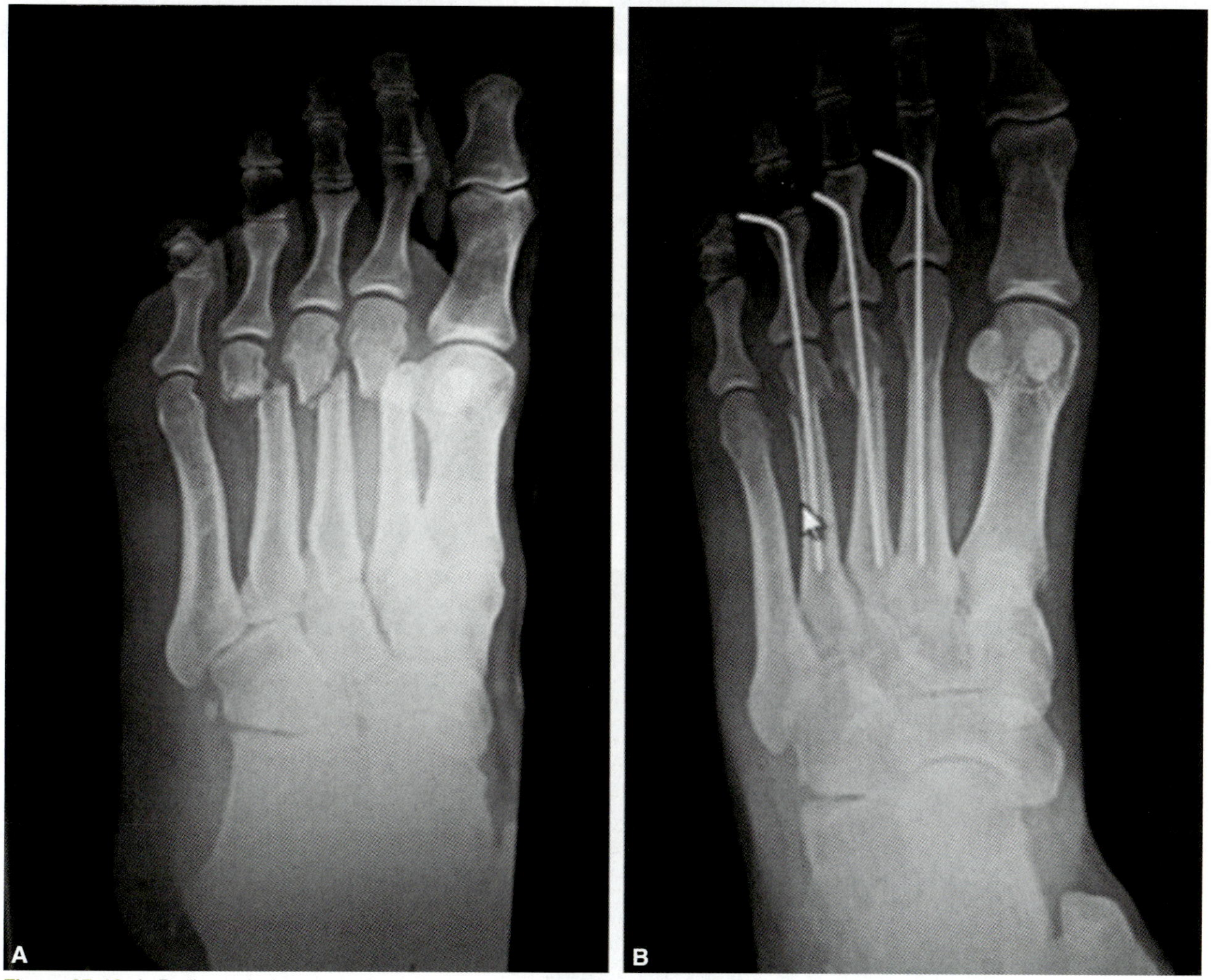

Figure 27-12. A, Radiograph demonstrating transverse fractures of the second, third, and fourth metatarsal necks with complete displacement. B, Postoperative image after open reduction and internal fixation of the fractures through K-wire fixation. From Cuttica DJ, Putnam RM. Metatarsal fractures: what should be fixed and how to fix it. *Tech Foot Ankle Surg*. 2014;13(4):177-183. doi:10.1097/BTF.0000000000000043.

- The goal is to restore the parabola of metatarsal heads.
- With a dental pick, scalpel, or periosteal elevator, remove debris from fracture site to expose ends of fracture fragments.

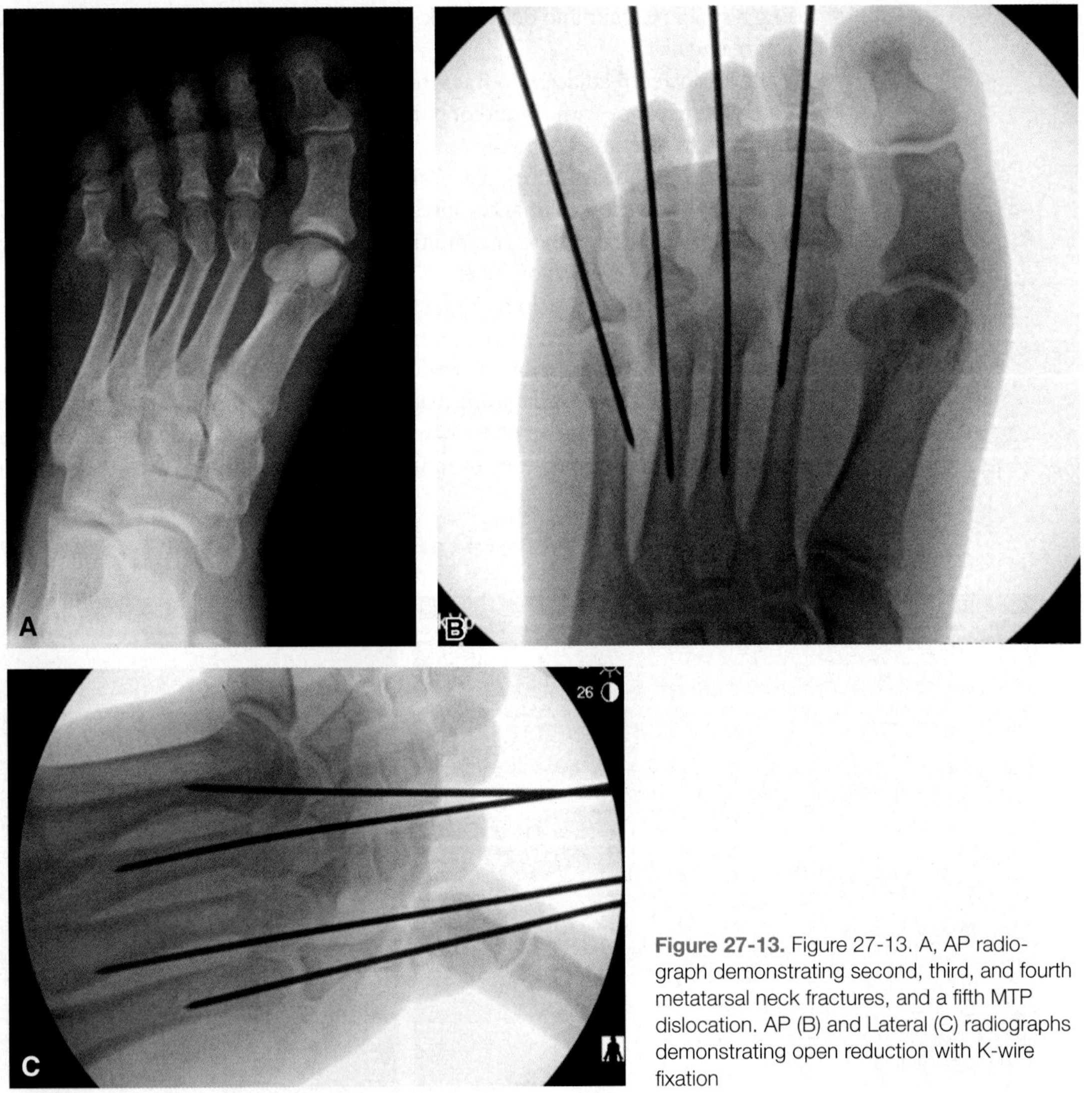

Figure 27-13. Figure 27-13. A, AP radiograph demonstrating second, third, and fourth metatarsal neck fractures, and a fifth MTP dislocation. AP (B) and Lateral (C) radiographs demonstrating open reduction with K-wire fixation

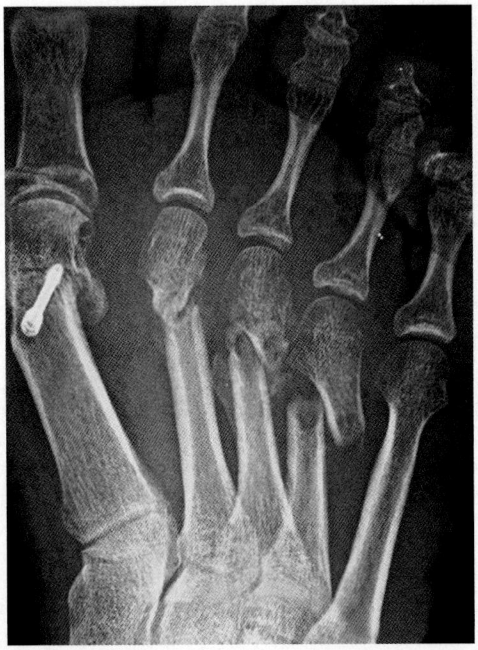

Figure 27-14. Second, third, and fourth metatarsal nonunion after minimally invasive osteotomy. From Khazen G, Wagner P, Wagner E. Lesser metatarsal complications after MIS surgery. *Tech Foot Ankle Surg*. 2017;16(1):28-33. doi:10.1097/BTF.0000000000000147.

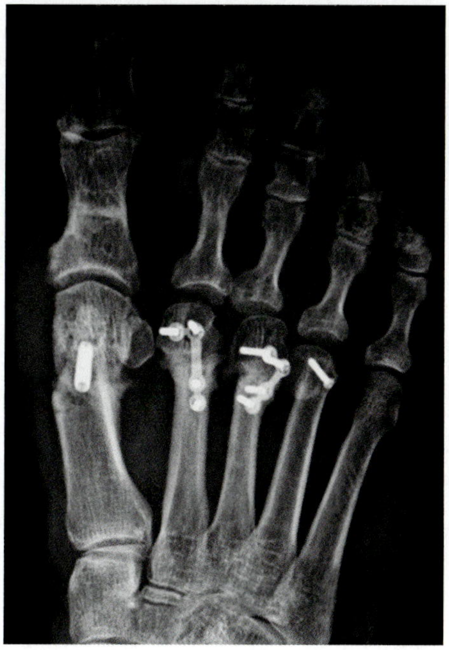

Figure 27-15. Revision surgery with bone graft and plate fixation for second and third metatarsal nonunion after minimally invasive osteotomy and fourth metatarsal Weil osteotomy. From Khazen G, Wagner P, Wagner E. Lesser metatarsal complications after MIS surgery. *Tech Foot Ankle Surg*. 2017;16(1):28-33. doi:10.1097/BTF.0000000000000147.

- Manual traction to restore anatomic length and rotation across fracture site
- Hold reduction with pointed forceps, and provisionally fix with K-wires placed perpendicularly across the fracture site, out of the plane of plate fixation.
- Permanent fixation:
  - Simple, oblique fractures—may be fixed with one or two lag screws, with optional addition of neutralization plate
  - Simple, transverse fractures—use an L- or a T-plate in compression via eccentrically placed screws.
  - Comminuted fractures—bridge multiple fracture fragments via an L- or a T-plate, ensuring preservation of length, alignment, and rotation.
- Final fixation may also be obtained via K-wires placed percutaneously distal to proximal through the distal phalanges and across the metatarsal fractures. K-wires should pass into the cuneiforms or out through a proximal metatarsal cortex for added stability.

Fifth Metatarsal

Fractures of the fifth ray are often amenable to nonoperative treatment given the flexibility of the lateral column of the foot. However, significant disruptions of the parabola of the forefoot, and especially plantar deviation of the metatarsal neck, must be adequately corrected.

- Long oblique fractures of the shaft extending into the neck may be treated with a minimum of two lag screws, placed perpendicularly across the fracture (the length of the fracture must be twice the transverse width of the metatarsal shaft).
- Transverse or comminuted fractures may be addressed with an L- or a T-plate similar to that used in the central metatarsals.

Postoperative Protocol

- Place in bulky Jones splint; no weight-bearing.
- Sutures out in 2 weeks, with transition to Controlled Ankle Motion (CAM) boot, and heel weight-bearing typically allowed unless fracture fixation tenuous or grossly unstable
- K-wires, if present, removed at 4 to 6 weeks
- Physical therapy initiated after removal of K-wires
- CAM boot discontinued after 6 to 8 weeks

Chapter 28
Lisfranc Injuries

CASEY M. O'CONNOR
JILLIAN KAZLEY

Sterile Instruments/Equipment

- Tourniquet
- Large pointed bone reduction clamps
- Dental picks and Freer elevator
- Implants
    - Mini- and small-fragment screws (2.0/2.4/2.7/3.5 mm)
    - Autograft, cancellous allograft, or other bone substitutes for fusion
- 1.6-mm K-wires and wire driver/drill
- C-arm

Positioning

- The patient is positioned in the supine position.
- A bump should be placed under the ipsilateral hip for correct position of the foot.
- A tourniquet should be placed on the ipsilateral side of the injury.

Surgical Approach

- Dorsomedial approach—the incision is centered between the first and second tarsometatarsal (TMT) joints (Figure 28-1).

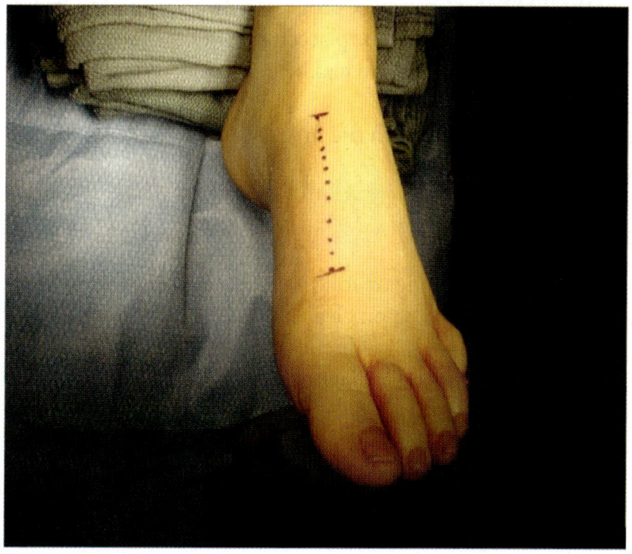

Figure 28-1. Dorsomedial incision of the midfoot. From Schiff AP, Gross CE, Pellegrini MJ, Hamid KS, Easley ME. Open reduction and internal fixation of the Lisfranc fracture-dislocation. In: Easley ME, Wiesel SW, eds. *Operative Techniques in Foot and Ankle Surgery*. Philadelphia, PA: Wolters Kluwer; 2017:chap 132:Tech Figure 3A-C.

  - This approach will provide access to the first to third TMT joints.
  - Deep dissection is performed between the extensor hallucis longus and extensor hallucis brevis tendons.
  - The extensor hallucis brevis is retracted laterally, at which point the deep peroneal nerve and dorsalis pedis artery can be identified and protected.
  - The first TMT capsule can be incised and subperiosteal dissection carefully performed to avoid injury.
- The dorsolateral approach may be used if access to the fourth, fifth, or the lateral aspect of the third TMT joint is needed. The incision is centered between the fourth and fifth TMT joints.
  - There should be at least a 3-cm skin bridge when using a dual-incision approach.
  - Deep dissection should be performed between the extensor digitorum brevis and the extensor digitorum communis tendons.
- Medial approach—a medial incision can be used for hardware placement from the first to the base of the second metatarsal.

Reduction and Fixation Techniques

Current best evidence supports the use of open reduction internal fixation (ORIF) for fractures or avulsion Lisfranc injuries compared to purely ligamentous injuries treated with primary fusion.

Closed Reduction

- May be done before ORIF to approximate the fracture
- Axial traction applied to the great toe and other affected TMT joints either by hand or with the aid of finger traps

External Fixation

- Unicolumnar frame—a 4.0 Schanz pin through the calcaneus and another at the base of the fourth and fifth metatarsal bases to maintain lateral column length
- This can be used for temporary fixation because the soft tissues improve or can be used as definitive fixation for the lateral TMT joints.
- Bicolumnar frame—a 5.0 Schanz pin is placed medial to lateral; a 4.0 Schanz pin is again placed at the base of the fourth and fifth metatarsal bases; and a 4.0 Schanz pin is placed in the medial aspect of the first metatarsal head.

Open Reduction Internal Fixation

- Depending on the severity of the injury and the joints involved, injuries can be approached through either a dual or single incision.
- Internal fixation of the TMT joint complex progresses from medial to lateral.
- Provisional reduction and fixation should be placed across all the involved joints primary to implant use.
- Use of 4.0-, 3.5-, or 2.7-mm screw fixation can be performed during ORIF and is dependent on surgeon preference and bone purchase.
- It is surgeon preference to approach with the first or second TMT joint first. We discuss initial reduction of the second metatarsal.

Reduction and Fixation of the Second Metatarsal

- It is essential that any interposed bone or soft tissue be removed from the second, third, or fourth TMT articulations. Emphasis is placed on clearing the space between the second metatarsal and medial cuneiform for correct anatomic reduction.
- Proper debridement is done at these joints with the assistance of different retractors. The use of a lamina spreader, Hintermann distractor, or Schanz pins can help adequately expose the joints.
- Using a large pointed reduction clamp placed on the lateral aspect of the base of the second metatarsal and the medial aspect of the medial cuneiform, the second metatarsal–medial cuneiform articulation can be reduced (Figure 28-2).
- If there is difficulty with anatomic reduction, ensure the space between the second metatarsal and medial cuneiform is cleared of interposed tissue.

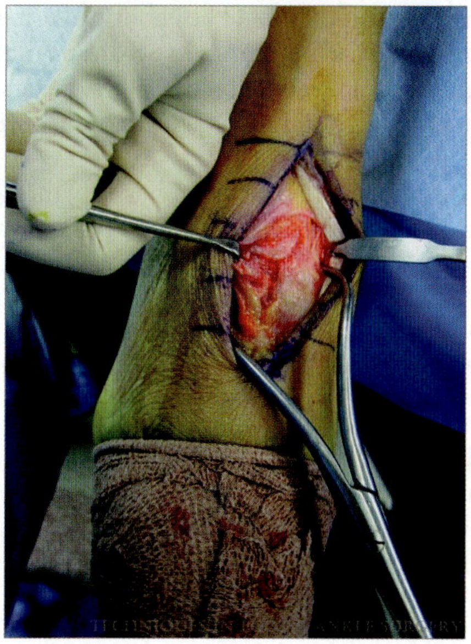

Figure 28-2. Reduction of the second tarsometatarsal joint with a large pointed reduction using the dorsomedial approach. From Schiff AP, Gross CE, Pellegrini MJ, Hamid KS, Easley ME. Open reduction and internal fixation of the Lisfranc fracture-dislocation. In: Easley ME, Wiesel SW, eds. *Operative Techniques in Foot and Ankle Surgery*. Philadelphia, PA: Wolters Kluwer; 2017:chap 132:Tech Figure 4.

- Provisional fixation can be held using 1.6-mm K-wires, making sure to not block your screw trajectory.
- Using lag by technique fixation, a 3.5-mm fully threaded cortical screw or a partially threaded screw should be placed from the medial cuneiform to the base of the second metatarsal to provide compression. This trajectory is that of the Lisfranc ligament and may be referred to as the Lisfranc screw.
- Fluoroscopic examination with the three standard foot films should be obtained to ensure anatomic reduction of the TMT articulations after placement of the Lisfranc screw.

With newer implant designs and variations in surgical techniques, the goal of ORIF is to establish anatomic reduction.

Reduction and Fixation of the First Metatarsal

In a situation where there is significant comminution of the base of the second metatarsal, the first TMT joint may need to be reduced to create a stable medial buttress (Figure 28-3).

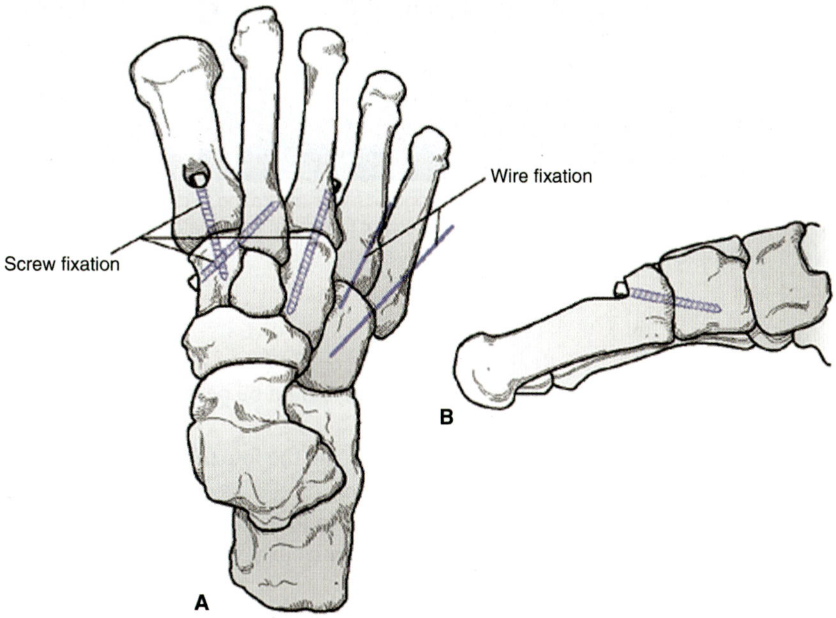

Figure 28-3. Demonstrates preferred fixation method for open reduction internal fixation of the first, second, and third tarsometatarsal joints (A). Note the trajectory of the screw crossing the first TMT joint (B). From Schiff AP, Gross CE, Pellegrini MJ, Hamid KS, Easley ME. Open reduction and internal fixation of the Lisfranc fracture-dislocation. In: Easley ME, Wiesel SW, eds. *Operative Techniques in Foot and Ankle Surgery*. Philadelphia, PA: Wolters Kluwer; 2017:chap 132:Tech Figure 5F.

- Reduction of the first TMT to the medial cuneiform should be performed using either a small reduction clamp placed around the first metatarsal head or inserting a Schanz pin into the first metatarsal.
- The Schanz pin can be used as a joystick to guide reduction of the first metatarsal.
- Provisional fixation of the base of the first metatarsal should be established with K-wire fixation into the medial cuneiform.
- Lag by technique with 3.5-mm fully threaded cortical screw or partially threaded screw should be performed for fixation from the base of the first metatarsal into the plantar medial aspect of the medial cuneiform.
- Using a countersink or a washer can be helpful to prevent propagation of a fracture line.

Reduction and Fixation of the Third, Fourth, and Fifth Metatarsals

- Fluoroscopy should be used to assess the third, fourth, and fifth TMT after successful reduction and fixation of the first and second TMT (Figure 28-4 and 28-5).
- The third TMT can be addressed similar to the first and second TMT joints described earlier. The medial aspect of the third TMT can be accessed via the dorsal medial approach. A dorsal lateral approach can be used if exposure of the lateral aspect of the third TMT is needed for reduction.

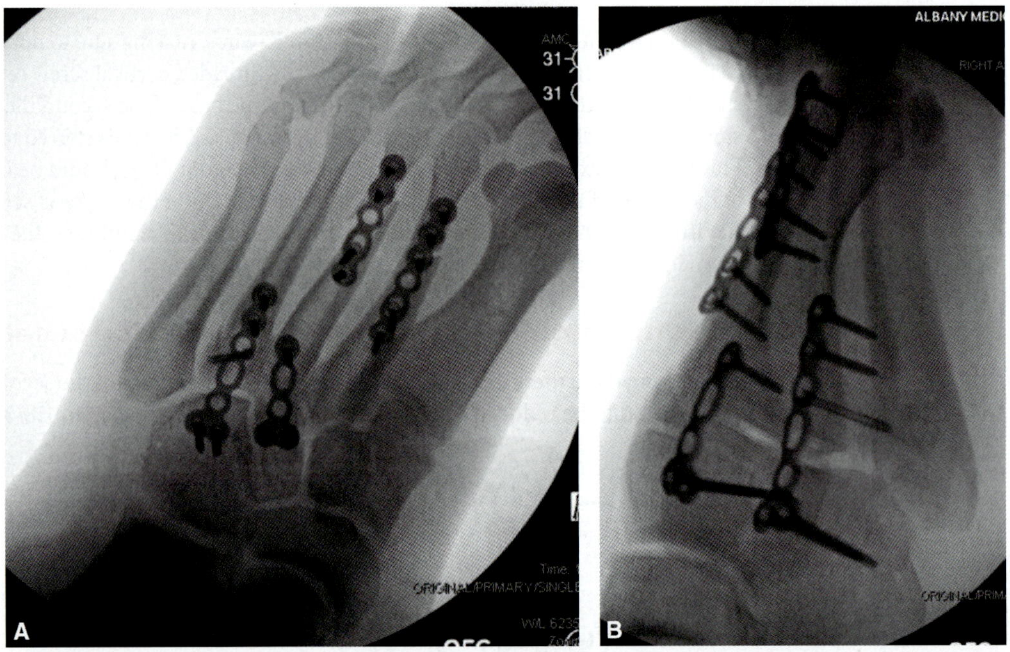

Figure 28-4. AP (A) and lateral (B) radiographs demonstrating third and fourth tarsometatarsal joint fixation with 2.4 mm plates (Arthrex, Naples, FL). Plating of the fourth tarsometatarsal joint was used because of a fourth MT base fracture necessitating more robust fixation.

- Placement of a lag screw by technique again should be performed from the base of the third metatarsal into the middle or lateral cuneiform.
- Often, during reduction of the third metatarsal, the fourth and fifth metatarsals are indirectly reduced without the need for further fixation.
- If reduction of the third metatarsal does not induce an indirect reduction, then reduction of the fourth and fifth should be performed percutaneously with K-wire fixation or the dorsal lateral incision can be used.
- Fixation of the fourth and fifth metatarsals should be established with K-wire fixation into the lateral cuneiform and cuboid, respectively.
- If a lateral frame was used initially for reduction and lateral column length, then the frame can remain until healing at 6 weeks with no need for additional K wires.

The lateral TMT joints do not need the same rigid fixation as the first to third TMT joints, which provide the majority of the dorsal–plantar stability.

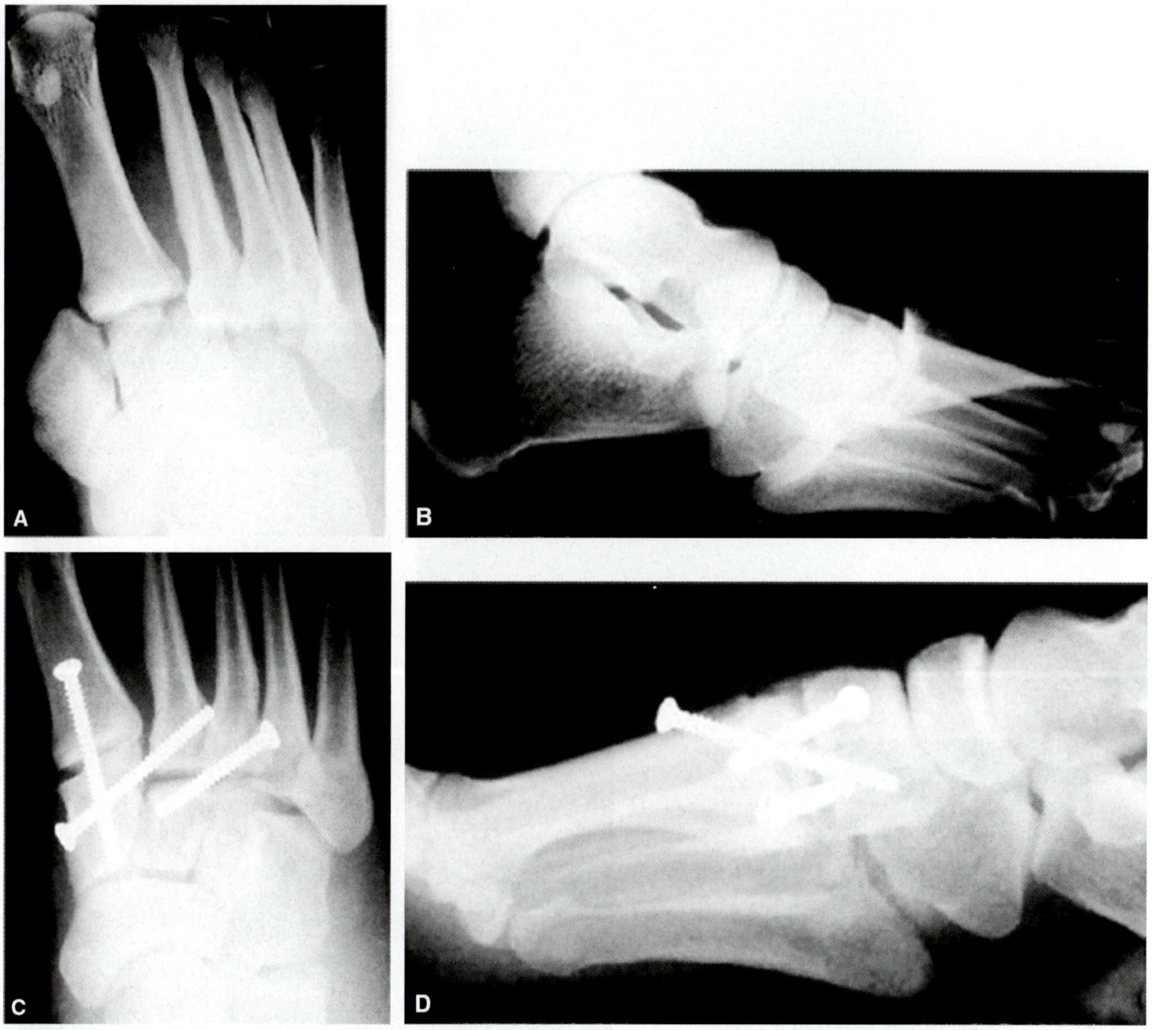

Figure 28-5. AP (A) and lateral (B) radiographs demonstrating a homolateral Lisfranc injury. Fixation of the first, second, and third tarsometatarsal (TMT) joints, as seen on AP (C) and lateral (D) radiographs, demonstrates anatomic reduction of the first, second, and third TMT joints and adequate indirect reduction of the fourth and fifth TMT joints. From Schiff AP, Gross CE, Pellegrini MJ, Hamid KS, Easley ME. Open reduction and internal fixation of the Lisfranc fracture-dislocation. In: Easley ME, Wiesel SW, eds. *Operative Techniques in Foot and Ankle Surgery*. Philadelphia, PA: Wolters Kluwer; 2017:chap 132:Tech Figure 6C.

Variations in Technique

- It is surgeon preference to approach the first or second TMT joint first, although provisional fixation of both should be obtained before screw placement (Figures 28-6 and 28-7).
- The first TMT joint can be fixed with crisscross screw placement.
  - The first screw is placed in a retrograde manner from the lateral aspect of the first metatarsal, aiming from dorsal to plantar into the medial cuneiform.
  - The second screw placement is anterograde from the medial cuneiform to the plantar prominence of the first metatarsal.
- Best evidence demonstrates that cannulated screw placement may be easier with an inexperienced surgeon. However, compared to solid screws, cannulated screws are weaker with respect to resisting bending moments and more cost inefficient.
- In patients with significant periarticular comminution or if the surgeon preference is to avoid intra-articular penetration, a mini-fragment plate can be used with the bridge plating technique.

Midfoot Arthrodesis

Indications for primary fusion include purely ligamentous injury, symptomatic midfoot arthritis, failed ORIF, or extensive comminution.

- If fusion is chosen, it is a partial arthrodesis still favoring K-wire fixation of the lateral fourth and fifth TMT joints as described earlier.

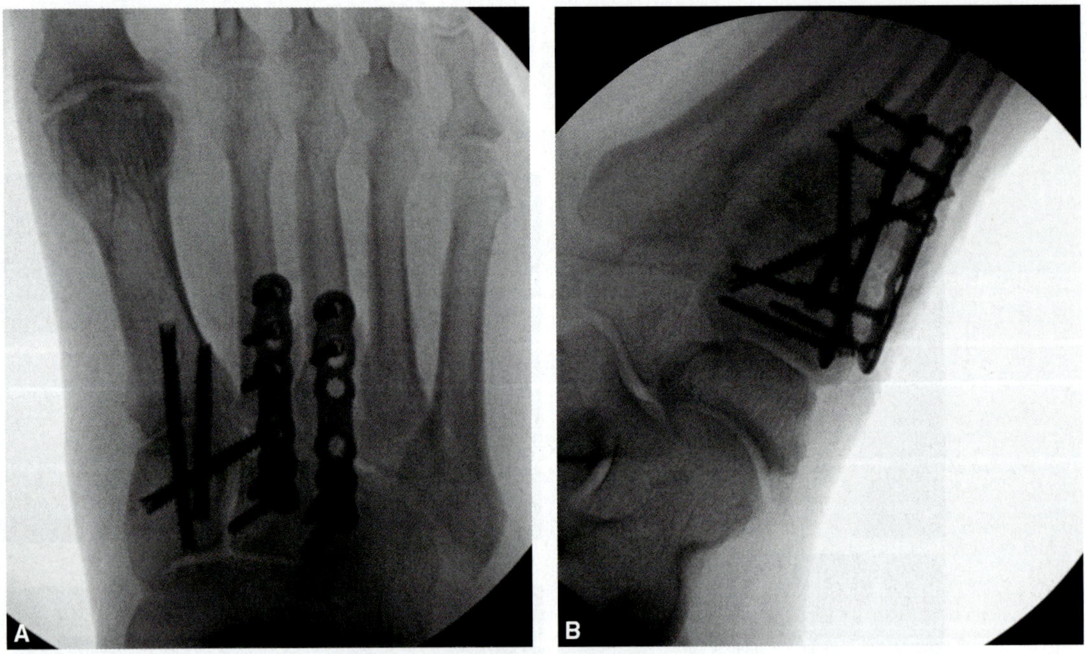

Figure 28-6. AP (A) and lateral (B) radiographs demonstrating first tarsometatarsal joint fixation with headless crossed screws.

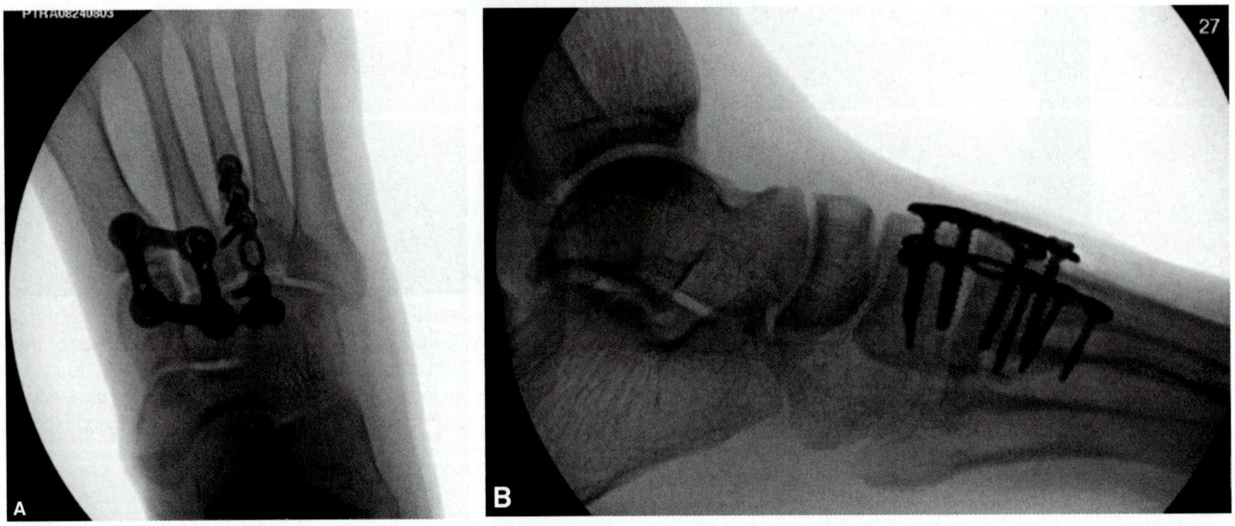

Figure 28-7. AP (A) and lateral (B) radiographs demonstrating the use of a Lisfranc specific plate (Arthrex, Naples FL) to stabilize the first and second tarsometatarsal joints. Another plate was used to address the third tarsometatarsal joint.

- Complete joint exposure using lamina spreader is necessary, with Schanz pin for temporary external fixation or Hintermann distractor use to allow adequate debridement.
- To promote fusion, all of the articular surfaces of the cuneiforms and metatarsal base must be removed.
  - Removal of the articular surface can be done with the help of curettes, rongeurs, and osteotomies.
  - The fusion surface can then be prepared with holes created by a K-wire or small drill bit.
- Assessment and reduction of the Lisfranc injury is the same as described earlier.
- Screws alone may be used or a plate may be used to augment fixation.
- Screw fixation is performed as described earlier.
- Before definitive screw or plate fixation, bone graft is often added to aid in fusion.
  - Autograft may be taken from the calcaneus or proximal/distal tibia. Allografts such as demineralized bone matrix may be used as well depending on surgeon preference.
  - A small amount of bone graft is placed between the fusion sites.
- Plate fixation may be used to augment the rigid fixation.
  - Plates may just bridge the first or second TMT separately or new plates may address both with one implant.

Chapter 29
Navicular Fractures

ERIC PERLOFF
JOSEPH YOUNG
ANDREW J. ROSENBAUM

Sterile Instruments/Equipment

- Tourniquet
- Pointed reduction clamps
- Dental pick
- Freer elevator
- Kirschner wire and wire driver
- Small fragment distractor
- Implants
    - 2.7- or 3.5-mm cortical lag screws
    - 2.0-, 2.4-, or 2.7-mm navicular plates

Positioning

- The patient is placed supine with a bump under the ipsilateral hip.
- A calf or thigh tourniquet is used.
- The patient is draped and prepared in a sterile manner.

Surgical Approaches

Anteromedial and Dorsolateral Approach to Navicular Fractures

- Anteromedial is usually sufficient to be utilized for type 1 navicular fractures. This approach for the navicular was originally described by Sangeorzan et al.[1]
    - Allows access to the medial navicular body and navicular tuberosity
- A second dorsolateral is often necessary for type 2 and 3 fractures, fractures with additional lateral column involvement, or in injuries with a large dorsolateral fragment.[2]
- In the anteromedial approach, a line is demarcated 1 cm below the tip of the medial malleolus, through the navicular, toward the first metatarsal head (Figure 29-1).
- The tibialis anterior (TA) tendon should be retracted dorsally and the posterior tibialis (PT) plantarly.[3]
- Dissect the periosteum to allow visualization of the navicular bone.
- Capsulotomies of the TN joint can be made from this approach to assess the joint surface.

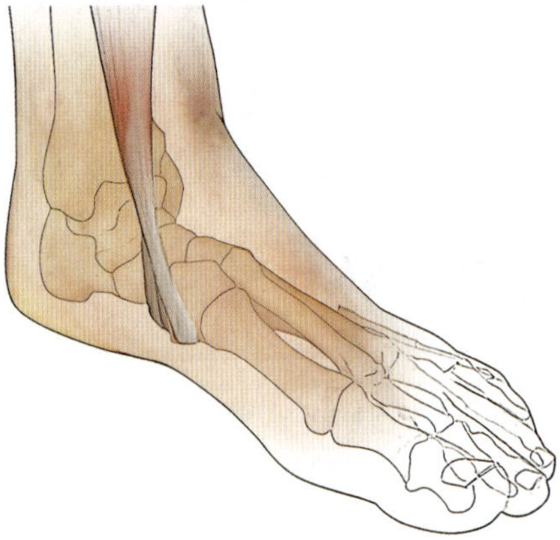

Figure 29-1. Illustration demonstrating the starting point and plane for the anteromedial approach. Incision is made 1 cm below the tip of the medial malleolus, extending through the navicular prominence. Reprinted with permission from Teasdall R, Allen PG. Surgical fixation of navicular body fractures. *Tech Foot Ankle Surg*. 2007;6(2):108-112. doi:10.1097/01.btf.0000235416.51876.36.

- If access to the lateral aspect navicular is needed, an additional incision can be made on the dorsolateral surface.[4]
  - Location of incision should be determined via fluoroscopy.[4]
- Incision is made between the planes of the extensor hallucis longus (EHL) and extensor digitorum brevis (EDB).[3]
  - In this approach, one must locate the motor branch of the deep peroneal and the superficial peroneal sensory nerves.[3]

Dorsomedial Approach to Navicular Fractures

- Allows access to the central third of the navicular bone
- Palpate and demarcate the TA and EHL tendons.
- Incision is made between interval of the TA and EHL tendons directly over the fracture.[5]
- The TA tendon should be retracted medially and the EHL tendon and neurovascular structures laterally to expose the periosteum.[5]
- Incise and dissect the periosteum to expose the body of the navicular.
- If necessary to expose the TN joint, the incision can be extended in the proximal direction and a small capsulotomy can be performed.
- Identify the fracture site, and remove sclerotic bone and debris using a rongeur and dental pick.

Reduction and Fixation Techniques

- In type 1 fractures, longitudinal traction and plantarflexion are often sufficient to obtain reduction, which can then be held with K-wire fixation.[6]
  - Reduction can be held via Weber clamps as well; stab incisions are placed in locations to allow clamping perpendicular to the fracture fragments.
- If further restoration of the medial column length is necessary, or adequate visualization of the TN joint cannot be obtained, a small distractor can be utilized (Figure 29-2).[6]
  - Proximally, the mini-distractor is placed in the base of the neck of the talus.
  - The mini-distractor is placed in the medial cuneiform distally.
- Autologous bone graft may be harvested and used to restore joint congruity or bone defect.

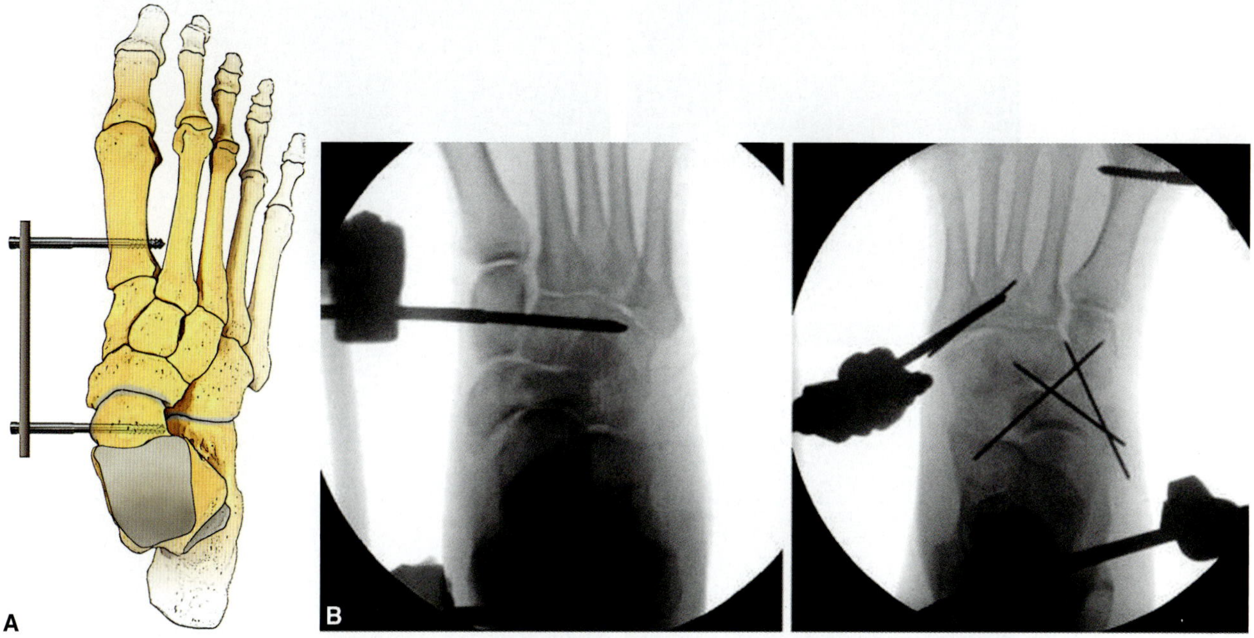

Figure 29-2. Illustration (A) and intraoperative images (B) showing external fixation of a navicular fracture. Pin inserted into the cuneiforms and talus for medial column distraction. A, Reprinted with permission from Teasdall R, Allen PG. Surgical fixation of navicular body fractures. *Tech Foot Ankle Surg*. 2007;6(2):108-112. doi:10.1097/01.btf.0000235416.51876.36. B, Reprinted with permission from Ramadorai MU, Beuchel MW, Sangeorzan BJ. Fractures and dislocations of the tarsal navicular. *J Am Acad Orthop Surg*. 2016;24(6):379-389. doi:10.5435/JAAOS-D-14-00442.

Cortical Lag Screw Technique

- In type 1 fractures, the single anteromedial incision is often sufficient for reduction.[3]
  - One to two 2.7- or 3.5-mm cortical lag screws can be utilized.
  - Insert the screws in a dorsal-to-plantar direction, causing compression of the fracture.[2]
  - Confirm placement using fluoroscopy (Figure 29-3).
- Ensure screw does not penetrate medial cortex because this may impinge the PT tendon.
- Noncomminuted or displaced type 2 fractures often require a dorsal approach directly over the fracture site to allow visualization of the fracture and TN joint.
  - Two 2.7- or 3.5-mm cortical lag screws can be placed through stab incisions.

Plate Fixation

- Comminuted type 2 or type 3 fractures often require plate fixation.
  - Type 3 often have a displaced dorsomedial fragment and a comminuted plantar lateral fragment that is not amenable to screw fixation.[2]
- Identification of the lateral plantar fragment is critical, using point-reduction clamps; the fragments can often be stabilized and compressed against this piece if it is not comminuted.
- Defects can be filled using autologous bone grafting.
- Anatomically shaped, low-profile 2.0-, 2.4-, or 2.7-mm navicular plates can be used.[2,4]
- Screws closest to the talus should be directed toward the forefoot to avoid entering the TN joint because of the concavity of the navicular surface at the TN joint.[7]

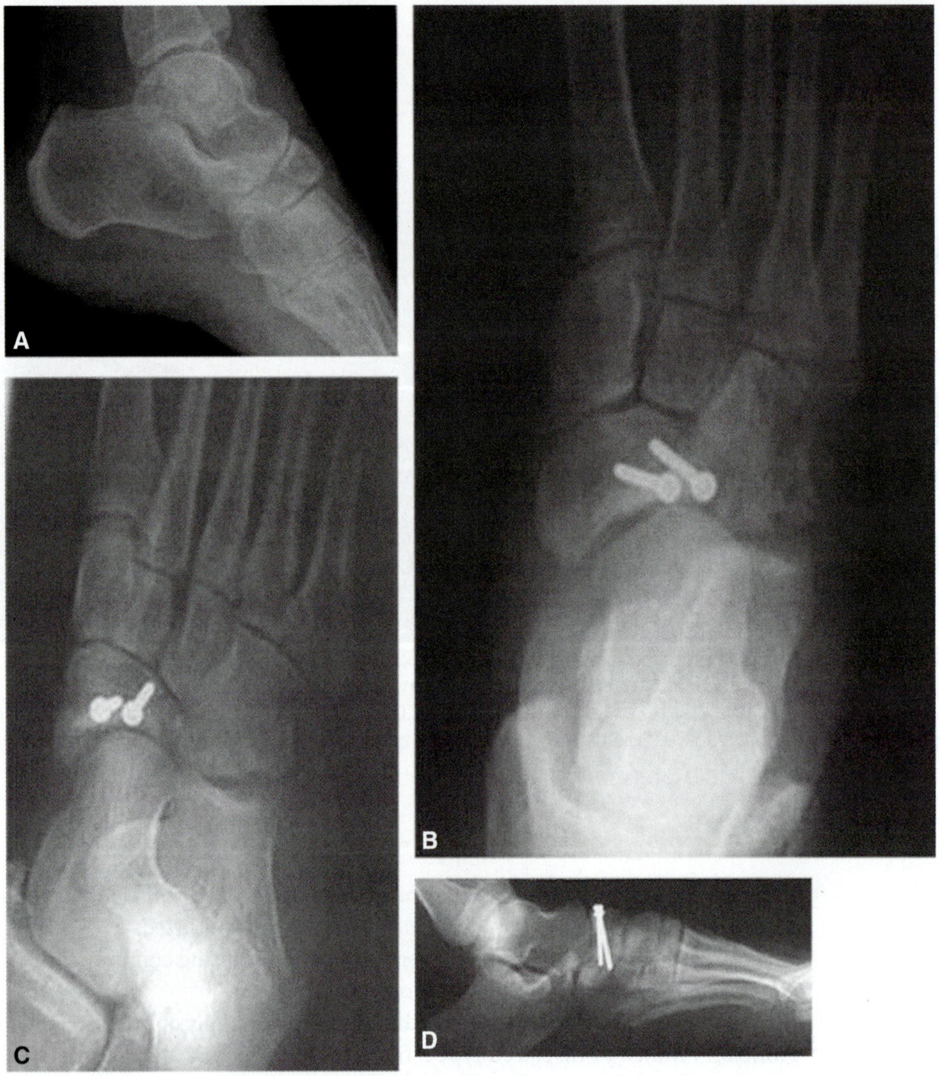

Figure 29-3. Shows preoperative (A) and postoperative AP (B), oblique (C), and lateral (D) films with placement of lag screws through a navicular fracture. Reprinted with permission from Teasdall R, Allen PG. Surgical fixation of navicular body fractures. *Tech Foot Ankle Surg*. 2007;6(2):108-112. doi:10.1097/01.btf.0000235416.51876.36.

Naviculocuneiform (NC) Joint Fusion

- Fixation across the NC joint can also be performed if reduction of the navicular cannot be obtained because of comminution.[2,4]
  - The NC joint has little function and motion, and can often be sacrificed.
- Two or three 2.7- or 3.5-mm cortical screws can be used.
- In a proximal and medial starting positing, the first screw is placed from the navicular extending into the lateral cuneiform.[4]
- Another screw is placed plantar to the first and is drilled from the lateral aspect of the navicular into the medial cuneiform.[4]
- If a third screw is needed, a starting positing in the medial cuneiform can be used, drilled in a retrograde and lateral direction into the lateral aspect of the navicular.[4]

References

1. Sangeorzan BJ, Benirschke SK, Mosca V, Mayo KA, Hansen ST Jr. Displaced intra-articular fractures of the tarsal navicular. *J Bone Joint Surg*. 1989;71(10):1504-1510.
2. Ramadorai MU, Beuchel MW, Sangeorzan BJ. Fractures and dislocations of the tarsal navicular. *J Am Acad Orthop Surg*. 2016;24(6):379-389.
3. Rosenbaum AJ, Uhl RL, DiPreta JA. Acute fractures of the tarsal navicular. *Orthopedics*. 2014;37(8):541-546.
4. Banerjee R, Nickisch F, Easley M, DiGiovanni CW. Foot injuries. In: Browner B, Levine A, Jupiter J, Trafton P, Krettek C, eds. *Skeletal Trauma*. Vol. V. Philadelphia, PA: W. B. Saunders; 2009.
5. Schmid T, Krause F, Gebel P, Weber M, Operative treatment of acute fractures of the tarsal navicular body: midterm results with a new classification. *Foot Ankle Int*. 2016;37(5):501-507.
6. Teasdall RD, Allen PG. Surgical fixation of navicular body fractures. *Tech Foot Ankle Surg*. 2007;6(2):108-112.
7. Clements JR, Dijour F, Leong W. Surgical management navicular and cuboid fractures. *Clin Podiatr Med Surg*. 2018;35(2):145-159.

References

Chapter 30
Calcaneus Fractures

AFSHIN A. ANOUSHIRAVANI

Instruments and Equipment

- Beanbag
- Tourniquet
- Large pointed bone reduction clamps (Weber clamps)
- Laminar spreader
- Dental picks and Freer elevators
- Hintermann distractor
- Hohmann retractor (small)
- Rongeur (small)
- Self-retaining retractor (small, sharp)
- Senn–Miller retractors (17 cm)
- Shoulder hook
- Schanz pins (2.5–4.0 mm)
- Femoral distractor (small)
- Wire driver/drill with K-wires and appropriate drill bits
- Implants
  - Mini- and small-fragment screws and mini-fragment plates (2.0/2.4/2.7/3.5 mm)
  - Calcaneal plates, locking or non-locking
  - Autograft, cancellous allograft, or other substitutes for bone defects

Patient Positioning

- The patient is positioned in the lateral decubitus position (Figure 30-1).

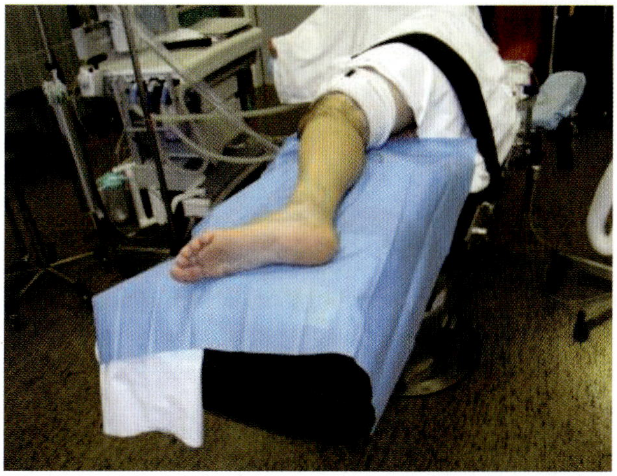

Figure 30-1. Patient positioning—lateral decubitus. Reprinted from Pfeffer GB, Easley ME, Hintermann B, et al. *Operative Techniques: Foot and Ankle Surgery*. 2nd ed. Philadelphia, PA: Elsevier; 2018. Figure 39.4. Copyright © 2018 Elsevier. With permission.

- The patient's torso should be secured with a beanbag and the operative extremity supported on a well-padded bump of folded towels.
- Special care is taken to pad all bony prominences, including the greater trochanter, fibular head, and elbow, thereby protecting the peroneal and radial nerves, respectively.

Indications and Contraindications for Surgical Intervention

Indications

- Intra-articular calcaneal fractures with ≥2-mm step-off of the posterior facet
- Intra-articular calcaneal fractures with Bohler angle <15° on lateral radiograph of the foot or ankle
- Anterior process fractures with >25% involvement of the calcaneal–cuboid articulation
- Displaced fractures of the calcaneal tuberosity
- Fracture dislocations
- Open calcaneal fractures

Contraindications

- Severe peripheral vascular disease
- Excessive swelling
- Poorly controlled diabetes
- Tobacco use
- Noncompliant patient

Surgical Approach[1]

Operative treatment of closed fractures can be performed with an extensile lateral incision, a lateral incision over sinus tarsi, medial, or posterior incision allowing access to the various facets and regions of the calcaneus (Figure 30-2).

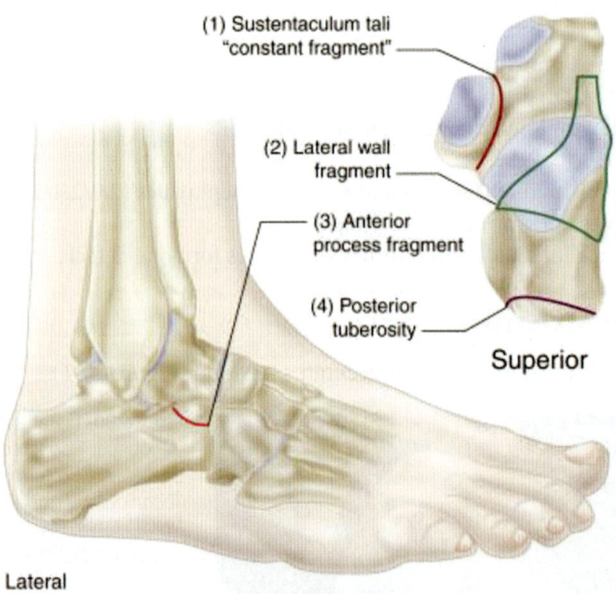

Figure 30-2. Frequently fractured anatomic landmarks on calcaneus. Reprinted from Pfeffer GB, Easley ME, Hintermann B, et al. *Operative Techniques: Foot and Ankle Surgery*. 2nd ed. Philadelphia, PA: Elsevier; 2018. Figure 37.5. Copyright © 2018 Elsevier. With permission.

Extensile Lateral Approach

- Most common approach used for displaced intra-articular calcaneal fractures
  - Distal fibula and calcaneus are well outlined, as illustrated in Figure 30-3.
  - Must be careful near posterior and plantar outlines, calcaneocuboid joint, lateral neck, and sinus tarsi
  - The incision is marked at the level of the ankle joint, coursing just anterior to the Achilles tendon—if necessary, the distal aspect of the incision may be extended superiorly.
  - Once the incision is made, careful dissection of the proximal and distal aspects of the incision will avoid transection of the peroneal tendons and sural nerve.
  - Soft tissues are sharply removed with a scalpel or rongeur, providing adequate visualization of the fracture site.

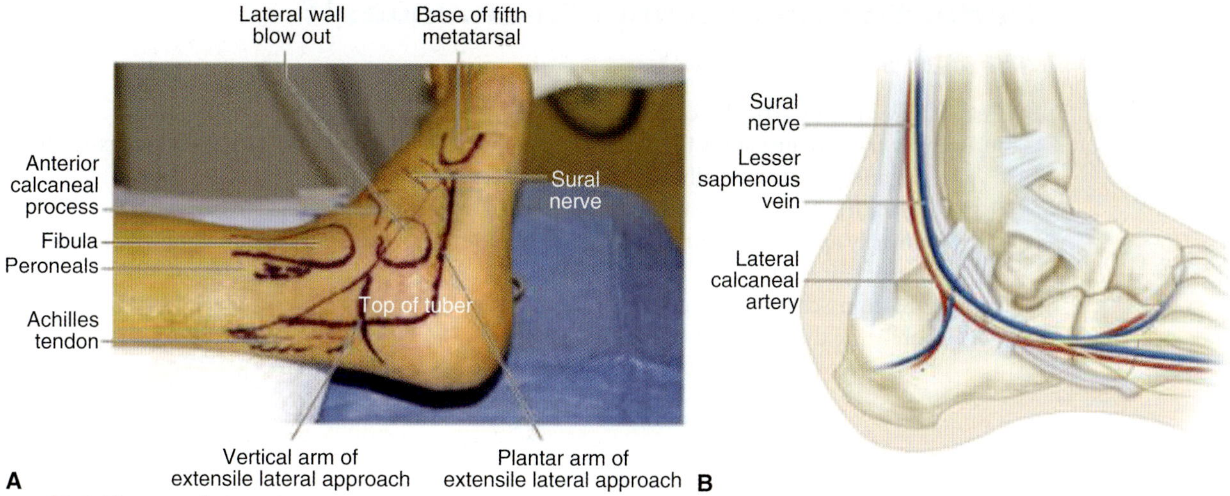

Figure 30-3. The extensile lateral approach incision placement. (A) The posterior arm begins midway between the fibula and Achilles tendon. The horizontal arm is in line with the base of the fifth metatarsal. The neurovascular structures (B) are elevated with the lateral flap during the exposure. Reprinted from Pfeffer GB, Easley ME, Hintermann B, et al. *Operative Techniques: Foot and Ankle Surgery*. 2nd ed. Philadelphia, PA: Elsevier; 2018. Figure 36.5AB. Copyright © 2018 Elsevier. With permission.

Lateral Incisions Over Sinus Tarsi

- A minimally invasive approach used to obtain reduction and percutaneous fixation of displaced intra-articular calcaneal fractures
  - A slightly curved incision from the tip of the fibula to the sinus tarsi is made (Figure 30-4). Must be careful near posterior and plantar outlines, calcaneocuboid joint, lateral neck, and sinus tarsi.
  - A 2.5-mm K-wire is placed into the talar neck and lateral tuber of the calcaneus and distracted by a Hintermann distractor exposing the subtalar joint.

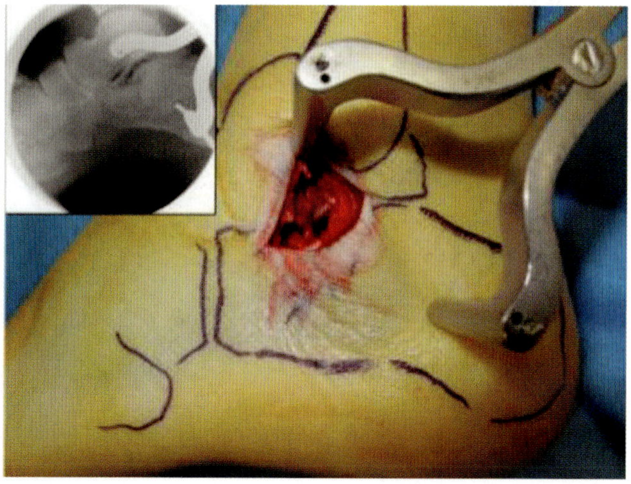

Figure 30-4. Lateral sinus tarsi approach to the calcaneus. Reprinted from Pfeffer GB, Easley ME, Hintermann B, et al. *Operative Techniques: Foot and Ankle Surgery*. 2nd ed. Philadelphia, PA: Elsevier; 2018. Figure 39.5. Copyright © 2018 Elsevier. With permission.

Medial Incision

- Commonly used to expose the sustentaculum tali
  - The incision is made 2 cm below the medial malleolus, 2 cm proximal to the navicular, and is approximately 5 cm in length.
  - The posterior tibial tendon, neurovascular bundle, and flexor hallucis tendon are identified and retracted.
  - The retinaculum is incised revealing the sustentaculum.

Reduction and Fixation Techniques[1,2]

Joint Depression Fractures

- Essex-Lopresti intra-articular calcaneal fracture classification
  - Primary fracture line splits the calcaneus obliquely through the posterior facet and exists antero-laterally and posteromedially.
  - Secondary fracture line exists superiorly behind the posterior facet.
    - Primarily approached through an extensile lateral approach in combination with a medial approach, if necessary
    - A 4.5-mm Schanz pin is inserted into the lateral or posterior aspect of the posterior tuber, mobilizing the fragment (Figure 30-5).

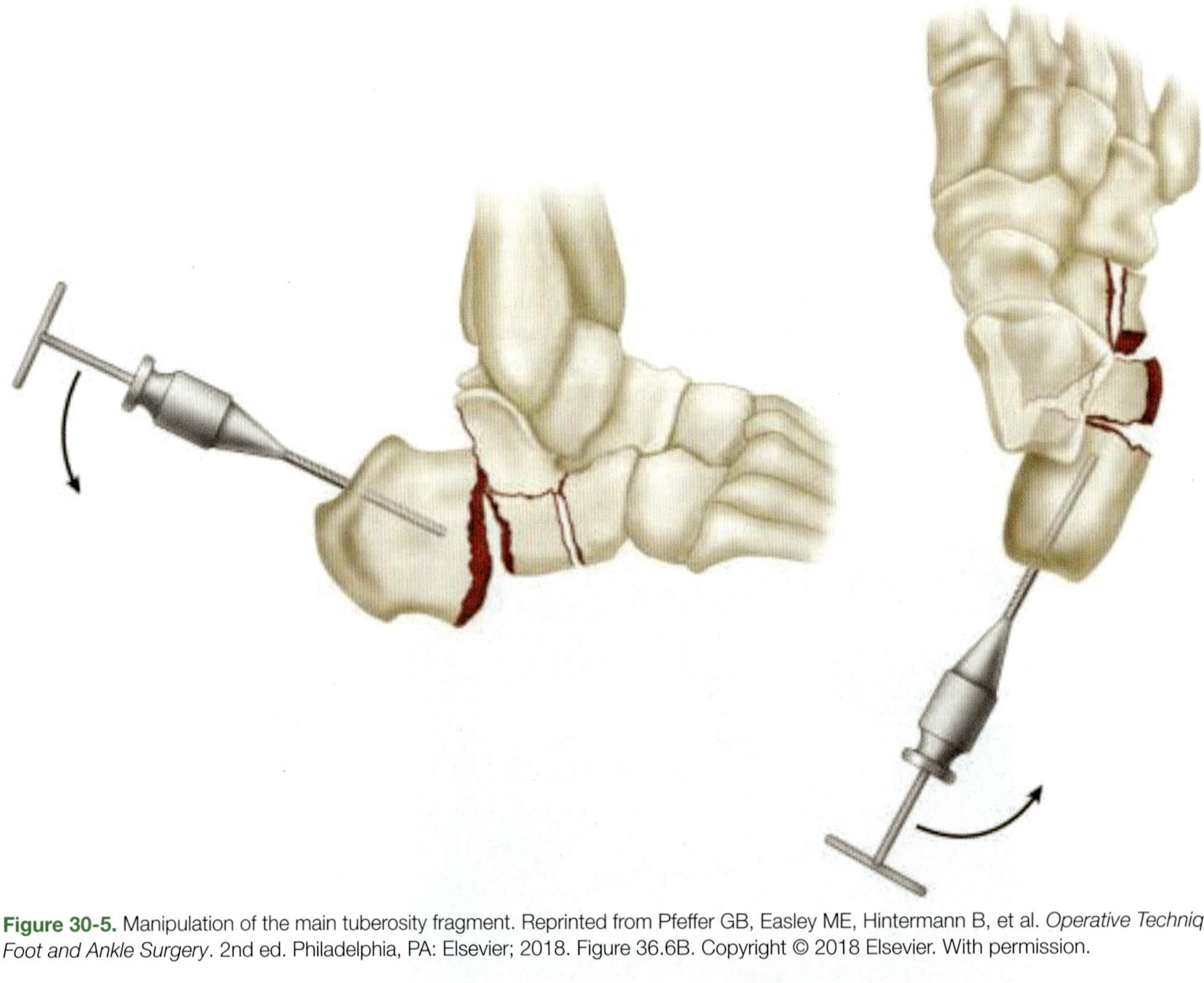

Figure 30-5. Manipulation of the main tuberosity fragment. Reprinted from Pfeffer GB, Easley ME, Hintermann B, et al. *Operative Techniques: Foot and Ankle Surgery*. 2nd ed. Philadelphia, PA: Elsevier; 2018. Figure 36.6B. Copyright © 2018 Elsevier. With permission.

    - Longitudinal traction and valgus force are then applied to the Schanz pin, enabling anatomic reduction of the lateral posterior fragment(s).
    - K-wires (1.8 mm) are inserted from the plantar aspect to hold the reduction (Figure 30-6).
    - Laminar spreader is inserted through the sinus tarsi and used to reduce the lateral neck restoring Bohler angle.
    - If the sustentaculum is also disrupted, a medial incision can be made to better visualize the fragments(s).
    - The subtalar joint is then reduced with K-wires in a stepwise manner from medial to lateral, as demonstrated in Figure 30-7.

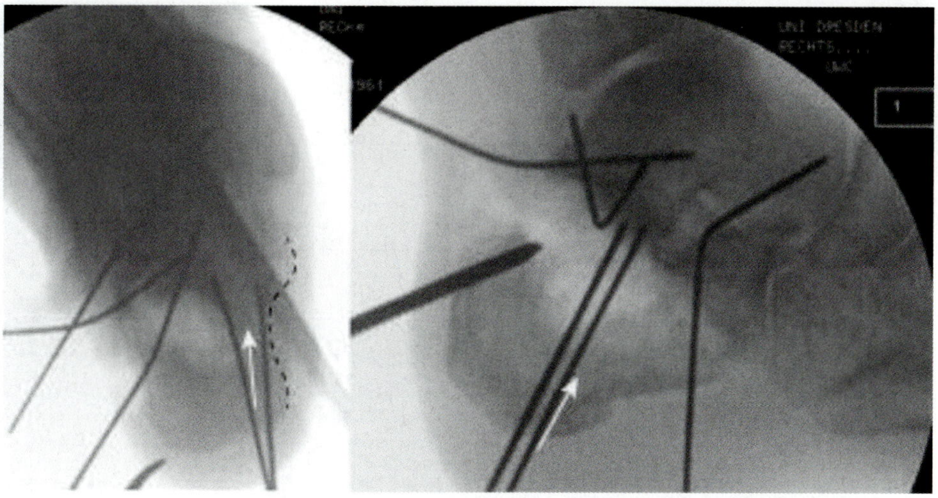

Figure 30-6. Percutaneous fixation of fracture. Reprinted from Pfeffer GB, Easley ME, Hintermann B, et al. *Operative Techniques: Foot and Ankle Surgery*. 2nd ed. Philadelphia, PA: Elsevier; 2018. Figure 36.7B. Copyright © 2018 Elsevier. With permission.

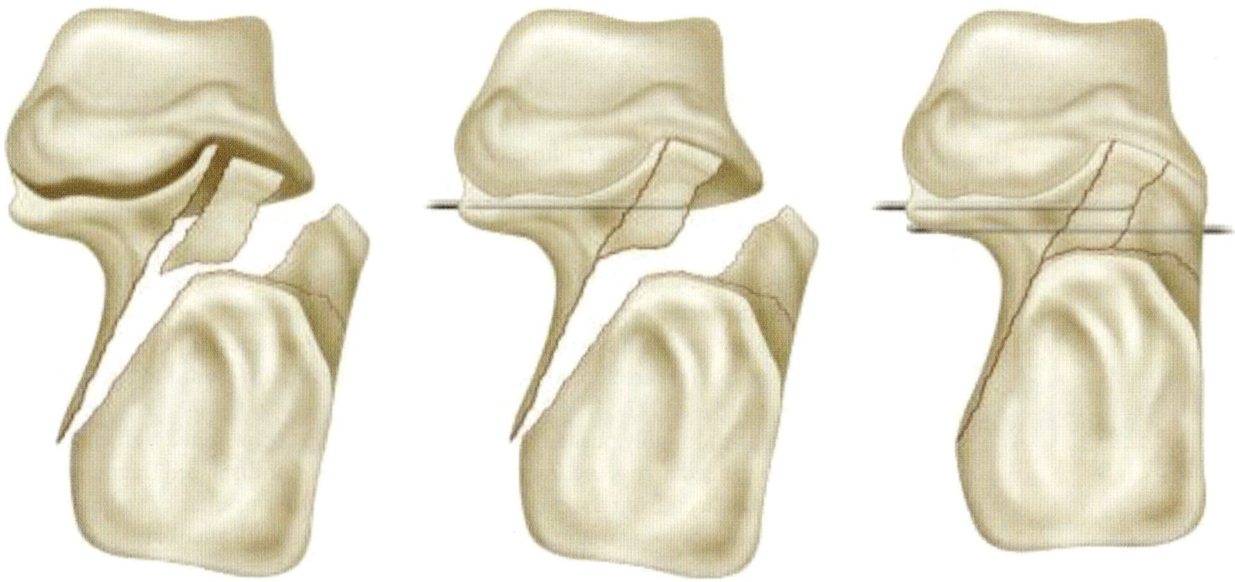

Figure 30-7. Stepwise reduction of the sustentaculum tali. Reprinted from Pfeffer GB, Easley ME, Hintermann B, et al. *Operative Techniques: Foot and Ankle Surgery*. 2nd ed. Philadelphia, PA: Elsevier; 2018. Figure 36.8. Copyright © 2018 Elsevier. With permission.

- Once reduced, the joint fragments are fixed with a small fragment screw that is directed toward the sustentaculum with the intent of maximizing bony purchase and stability.
- The tuberosity fragment is reconstructed to the posterior joint block with the help of a Schanz pin and K-wires are introduced from the tuberosity into the anterior process.
- The lateral wall is then folded back and should demonstrate a close to anatomic fit if proper reduction is obtained.
- An appropriately sized calcaneal plate is applied and contoured to the lateral aspect of the calcaneus. At least one of the screws through the plate compresses the sustentaculum fragment and a minimum of two screws are placed through the anterior process and tuberosity fragment each.
- Another type of fixation is percutaneously placed screws (Figure 30-8).
- Anatomic reduction, implant position, and screw length are assessed fluoroscopically with lateral, axial, and Broden views.
- The incision is closed using tension-free closure of the skin and subcutaneous layers, limiting the potential for tissue necrosis and wound dehiscence.

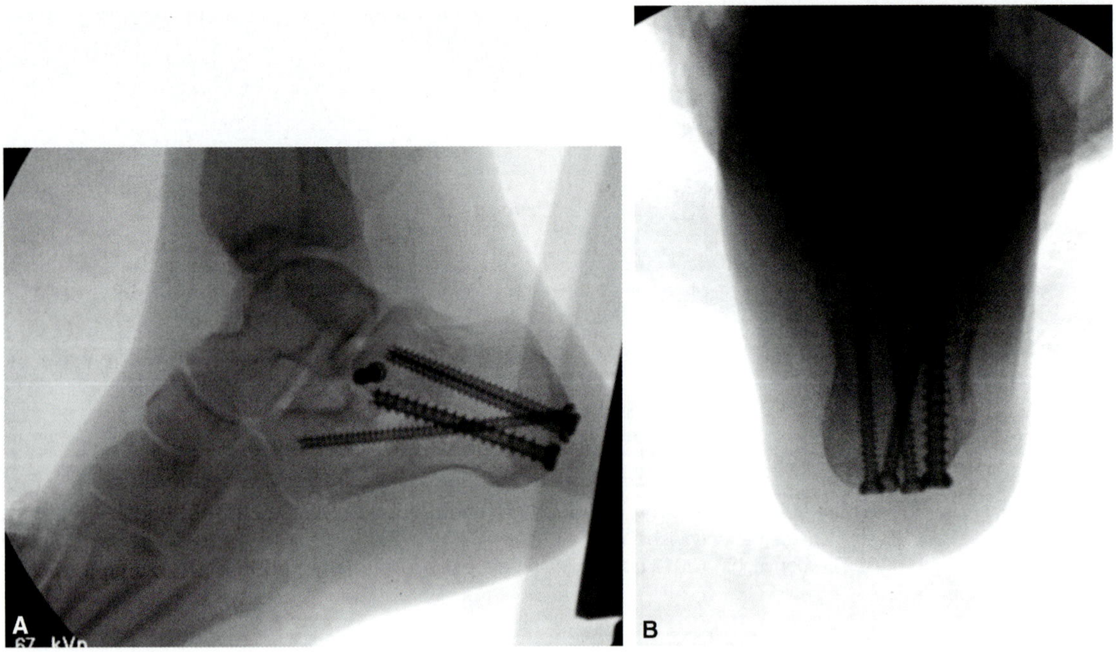

Figure 30-8. Lateral (A) and axial heel (B) views of an intra-articular calcaneus fracture fixed via a sinus tarsi approach with 6.7 and 4.5 mm cannulated screws (Arthrex, Naples FL).

Tongue-Type Fractures

- Essex-Lopresti intra-articular calcaneal fracture classification
  - Primary fracture line exists anterolaterally and posteromedially.
  - Secondary fracture line appears beneath the posterior facet and exists posteriorly through the tuberosity.
    - Tongue-type calcaneal fractures are amenable to fixation through the minimally invasive osteotomy (MIO) posterior approach.
    - A 4.5-mm Schanz pin can then be introduced into the posterior superior portion of the calcaneal tuberosity—special care should be taken to guide the pin downward to avoid penetrating the subtalar joint.
    - The Schanz pin is then forcibly pushed down to elevate the tip of the bone fragment.
    - Next, the pin is advanced across the fracture into the anterior nondisplaced fragment.
    - Additional pins are placed from the posterior superior and posterior inferior fragments into the adjacent anterior bony fragments, further stabilizing the calcaneus and preserving anteroposterior length.
    - 6.5-mm headless compression screws are then introduced over these pins, obtaining definitive interfragmentary fixation of the fracture site.
    - Anatomic reduction, implant position, and screw length are checked fluoroscopically with lateral, axial, and Broden views.
    - The incision is closed using tension-free closure of the skin and subcutaneous tissue to limit potential for necrosis and dehiscence.

Medial Process Fractures

- Occur following a fall from a height, resulting in an avulsion-type fracture off the medial aspect of the posterior calcaneus
  - A displaced medial process fracture can result in altered gait and a painful heel.
  - It is not uncommon for the heel pad to be displaced medially.
  - A modified oblique incision is made to reduce the medial process while taking special care not to violate the medial plantar nerve.
  - Once reduced, a properly sized H-plate is positioned, providing definitive fracture fixation.

Tuberosity Avulsion Fractures

- Often occur following forced dorsiflexion, resulting in violent contraction of the gastrocnemius–solus complex avulsing the fragment on the calcaneal tuberosity
    - A MIO posterior approach is indicated as described earlier, and preliminary anatomic reduction is achieved with pointed reduction forceps.
    - Two K-wires are then placed perpendicular to the fracture plane under fluoroscopic guidance.
    - Cannulated lag screws (with washers if osteoporotic) are then placed to achieve interfragmentary compression.
    - The incision is then reapproximated and closed—the foot is immobilized to prevent reinjury.

References

1. Pfeffer GB, Easley ME, Hintermann B, et al. *Operative Techniques: Foot and Ankle Surgery*. 2nd ed. Philadelphia, PA: Elsevier; 2018.
2. Gardner MJ, Nork SE, Barei DP, Kramer PA, Sangeorzan BJ, Benirschke SK. Secondary soft tissue compromise in tongue-type calcaneus fractures. *J Orthop Trauma*. 2008;22(7):439-445. https://insights.ovid.com/crossref?an=00005131-200808000-00001.

Index

Note: Page numbers followed by *f* indicate figures.

N

O

T

V

W